D0984716

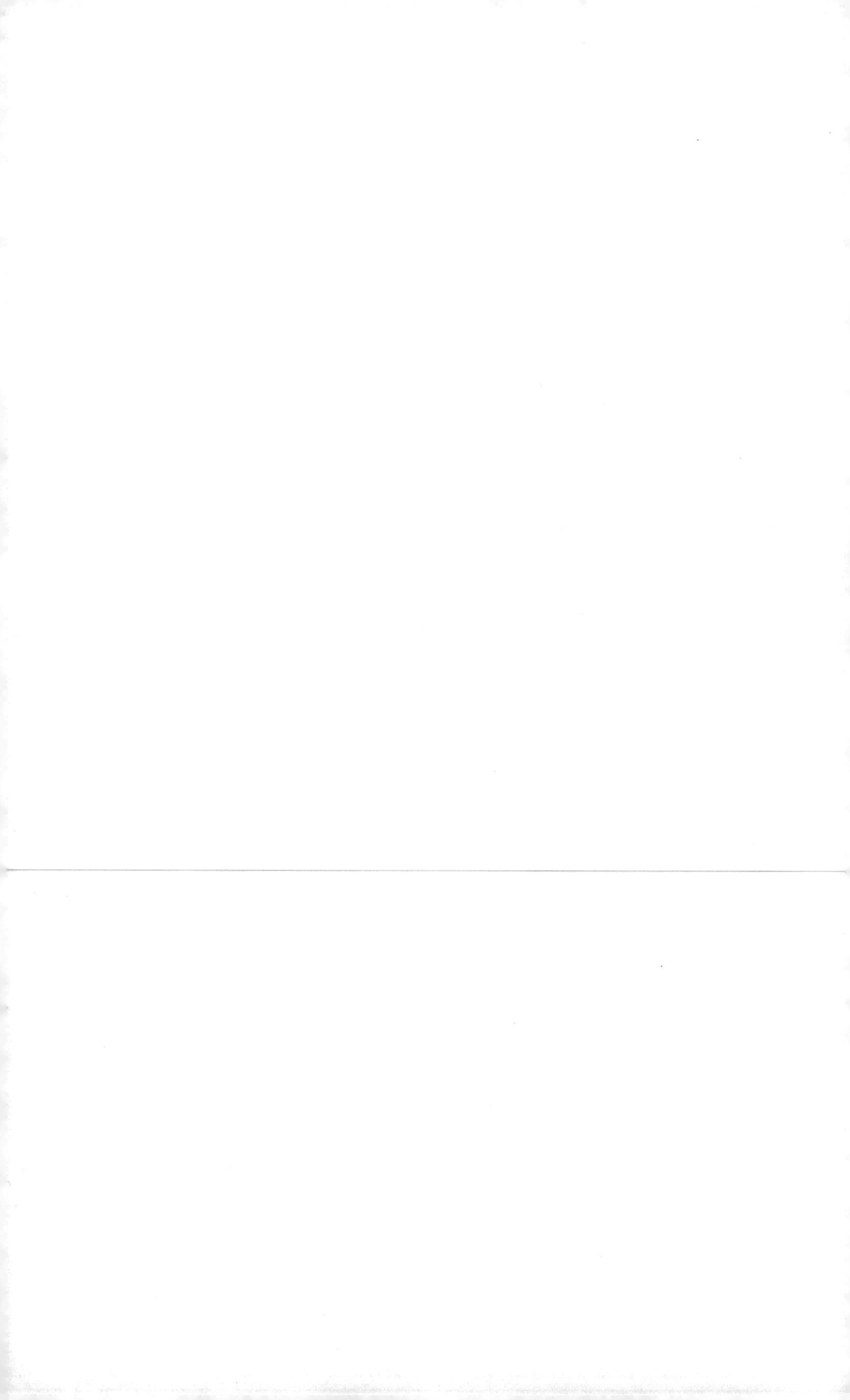

Ethics in Obstetrics and Gynecology

Ethics in Obstetrics and Gynecology

Laurence B. McCullough, Ph.D.
Frank A. Chervenak, M.D.

New York Oxford
OXFORD UNIVERSITY PRESS
1994

Oxford University Press
Oxford New York Toronto
Delhi Bombay Calcutta Madras Karachi
Kuala Lumpur Singapore Hong Kong Tokyo
Nairobi Dar es Salaam Cape Town
Melbourne Auckland Madrid

and associated companies in
Berlin Ibadan

Published by Oxford University Press, Inc.,
200 Madison Avenue, New York, New York 10016

Oxford is a registered trademark of Oxford University Press

Library of Congress Cataloging-in-Publication Data
McCullough, Laurence B.
Ethics in obstetrics and gynecology / Laurence B. McCullough and Frank A. Chervenak.
p. cm. Includes bibliographical references and index.
ISBN 0-19-506005-9
1. Gynecology—Moral and ethical aspects.
2. Obstetrics—Moral and ethical aspects.
I. Chervenak, Frank A. II. Title.
[DNLM: 1. Ethics, Medical. 2. Gynecology. 3. Obstetrics.
4. Physicians, Family. WQ 100 M478e 1994]
RG103.M287 1994
174'.2—dc20 DNLM/DLC
for Library of Congress 93-6426

9 8 7 6 5 4 3 2 1

Printed in the United States of America
on acid-free paper

for Linda
and
for Judy, Frank, and Joseph

Preface

This book is about ethics in obstetrics and gynecology. We wrote this book for physicians in gynecologic and obstetric practice, including gynecologists, obstetricians, and family physicians, as well as residents in training for the specialties of obstetrics and gynecology and family medicine. Medical students with an interest in either specialty will find the book useful to them as well. We also expect that patients will find this book to be of interest, in understanding how both physicians and patients should make ethically justified decisions about patient care. Professional ethicists and philosophers will find much that is of methodological and clinical interest.

There has been a good deal of skepticism about ethics as it relates to the clinical practice of obstetrics and gynecology. This skepticism has been justified, given the poor intellectual quality or lack of clinical applicability of some of the literature on the subject. Our aim in this book is to rebut this skepticism by providing intellectually rigorous, clinically based frameworks for obstetric and gynecologic ethics. When fair-minded readers finish this book, we hope they will abandon this skepticism and come to see clinical ethical judgment and decision making as fundamental clinical skills in the practice of obstetrics and gynecology. We believe that the practice of obstetrics and gynecology without these skills jeopardizes the integrity of the profession of medicine and the interests of patients, their families, and society.

The primary and unique emphasis of this book is on preventive ethics. Other books in bioethics emphasize the resolution of ethical conflicts after they have occurred. We are convinced that this approach no longer suffices in clinical practice. Ethical conflicts occur too frequently in clinical practice, and thoughtful physicians can act effectively to prevent ethical conflict. By making preventive ethics strategies routine in the care of female and pregnant patients, physicians in gynecologic and obstetric practice can go a long way toward improving the quality of patient care and the morale of both physicians and patients.

The task of clinical ethical judgment in gynecologic and obstetric practice is to join scientific information about diagnosis and treatment to the particular circumstances of the female or pregnant patient. The first step in doing so is the cultivation of the virtues that direct and move the physician to protect and promote the interests of each individual patient. The second step is to interpret those interests into action guides for clinical practice via ethical principles. These first two steps are accomplished in Part I of this book. Part I, by providing a general framework for bioethics in clinical practice and frameworks for both gynecologic and obstetric ethics in the clinical setting, lays the foundation for the rest of the book. Indeed, subsequent chapters rely heavily on these frameworks. As an aid to the reader, we provide a glossary of terms at the end of Chapter 7, which can be easily referred to as the reader turns to subsequent chapters. (See pp. 267–68.)

The third step is to employ the clinical strategies of preventive ethics—informed consent, negotiation, respectful persuasion, and the proper use of ethics committees—in patient care. This step is accomplished in Part II of this book.

The fourth and final step is to employ, only as a fallback strategy in those rare cases when preventive ethics strategies are not successful, the clinical strategies of managing ethical conflict through the ethically justified exercise of institutional and state power. This step is accomplished in Part III of this book.

Together the three parts of this book provide the physician in gynecologic and obstetric practice with a comprehensive approach to gynecologic and obstetric ethics that involves the *identification, prevention,* and *management* of ethical conflict and crisis in clinical practice. No other book or approach provides such a comprehensive, clinically practical account of ethics in obstetrics and gynecology, which is a continually evolving field.

Houston L.B.M.
New York F.A.C.
March 1993

Acknowledgments

We benefited considerably from the comments, criticisms, and suggestions from a number of colleagues as we undertook the writing of this book. We gratefully acknowledge the contributions of Baruch A. Brody; Stuart Campbell; H. Tristram Engelhardt, Jr.; B. Andrew Lustig; E. Haavi Morreim; and the two reviewers for Oxford University Press, Jonathan D. Moreno and Thomas Elkins, toward the improvement of our work. We want especially to thank Stephen Wear for his very close and critical reading of the penultimate draft. We owe a special debt of gratitude to our editor at Oxford University Press, Edith Barry, whose patience we very much appreciate and whose editorial criticisms were always valuable. We owe a great deal to these colleagues for the strengths of this book; we take full responsibility for any shortcomings that might remain.

We would also like to express our gratitude for the irreplaceable support for this work that we have received from Baruch A. Brady and the Center for Ethics, Medicine, and Public Issues of the Baylor College of Medicine, and from William Ledger and the Department of Obstetrics and Gynecology, The New York Hospital-Cornell University Medical Center.

Pearlena Duncan-Hackle and Delores Smith provided skillful and much appreciated wordprocessing assistance in the preparation of successive drafts of the text.

Finally, we spent many weekends and nights in the writing of this book, time that our families generously gave us. In gratitude for their many sacrifices as we have worked on this project over the past several years, we dedicate this book to them.

Portions of chapters of this book have appeared previously and are included with permission: Frank A. Chervenak and Laurence B. McCullough, "Cephalocentesis," in *Ultrasound in Obstetrics and Gynecology,* Frank A. Chervenak, Glenn C. Isaacson, and Stuart Campbell (eds.), Boston, Little, Brown and Company, 1993, pp. 1339–44, with permission from Frank A. Chervenak (Chapter 6); Frank A. Chervenak and Laurence B. McCullough, "Ethical Analysis of the Intrapartum Management of Pregnancy Complicated by Fetal Hydrocephalus with Macrocephaly," *Obstetrics and Gynecology* 68 (1986): 720–25 (Chapter 6) and "An Ethically Justified, Clinically Comprehensive Management Strategy for Third Trimester Pregnancies Complicated by Fetal Anomalies," *Obstetrics and Gynecology* 75 (1990): 311–16, reprinted with permission from the American College of Obstetricians and Gynecologists (Chapter 6); Frank A. Chervenak and Laurence B. McCullough, "The Fetus as Patient: Implications for Directive versus Non-Directive Counseling for Fetal Benefit," *Fetal Diagnosis and Therapy* 6 (1991): 93–100, with permission from S. Karger, AG, Basel (Chapter 6); Frank A. Chervenak and Laurence B. McCullough, "An Ethically Based Standard of Care for Fetal Therapy," *Journal of Maternal-Fetal Investigation* 1 (1991): 185–90, with permission from Springer-Verlag (Chapter 6); Frank A. Chervenak, Laurence B. McCullough, and Ronald J. Wapner, "Selective Termination to a Singleton Pregnancy is Ethically Justified," *Ultrasound in Obstetrics and Gynecology* 2 (1992): 84–87, with permission from Parthenon Publishing (Chapter 5); Frank A. Chervenak and Laurence B. McCullough, "How to Critically Evaluate Positions on Obstetric Ethics," *The Journal of Reproductive Medicine* 38 (1993): 281–84, with permission from *The Journal of Reproductive Medicine* (Chapter 1); Frank A. Chervenak and Laurence B. McCullough, "Justified Limits on Refusing Intervention," *Hastings Center Report* 21 (1991): 12–18, with permission from *Hastings Center Report* (Chapters 1 and 7); Frank A. Chervenak and Laurence B. McCullough, "Clinical Guides to Preventing Ethical Conflicts between Pregnant Women and Their Physicians," *American Journal of Obstetrics and Gynecology* 162 (1990): 303–307 (Chapter 4) and "Does Obstetrics Ethics Have Any Role to Play in the Obstetrician's Response to the Abortion Controversy?," *American Journal of Obstetrics and Gynecology* 163 (1990): 1425–29 (Chapters 3, 5, and 6), Frank A. Chervenak, Laurence B. McCullough, and Judith L. Chervenak, "Prenatal Informed Consent for Sonogram (PICS): An Indication for Obstetrical Ultrasound," *American Journal of Obstetrics and Gynecology* 161 (1989): 857–60 (Chapter 6), Laurence B. McCullough, John H. Coverdale, Timothy L. Bayer, and Frank A. Chervenak, "Ethically Justified Guidelines for Family Planning

Interventions to Prevent Pregnancy with Female Chronic Mental Patients," *American Journal of Obstetrics and Gynecology* 167 (1992): 19–25 (Chapter 5), with permission from Mosby-Year Book, Inc.; and Laurence B. McCullough, "An Ethical Model for Improving the Patient-Physician Relationship," *Industry* 25 (1988): 454–65, with permission from *Inquiry*.

Contents

I *The Identification of Ethical Conflict and Crisis in Gynecologic and Obstetric Practice*

1 | A Framework for Bioethics in the Clinical Setting

Introduction: The Aim of This Book

The modern practice of gynecology and obstetrics requires physicians in gynecologic and obstetric practice to be prepared to deal effectively with ethical conflicts that they confront in the clinical setting. Ethical conflicts occur when the circumstances of a case force a choice between two well-founded obligations. For example, when a pregnant woman refuses cesarean delivery for the management of severe fetal distress, there exists a conflict between the ethical obligation to respect her decision and the ethical obligation to protect the fetus and child it is about to become from the adverse effects of severe fetal distress. When a woman refuses surgical management of uterine cancer, there exists a conflict between the ethical obligation to prevent unnecessary mortality and morbidity and the obligation to respect the patient's choice.

Some ethical conflicts involve fundamental and apparently irresolvable differences in ethical obligations. For example, a pregnant woman may refuse cesarean delivery for the intrapartum management of a pregnancy complicated by well-documented, complete placenta previa[1] and insist on vaginal delivery instead. On the one hand, there is an ethical obligation to the at term fetus to prevent its unnecessary death and to prevent the mortality and morbidity risks for the pregnant woman of vaginal delivery. On the other hand, forcing cesarean delivery on a woman who has refused it constitutes a very serious invasion of her body and freedom. When a patient who has agreed to surgical management of uterine cancer refuses to permit the intraoperative administration of blood products on religious grounds, the physician must choose between failing to prevent unnecessary mortality and morbidity and doing violence to a patient's religious beliefs and values. In both cases, the first alternative is unreasonable from a clinical perspective while the second alternative is unreasonable from the patient's perspective. Yet some choice must be made; doing nothing is not an option. Hence, rarely, some ethical conflicts count as ethical crises.

The purpose of this book is to equip the reader with the intellectual and clinical tools to deal effectively with ethical conflicts and crises in clinical practice. The usual approach in the bioethics literature involves proposing and defending strategies for resolving ethical conflicts. This book differs in that it emphasizes the *prevention* of ethical conflict in gynecologic and obstetric practice and, when prevention fails, the *management* of ethical crises. Ethical conflicts and crises both occur too frequently in clinical practice. It will be better for all concerned—patients, their families, the physicians who care for them, health care institutions, and society—if the incidence of ethical conflicts and crises were reduced, substantially reduced.

This much-needed reduction in the incidence of ethical conflicts and crises and the consequent improvement in the quality of gynecologic and obstetric medical care constitute the overall goals of this book. We intend to accomplish these goals in three steps. First, we provide ethical frameworks for the identification of ethical conflicts and crises in gynecologic and obstetric practice in terms of a framework for bioethics in the clinical setting (Part I of this book). We then develop and defend clinical strategies for the prevention of ethical conflicts and crises in gynecologic and obstetric practice (Part II of this book). Finally, because the prevention of ethical crises may sometimes fail, we develop and defend clinical strategies for the management of those ethical crises that do occur in gynecologic and obstetric practice (Part III of this book). The three parts of this book, taken together, aim at a comprehensive account of gynecologic and obstetric ethics.

The Aims of This Chapter

Because gynecologic and obstetric ethics are subspecialties of bioethics, clarifying the nature of bioethics is the necessary first step of the inquiry that we undertake in this book. Therefore, in this first chapter we provide an account of what bioethics is, describe the methodology that we shall employ, introduce the reader to a framework for bioethics in the clinical setting, and distinguish this framework from others in the literature.

Doing so sets the stage for the second and third chapters: describing and defending frameworks for both gynecologic and obstetric ethics in the clinical setting. These frameworks make possible the identification of ethical conflict in gynecologic and obstetric practice.

What Bioethics Is

Bioethics is the disciplined study of the morality of health care,[2] including the morality of: physicians; patients; the institutions[3] of health care that organize, deliver, or pay for health care; and health care policy. Morality concerns the beliefs and practices of human beings and social institutions about right and wrong behavior and about good and bad character. Right and wrong behavior concerns what we ought and ought not to do in our behavior toward each other and toward institutions and in the behavior of institutions toward each other and toward us. Good and bad character concerns the traits of character that we ought to cultivate, the virtues, and the traits of character that we ought not to cultivate and ought to eliminate when they come to exist in our lives, the vices.[4]

We understand virtues to be those traits of character that blunt mere self-interest and therefore direct our concern to the interests of others. In other words, the virtues both move us to focus our main concern on and, crucially, to promote and protect the interests of others. Virtues both motivate us and generate distinctive obligations. Their essentially *other*-regarding nature and motivating force make the virtues basic to what morality ought to be in medicine, because on the basis of the virtues the physician creates the obligation to protect and promote the patient's interests. We understand the vices to be those traits of character that unleash mere self-interest, so that we become blinded to the interests of others and thus become unmoved to act in a way that protects and promotes the interests of others. The vices generate no obligations. Their exclusively *self*-regarding nature makes the vices antithetical to what morality ought to be in medicine, because the vices undercut the physician's obligation to protect and promote the patient's interests.

Methodological Considerations

Before setting out and defending a framework for bioethics in the clinical setting, in terms of which frameworks for gynecologic and obstetric ethics will be developed, we want to make some comments on methodology in bioethics. We do so because bioethics is marked by methodological disputes. These concern the content or subject matter of bioethics, the starting point for bioethics, the relationship between philosophical ethical theory and bioethics, and the result that should be expected from inquiries such as the one we undertake in this book. In this section we will clarify our view in this book for each of these four methodological considerations.

The Content or Subject Matter of Bioethics

We understand the subject matter of bioethics to comprise well-argued answers to the question: What ought morality to be in health care? "Health care", in turn, is meant to include the morality of physicians, patients, institutions of health care, and health care policy (locally, regionally, nationally, and internationally). At present, the morality of physicians and the morality of health care policy dominate the bioethics literature.

This book can be distinguished from others in bioethics because it emphasizes the morality of *both* physicians *and* patients. Thus, the frameworks for gynecologic and obstetric ethics that we will defend address the ethical obligations of *both* the physician *and* the female patient and pregnant woman. The ethical obligations of patients constitute an essentially neglected topic in bioethics.[5] Our focus is thus on bioethics in clinical practice. Ours is not a book, however, on clinical ethics, as that term is used by some, namely, to indicate that clinical ethics is an autonomous intellectual discipline.[6] To the contrary, clinically oriented bioethics should correctly be understood to be a field with disciplinary roots in both philosophy and medicine.

We do not equate the subject matter of bioethics with health care policy or policy considerations, as some do, with the result that bioethics becomes a subspecialty of political philosophy.[7] This approach to bioethics abstracts from the micro-level of the physician-patient relationship to the macro-level of public policy. The macro-level approach focuses on what morality ought to be in health care policy—and, to some extent, on what morality ought to be for health care institutions—as the main subject matter of bioethics. In addition, the macro-level approach tends to treat all ethical conflicts between physicians and patients as ethical crises, where the central issue becomes constraints on the use and abuse of power of the state to coerce beliefs and behaviors on the part of patients. The ethics of power is a crucial, though much overlooked, topic in bioethics.[8] We shall address this topic, but in the concrete context of an inquiry into what morality ought to be for physicians and patients, when that morality is affected by institutions of health care and health care policy.

The Starting Point for Bioethics in the Clinical Setting

If one takes the view that the subject matter of bioethics is to be equated to health care policy, then one is justified in starting bioethics where, for example, Engelhardt does: asking after the necessary conditions for the possibility of a peaceable community, where conflicts of power should be negotiated by the transmutation of power into the discourse of reason, rather than resolved through the application of power.[9]

In our view, the main problem with this starting point is that it makes bioethics an almost purely abstract enterprise. To inquire into the *possibility* of something is to inquire into an idea, for possibilities possess only the ontological status (i.e., type of being) of ideas. To inquire into the *necessary conditions* of an idea results in conceptual clarity only. Whether such clarity is applicable and adequate to concrete human relationships, such as that between physicians and their patients, and to concrete social institutions, such as group practices and hospitals, cannot be determined solely on the basis of conceptual clarity. The applicability of conceptual clarity to clinical practice must be independently established. To establish applicability, one needs to establish the individually necessary and jointly sufficient material conditions of concrete human relationships, such as the physician-patient relationship. These conditions are provided by the virtues. The virtues constitute the starting point of bioethics because they provide intellectual warrant or justification for the physician-patient relationship as fundamentally moral, or other-regarding, in character,[10] because the virtues are the basis of the obligation to protect and promote the interests of the patient.

The Relationship Between Philosophical Ethical Theory and Bioethics

Once the starting point for bioethics in the clinical setting has been identified, an important, indeed, fundamental, methodological question immediately arises: How should one proceed from that starting point through the subject matter of bioethics in the clinical setting? Baruch Brody has recently provided a succinct categorization of the two basic answers that have been made in response to this question: the "upwards-down model" and the "downwards-up model."[11]

An "upwards-down model" works through the subject matter of bioethics in terms of an ethical theory that is assumed to be adequate, without revision, to the task. Ethical theory is thought of as akin to Newtonian physics, which is taken to be a correct and adequate theory because it allows us to deduce answers to our questions. The classic example is Clouser's "Bioethics" entry in the *Encyclopedia of Bioethics*. "What constitutes one's view of the 'same old ethics' . . . is simply carried over to the biomedical arena."[12] Ethical theory is already assumed to be adequate and is simply applied to the clinical setting. This methodology has been dubbed the "engineering model" by Caplan[13] and subjected to serious criticism. Any particular theory, when employed deductively, is shown to be inadequate sooner or later.[14] To this criticism we would add that adherents of this model tend to address only one half of morality in health care, for example, right and wrong behavior, and do so at the expense of the virtues[15] (or the virtues at the expense of right or wrong behavior).[16] As a consequence, the connections between the two are strained, at best, and artificial, at worst, and so the "engineering model" fails to provide a coherent account of bioethics in the clinical setting.

In our view, the "downwards-up model" has a great deal to recommend.[17] It does not assume the existence of an already applicable and adequate ethical theory in the abstract, but seeks to develop theoretical concerns out of concrete human relationships and social institutions, the physician-patient relationship and the clinical setting in particular. On the engineering model, ethical principles tend not to be concrete action guides, as they should. Clouser and Gert's criticism of "principlism" is apropos here: because of their abstractness, principles derived in an engineering model for bioethics tend to be little more than "chapter headings for discussion of some concepts which are often only superficially related to each other."[18] On a downwards-up model, by contrast, and as we intend to show, it is possible to articulate ethical principles as genuine action guides, as "specific directive[s] for action"[19] in the form of "clear, coherent, comprehensive, and specific rules for action."[20]

Our approach in this book is not casuistical, an important and powerful methodology for bioethics.[21] We do not start with cases—analyzed either in terms of rules with "triangulation" to new cases[22] or analyzed in terms of intuitions with extrapolation to principles.[23] Instead, in a variant of the downwards-up model, we start with the individually necessary and jointly sufficient material conditions for the physician-patient relationship and develop the meaning, scope, and implications of the principles of beneficence and respect for autonomy on this basis.[24]

The Result That Should be Expected

Our final methodological consideration concerns the result to be expected from a "downwards-up model" for bioethics. This can be concisely stated: a rigorous, clinically applicable and adequate account, based on the virtues of self-effacement, self-sacrifice, compassion, and integrity, of the ethical principles of beneficence and respect for autonomy that explains the basis, meaning, scope, and implications of those principles in clinical practice.

The account that we shall offer is defensible because it is subject to the methodological requirements of philosophical reasoning: clarity, consistency, coherence, applicability, and adequacy. These are traditional criteria for rigorous philosophical reasoning.[25] In the absence of clarity, consistency, and coherence, analysis of ethical conflicts and arguments about their identification, prevention, and management cannot be undertaken in any reliable fashion. In the absence of applicability and adequacy, even the most rigorous analysis and argument will have no demonstrable relevance to the actual moral behavior and character of physicians and patients. These five criteria are individually necessary and jointly sufficient methodological conditions for practical philosophical reasoning in bioethics.

Clarity requires that terms and concepts be provided precise meaning. Consistency requires that those terms always be used with precise meaning and that reasoning be free of contradiction. Coherence requires that approaches to bioethics be cohesive internally. Applicability requires that bioethics results in comprehensive, clinically relevant guides to behavior and character. Finally, adequacy requires that gynecologic and obstetric ethics guide physicians not only in identifying and managing ethical conflicts, but also in preventing ethical conflicts, in clinical practice. Applicability concerns present practices and policies, while adequacy concerns future practices and policies.

We choose the term "basis" deliberately because this book is not about the *foundations* of ethical principles or the *foundations* of bioethics.[26] At the same time, we do not go as far as some and take the view that philosophy must get by with no foundation or basis whatever for principles.[27] Instead, we believe that for any account of the ethics of concrete relationships, such as the physician-patient relationship, some grounds must be provided for that account, some reason for the plausibility of the account.[28] "Basis" captures the sense of what we intend to provide well enough. It "works, and for as long."[29]

The meaning of ethical principles is found in the content of the principles of beneficence and respect for autonomy in the clinical setting. Despite its ancient pedigree, especially in the history of medical ethics, there has been scant effort to articulate the content of the principle of beneficence, particularly in relationship to the "interests" of patients. The same can be said for the meaning of respect for autonomy in relationship to the interests of patients. An original contribution of this book to bioethics is to clarify these principles in terms of an account of three types of patients' interests and in the form of concrete action-guides for the care of patients.

The scope of these two principles is found in the limits of the areas of human interests to which they apply. This is an especially important consideration for beneficence (which should not be equated with paternalism), the limited scope of which we underscore throughout this book. The failure to appreciate its limited scope has caused fundamental misunderstanding of beneficence, both by those who argue that it cannot be a lexically ordered principle in bioethics[30] and by those who defend other versions of the principle.[31] Similarly, we shall argue that respect for autonomy has a limited scope, even when exercised in refusal of health care interventions.

The implications of beneficence and respect for autonomy concern what each, considered alone, requires, as well as what their limits should be when considered together. The latter concerns the relative significance of the principles and how they are related to each other.

Having clarified what bioethics is and having situated ourselves methodologically, we are now in a position to introduce the reader to a framework for bioethics in the clinical setting.

A Framework for Bioethics in the Clinical Setting

A framework for bioethics in the clinical setting sets out and defends an account of the basis, meaning, scope, and implications of the ethical principles of beneficence and respect for autonomy in the physician-patient relationship. By doing so, a framework for bioethics explains the origin and meaning of the obligation to protect and promote the patient's interests. Beauchamp and Childress claim, correctly, that "the belief that there is an obligation to provide benefits is an unchallenged assumption in medicine,"[32] deeply rooted in the histories of the ethics of the health care professions.[33] This obligation, however, is not free floating, self-sustaining, and waiting to be discovered. Instead, it must be created and sustained by the physician, in order for the physician-patient relationship to come into existence as a moral relationship. The virtues account for this moral phenomenon. Thus, a framework for bioethics in the clinical setting finds its basis in four fundamental virtues—self-effacement, self-sacrifice, compassion, and integrity—because these virtues constitute the starting point for bioethics in the clinical setting.

This section therefore begins with an account of how these four virtues constitute the basis of a framework for bioethics in the clinical setting. These virtues direct the physician to protect and promote the interests of the patient. In the second part of this section we therefore provide an account of three different kinds of interests patients have: social-role, subjective, and deliberative. In the third part of this section we show how the ethical principle of beneficence interprets the social-role interests of an individual patient in clinical practice. In the fourth part of this section we show how the ethical principle of respect for autonomy interprets the subjective and deliberative interests of an individual patient in clinical practice. In the fifth part of this section we address the relative significance of beneficence and respect for autonomy in clinical judgment. In the sixth part of this section we address a crucial question for obstetric ethics: When is a human being a patient? In the seventh part of this section we provide a critique of the concept of patients as "strangers" to their physicians. Our framework for bioethics in the clinical setting firmly rejects this concept. Because the physician-patient relationship is situated in the context of third and fourth parties to that relationship, we address the physician's obligations to these parties in the eighth part of this section.

Four Basic Virtues: Self-Effacement, Self-Sacrifice, Compassion, and Integrity

The relationship between virtues and principles in bioethics, in our view, concerns how the former serve as the basis for the latter because four basic virtues—self-effacement, self-sacrifice, compassion, and integrity—constitute the individually necessary and jointly sufficient material conditions for creating and sustaining the physician-patient relationship as moral in character, that is, as fundamentally other-regarding.[34] Creating and then sustaining a moral relationship with patients by the physician involves, first, turning one's attention and concern away from oneself, away from one's own interests, to the interests of the patient and, second, routinely acting to protect and promote the patient's interests. The virtues of self-effacement and self-sacrifice move the physician to turn his or her attention to the patient. Sustaining a moral relationship with patients involves the physician in being moved over time to protect and promote the interests of patients and to do so with renewed dedication to patient after patient. These are what the virtues of compassion and integrity do in the physician's moral life. Self-effacement and self-sacrifice, on the one hand,

and integrity and compassion, on the other, are synergistic. Each pair refreshes and enriches the other. Thus, together the four create and sustain the obligation on the part of the physician to protect and promote the patient's interests.

Can one practice gynecology and obstetrics (or any other health care specialty) without being virtuous? "Perhaps" is the strongest possible answer, we believe, because, in the absence of these virtues, one's relationship with patients becomes entirely contractual: the physician delivers specified services and nothing more. This is a minimalist relationship, not just morally but also legally.[35] In the law, it is important to note, the physician-patient relationship is not simply contractual; it also has a fiduciary dimension.[36] A fiduciary is legally understood to be "a person holding the character of a trustee, in respect to the trust and confidence involved in it and the scrupulous good faith and candor which it requires" and also to be a "person having duty, created by his undertaking, to act primarily for another's benefit in matters connected with such undertaking."[37] In medicine the fiduciary holds the interests of the patient in trust. The physician, as fiduciary (1) must be in a position to know reliably the patient's interests, (2) should be concerned primarily with protecting and promoting the interests of the patient, and (3) should be concerned only secondarily with protecting and promoting the physician's own interests.

In a contractual relationship none of these three conditions apply. To be sure, the physician is to treat the patient as a person, an end in herself, as Kant's categorical imperative would demand.[38] This means that the physician is never to treat the patient as a means merely to the physician's own end. Protection against such abuse is provided by an insistence on informed consent, a process in which the physician provides the patient scientific and technical information in an impartial and complete fashion and then leaves the patient alone to decide for herself what is or is not to be done.[39]

Respect for the patient as a person entails respect for this power to decide and noninterference with its exercise. To be sure, respect for the patient as a person blunts the physician's self-interest. But respect for the patient as a person, in this Kantian sense, is abstract, because the power to decide is the same in all patients. Thus, in a contractual relation of this Kantian type, the physician is surely obliged to acknowledge the patient's autonomy, in the form of the power to decide, but not to go on to attend to the concrete, particular interests that provide the context in which the exercise of power is meaningful to the physician and patient. Unable to know what those interests are, the contractual, bureaucratic physician need not be moved to act to protect and promote them.[40] A contractual model of the physician-patient relationship is therefore unable to connect physicians and patients, to explain why and how it is that a physician cares for a particular patient. Some account must be given for how to fulfill the obligation to protect and promote *this* patient's interests, not interests abstractly, and thus for why the physician-patient relationship involves concrete, particular individuals, not abstractions, that is, (mere) concepts.

A Kantian, contractual account cannot explain how this occurs; an account based on virtues can. The physician's patient-directed concern becomes a concrete reality, rather than a possibility, when four fundamental virtues characterize the physician: self-effacement, self-sacrifice, compassion, and integrity. They are thus the individually necessary and jointly sufficient material conditions for creating and sustaining the obligation to protect and promote the patient's interests and thus making the physician-patient relationship a concrete moral, fiduciary relationship. Let us consider each virtue in greater detail.

Self-Effacement

The first of these fundamental virtues is self-effacement. This trait or habit of character inclines the physician to blunt mere self-interest and to focus attention on the interests of the patient. Self-effacement accomplishes this other-directed, moral concern by negating the adverse impact on the physician's attitude and behavior of possibly distracting differences between the physician and a particular patient in matters of socioeconomic class, education, race, gender, culture, religion, language, manners, hygiene, and the "weakness and bad behavior of patients, and the number of little difficulties and contradictions which every physician must encounter in his practice."[41] By negating the adverse affect of these factors on the physician, self-effacement erases or effaces them as far as the physician is concerned. The effect of self-effacement is thus to turn the physician's attention away from matters of mere self-interest toward the interests of the patient.

Self-effacement has a venerable history in medical ethics. In his *Medical Ethics* Thomas Percival addressed self-effacement as one of four cardinal virtues.[42] His term for it was "condescension." Unfortunately, this term jars the late-twentieth century ear, but it made good sense in his day. Percival practiced and conceived his medical ethics at a time when medical care was no longer delivered just in the privacy of the homes of the gentry, the socioeconomic class to which university-educated physicians themselves belonged. Medical care was also provided in public hospitals, called "infirmaries," that were expressly created for the care of the lower socioeconomic classes, especially the so-called "sick poor." In the setting of the infirmary the physician encountered patients outside the normal patterns of social intercourse, which in Percival's England were markedly class-conscious on both sides. It would not do, Percival seemed to have thought, to treat the sick poor, what we now call "public" or "clinic" patients, as someone's servant or cook or gardener. To see such individuals as patients, as individuals in need of the physician's ministrations, differences that would ordinarily have been an automatic feature of socially conditioned human relationships had to be negated. Percival's solution was to require the physician to "condescend," to put aside as unimportant to himself his comparatively lofty social standing, superior education, and comfortable life and descend to the level of the patient, of a sick individual. The result is that the physician's full attention can then be given to the patient.

In our time the vast majority of physicians come from the more comfortable socioeconomic classes and, by virtue of their salaries, enjoy at least upper middle class economic status. The challenge that Percival and his colleagues faced with the advent of the social institution of the infirmary remains a permanent challenge to physicians. This is especially the case for medical students and residents, who spend a great deal of their time in training in public institutions or with "public" or "clinic" patients. Moreover, in the United States, with our history of openness to immigrants, many of these patients are newly arrived—with or without legal documentation—and so their languages, customs, and expectations can diverge sharply from those of physicians and students caring for them. Self-effacement requires that such differences be set aside by the physician, so that he or she can come to see the patient as an individual, someone the protection and promotion of whose particular interests should be the physician's primary concern. Self-effacement requires a certain discipline, a discipline of patience and a steady focus on the patient's interests.

Self-Sacrifice

Taking care of patients is demanding as well as rewarding work. Taking care of patients can also be irritating, frustrating, and dangerous work. Demanding work and personal risk call for sacrifice on the part of the physician, sacrifice of time, energy, obligations to others, especially family, other interests, and even health and life. It is important to recall that the latter two were not newly introduced as concerns for physicians by the HIV epidemic. There have been epidemics before, as well as risk of infection for diseases such as hepatitis in its various classifications. In addition, physicians in the military in combat areas are at constant peril, given the fluidity and lethality of the modern battlefield—land, air, and sea alike. And, of course, physicians who staff emergency departments regularly face personal risk in the care of violent, often critically ill patients. Self-sacrifice requires physicians to accept risk to themselves and to be calm in that acceptance, so that mere self-interest is blunted in favor of protecting and promoting the interests of the patient.[43]

Compassion

Self-effacement and self-sacrifice direct the physician's attention and concern to the patient's interests. These two virtues thus begin the process of creating a moral relationship with the patient. These two virtues, however, do not continue or sustain that process, because they do not move the physician to protect and promote the interests of the patient. When the physician is moved to do so, the moral relationship with the patient is initially sustained. Compassion is the virtue that initially sustains the moral relationship with patients.

Like self-effacement, compassion enjoys a certain prominence in the history of medical ethics. John Gregory, the leading medical ethicist of the Scottish Enlightenment, followed his contemporary, the philosopher David Hume, in believing that each of us has a natural capacity to experience the very feelings that another experiences.[44] When we feel the pain or distress of another, our repugnance to that feeling moves us to act to relieve that pain or distress. Hume and Gregory call this capacity "sympathy" or "humanity":

> I come now to mention the moral qualities peculiarly required in the character of a physician: that sensibility of heart which makes us feel for the distresses of our fellow creatures, and which, of consequence, incites us in the most powerful manner to relieve them. Sympathy produces an anxious attention to a thousand little circumstances that relieve the patient; an attention that money can never purchase . . . If the physician possesses gentleness of manners and a compassionate heart . . . , the patient feels his approach like that of a guardian angel ministering to his relief; while every visit of a physician who is unfeeling, and rough in his manners, makes his heart sink within him, as at the presence of one, who comes to pronounce his doom.[45]

Two centuries later, we are less inclined to accept Gregory's (and Hume's) moral psychology, and so we require an alternative account. Reich has recently provided an excellent, clinically applicable account of compassion.[46] On Reich's account, compassion has three moments or phases, each in response to three moments or phases of another's suffering.

The first phase is mute suffering, "the experience of being speechless in the face of one's suffering."[47] The compassionate first response of the physician is therefore "silent empathy, silent compassion, an active response of being present in a way that encourages the patient to speak, to name her suffering."[48] The patient's suffering then enters a second phase, "expressive suffering," which can be a "lament" or, importantly, a "story."[49] The physician's response, "expressive compassion," again active, is to name the patient's suffering, for example, through the language of diagnosis and retelling the patient's story.[50] The third phase of suffering involves finding a "new identity in suffering," making sense of one's suffering and coming to terms with it.[51] The response of the physician is to undergo change with the patient, to suffer in response to the patient's suffering.[52] Being present to the patient, helping to shape the patient's experience through diagnostic language and therapeutic interventions, and suffering in response to and for the patient make together for a compassionate response to the patient.

Integrity

Integrity is the virtue that sustains a compassionate response and thus sustains over time the moral relationship to patients. Integrity concerns the coherence, the well-knitted-togetherness of the physician's moral life. Integrity has several dimensions. One is intellectual and practical: a lifelong commitment to excellence in the care of patients,[53] lived out in a commitment to well-formed clinical judgment. In the absence of this intellectual commitment, integrity vanishes. Another is aesthetic: a renewing of oneself, so that one can suffer in response to and for patients without being used up in the process. Suffering in response to and for patients involves an enormous expenditure of energy in response to events and experiences that are not pretty. It is as if a little bit of one's self is used up, requiring one to refresh or renew oneself. The commitment to intellectual and practical excellence is valuable precisely because it is so renewing of oneself. Another dimension of integrity is social: the commitment to a moral life in service to others. Here integrity connects to self-effacement and self-sacrifice through compassion. In this way, integrity brings the fundamental virtues together into sustained synergy. As a consequence, integrity moves the physician to fulfill his or her obligations in service to each patient, day in and day out, for a lifetime. Any threat to integrity is thus a threat to the existence of the physician-patient relationship.

Limits on the Virtues: Legitimate Self-Interest

These four fundamental virtues have limits on the obligations that they generate. Self-effacement and self-sacrifice can become tyrannical, destructive traits of character if they are taken to be absolute, without limits of any kind. Some have asserted what amounts to such a view in discussing the responsibility of physicians to care for HIV-infected patients. For example, one leading scholar of bioethics claims: "To refuse to care for AIDS patients, even if the danger were much greater than it is, is to abnegate what is essential to being a physician."[54] This sort of claim shows a misunderstanding of self-sacrifice and of the virtues generally. They *blunt* self-interest but, in doing so, they do not *eliminate* all self-interest as mere self-interest or, more harshly, selfishness. In other words, the mistake made in this claim is to fail to recognize the morally significant category of legitimate self-interest on the part of physicians and the compatibility of the physician's legitimate self-interest with such virtues as self-effacement and self-sacrifice.

THREE FORMS OF LEGITIMATE SELF-INTEREST. The concept of legitimate self-interest has not been given the careful consideration it should be accorded in approaches to bioethics that take the virtues seriously. In our view, legitimate self-interest comprises a variety of morally significant features of a physician's life as a whole, because self-interest can connect to integrity. The forms of legitimate self-interest range along a continuum: beginning with the individually necessary and jointly sufficient conditions for learning and practicing medicine well; extending through fulfilling serious, inescapable obligations to individuals in the physician's moral life other than patients; and to embracing those activities necessary for a coherent and meaningful life. Let us consider each in turn.

First, physicians properly claim a legitimate self-interest in the requisites in their own lives for learning and practicing with integrity the skills of good patient care: time to study and learn, time to reflect, adequate rest and an alert mind, to name a few that quickly and appropriately come to mind. That is, some forms of self-interest become legitimate self-interest when they constitute the individually necessary and jointly sufficient conditions for providing good patient care. This variety of legitimate self-interest, for example, justifies reasonable limits on duty hours for those in residency training programs.

Second, physicians are bound by serious, inescapable obligations to people other than patients, namely and particularly, spouses, children, lovers, family, friends, students, and colleagues. While the physician may have freely accepted such obligations, he or she is not morally free to abrogate those obligations. Fulfilling those obligations is a central feature of the physician's moral identity as a whole person and so they should properly be regarded as part of the physician's legitimate self-interest.

Finally, legitimate self-interest includes those personal traits and activities that each physician finds to be meaningful outside being a physician and outside the network of obligations to others. These are the activities that engage him or her as a "private" person and that also provide deep and lasting fulfillment and satisfaction; these activities make for a complete life or at least a life that is coherent and meaningful. They often support and sustain the first two forms of legitimate self-interest, connecting them together and to integrity. Religious beliefs and other forms of serious moral convictions are among this third type of legitimate self-interest.

We are now in a position to define mere self-interest—"selfishness" seems too harsh a term. Mere self-interest comprises those forms of self-interest that cannot be shown to be one of the above three forms of legitimate self-interest.

SELF-EFFACEMENT AND LEGITIMATE SELF-INTEREST. Self-effacement is directed as a virtue to blunting forms of self-interest that are in almost all cases forms of mere self-interest. These mere self-interests—for example, unreflective frustration with the so-called noncompliant patient or anger at bureaucratic hurdles that third party payers seem devoted to erecting in the physician's path—can be readily reined in by the virtue of self-effacement. Thus, for the most part, self-effacement is a virtue the moral demands of which should be regarded in clinical practice as routine and nonburdensome.

There may be some exceptions. A colleague of ours, a pediatric critical care physician, told of how he had finally had it with a grandmother who was interfering with her daughter's decisions about the patient, the woman's grandchild. This woman was also interfering, sometimes quite obtrusively, with the care of the child by nurses, physicians, and technicians. She was a general nuisance most of the time, something worse sometimes. Over many days, he said, he asked this woman to appreciate the difficulties she was causing, he tried to understand her needs and respond to them, and he asked her please not to do what she was doing.

Finally, one morning, after a particularly unpleasant event, he had told her, "Back off!"

This, of course, was an expression of anger. As such, it was clearly meant to focus this woman's mind and change her behavior. One might ask, "Are there unjustified expressions of anger on the part of the physician?" After all, isn't anger at the surrogates of pediatric patients—or at patients themselves—a form of mere self-interest that self-effacement is always supposed to blunt? Perhaps not, especially when such expressions of anger are undertaken as last-ditch efforts to get a patient's or a patient's surrogate's attention and change behavior that is at risk for adversely affecting the patient. Sometimes expressions of anger can succeed in accomplishing these goals when nothing else has.

If this line of reasoning makes sense, then the following can be said with some confidence: patients or patients' surrogates have no right to take umbrage at legitimate expressions of anger or other forms of legitimate self-interest rooted in the well-being of patients on the part of physicians. Indeed, patients and their surrogates are ethically obligated to attend to these forms of legitimate self-interest and act on them. After all, it seems, patients and their surrogates owe their physicians a certain level of serious attention and consequent intellectual and behavioral discipline. This is especially true when the stakes are high for patient care of allowing undisciplined thinking and behaviors to go unchecked. This theme will emerge to greater prominence in the course of the following chapters.

SELF-SACRIFICE AND LEGITIMATE SELF-INTEREST. The virtue of self-sacrifice also affects both mere and legitimate self-interest. If the care of a particular patient requires extra time or if the hospital requires paperwork to be completed in a timely fashion so that it can routinely collect payments and secure the financial base of its mission, expecting the physician to be self-sacrificing seems reasonable. When self-sacrifice involves risk to the physician's health or life, however, self-sacrifice aims at something more, the regulation of the physician's legitimate self-interest. This is because risks to health and life involve all three forms of legitimate self-interest described above. "Must legitimate self-interest always be sacrificed?" is a question that must be addressed in any adequate account of the virtue of self-sacrifice.

One thing seems clear from the outset: the virtue of self-sacrifice cannot be understood to be absolutely controlling of the physician's thought and behavior, as some would seem to have it.[55] This is because legitimate self-interest should always be taken into account by the physician in the process of determining the proper moral demands of the virtue of self-sacrifice.

There is no straightforward algorithm for negotiating conflicts between self-sacrifice and legitimate self-interest. In part, this is because there is no uniform set of legitimate self-interests that characterizes each and every physician. Some are married or in long-term relationships, others not. Some have or wish to have children; others not. Some have weighty obligations to family, for example, caring for a frail, elderly parent at home; others have the routine obligations to family. Some are devoted full-time to their profession; others cannot flourish without an occasional foray in a trout stream or an evening of Puccini or Mozart. As a consequence, the process of negotiating conflicts between self-sacrifice and legitimate self-interest will allow of some variability.

Some rules of thumb, though, seem reasonable. First, every effort should be made to reduce unnecessary impositions on legitimate self-interest in day-to-day clinical practice. We have in mind such matters as making universal infection control a reality, establishing rational and fair staffing and call schedules, and so on. Second, the physician needs to distinguish carefully between one's legitimate self-interest and mere self-interest. When in doubt the physician should favor the conclusion that the self-interest in question should be treated as mere self-interest, so that the physician's primary focus remains the patient's interests. Third, one's judgment of the resolution of conflicts between self-sacrifice and legitimate self-interest should be tested for its intellectual rigor and reliability against the considered judgment of colleagues and, perhaps, the views of thoughtful patients or the public.

Fourth, institutional practices and policies need to be carefully reviewed, to determine whether they impose a tyrannical concept of self-sacrifice, on the one hand, or encourage mere self-interest, for example, in remuneration for its own sake, to rule the roost, on the other hand. Both tyrannical self-sacrifice and mere self-interest, we believe, are threats to the moral life of the physician. Institutional third parties therefore have an ethical obligation to protect and promote both the virtues and the legitimate self-interests that are essential to the moral lives of physicians. In other words, institutional third parties have an obligation to respect the autonomy of the physician when that autonomy is exercised on behalf of the virtues of self-effacement and self-sacrifice or of legitimate self-interest connected to these two basic virtues. In our view, institutional third parties for the most part have yet to acknowledge this as among their ethical obligations. We are all of us, physicians and patients alike, at moral peril as the result.

Finally, if one reaches reliably the conclusion that a conflict between self-sacrifice and legitimate self-interest should be managed in favor of legitimate self-interest, this should be explained to the patient. After all patients, too, have a vital stake in sustaining the moral lives of their physicians. That is, respect on the part of the patient for the autonomy of the physician should include respecting the physician's legitimate self-interests. This would be a direct parallel to the physician's autonomy-based obligation to respect the patient's legitimate interests.

SELF-SACRIFICE AND HIV-INFECTED PATIENTS. The preceding discussion applies directly to an ethical issue of considerable contemporary significance, the nature and limits of the physician's obligation to care for HIV-infected patients. This is no small matter in obstetrics, for example, where occupational exposure to infected blood may occur with greater incidence than in some other specialties. We assume here that universal infection control reduces the risk of exposure to a manageable minimum. Intellectual integrity requires this assumption, because reliable current evidence supports it. We also assume that changes in technique, for example, using surgical techniques that are less blood-producing or suturing away from, rather than towards, one's hands make important contributions to this goal. Technological innovations can also make significant contributions to this goal. Every physician has an indisputable legitimate interest in institutional policies and practices that reduce the incidence of occupational exposure to a manageable minimum. Any institution that fails to have such policies and practices as a routine undermines that legitimate interest and thus fails to fulfill its minimum ethical obligation to physicians. Physicians who do not rigorously observe and follow such policies and practices similarly violate their obligations to other health care professionals.

Physicians are not, we believe, obligated to take unreasonable risks to their health and lives. To expect them to do so as a matter of course[56] transforms the virtue of self-sacrifice into a vice, namely, tyrannical self-sacrifice or false heroism,[57] because such an expectation presumes that self-sacrifice generates an absolute obligation. We expect no such obligation of others who routinely face risks to health and life. For example, no military officer is obligated to defend a position "to the last man." Such a deed is not part of the routine moral life of military personnel.[58] This aspect of military ethics has been overlooked by those who draw analogies to the military as the basis for arguments to accept serious risk to self in the care of HIV-infected patients.

There is no accepted algorithm for determining when risk to self becomes unreasonable. Nonetheless, it is reasonable to insist that a rigorous process be applied in reaching and testing such a judgment. First, the incidence of risk must be such that it is at a level where most would argue that the level is significant, in contrast to the present incidence of less-than-1-percent. Second, it must be the case that no known or experimental equipment or procedures could reasonably be expected to reduce that incidence to a manageable minimum. Third, any claim that a significant risk should count as an unreasonable risk must be subject to rigorous peer review. An individual physician's impressions or beliefs, however forcefully asserted, fail this crucial test of intellectual integrity.[59]

Should the incidence of risk of a particular procedure or setting be someday reasonably judged to be irreversibly unreasonable for a particular procedure or setting, institutional policy and practice should be to call for volunteers, because the obligation to be self-sacrificing no longer exists. These individuals should be fully indemnified, for disability as well as loss of life, for occupational HIV infection. Here an analogy to a military tradition is appropriate: calling for volunteers for dangerous missions, where the danger is "above and beyond the call of duty," what philosophers term "supererogatory."

Notice that disclosure of HIV+ status by the patient to the physician is not a factor in the physician's obligation to accept routine, reasonable risks of exposure to HIV infection. It is, however, a factor when the physician's risk is reliably judged to be unreasonable. Thus, the patient has an ethical obligation vis-à-vis the physician's legitimate interest in avoiding unreasonable risks to disclose HIV+ status. This also applies when documented exposure to a known sector for HIV infection occurs. In both cases, the patient is obligated to her physician to disclose her HIV serostatus and consent to testing.

Obviously, in the case of reasonable risk of exposure, it is surely to the advantage of the patient to disclose her HIV+ status, so that appropriate changes in the management plan to benefit and protect the patient can be made. Physicians are thus justified on these grounds in asking for information about HIV status. But, given current scientific information regarding the occupational risk of HIV infection, there is no ethical justification for universal mandatory screening, only mandatory screening for procedures involving risks reliably judged to be unreasonable (a condition not met at present by any gynecologic or obstetric procedure or setting) or when documented occupational exposure has occurred. The latter is justified because the patient has no right in any ethical theory to expose the physician to gratuitous, unconsented-to harm.

Does the physician have an ethical obligation to the patient to disclose that the physician is HIV+, when this is the case? This is a matter of considerable and ongoing controversy.[60] Such disclosure to patients, we believe, is an essential element in efforts to reduce the exposure of the patient to HIV from procedures which could cause physician-to-patient infection and to protect the patient from HIV-related cognitive or physical disability on the physician's part. This would also seem to be information to which the patient is entitled under the reasonable person standard of disclosure in informed consent.[61] A theoretical or only slight risk of an event of serious nature, namely, serious illness followed by premature death, seems significant in our understanding of this standard. This is because a reasonable person can surely count the qualitative significance of a disastrous event in her life as much as or even more than its incidence of occurrence. Hence, disclosure of HIV+ status by the physician to the patient would seem to be obligatory. The same would apply to disclosure of alcohol or drug abuse that impairs the physician's clinical judgment and skills.

Some physicians worry that such disclosure means the end of their professional life and livelihood.[62] This need not be the case, however. At least five roles for the physician remain entirely unaffected by HIV+ status, assuming that the physician is medically fit, that is, not disabled under the law, to perform these tasks. First, the physician can participate in patient care in ways that involve no risk of infectious contact with the patient, for example, observing during a complicated cesarean delivery to assist less experienced colleagues with advice and guidance. Second, the physician, especially the highly experienced physician, can play a valuable role in consulting and helping to plan management alternatives in complicated cases. Third, the physician can teach students, residents in training, and colleagues. Fourth, the physician can conduct research that involves no exposure of patients to HIV infection from the physician. Finally, the HIV+ physician could volunteer for those procedures and settings that might in the future be shown to involve well-documented unreasonable risks of exposure to HIV infection.

COMPASSION AND LEGITIMATE SELF-INTEREST. Compassion has its limits, as well. Gregory saw this when he wrote:

> Men of the most compassionate tempers, by being daily conversant with scenes of distress, acquire in process of time that composure and firmness

> of mind so necessary to the practice of physic. They can feel whatever is amiable in pity, without suffering it to enervate or unman them.[63]

This is, of course, a familiar problem to the experienced physician, resident, and medical student alike. There are limits to compassion, namely, when one's suffering becomes such that it turns one's attention away from the patient and to oneself. This can happen, usually involuntarily. Hence the importance of integrity, for it provides the intellectual, aesthetic, and social resources with which to renew compassion, to suffer again with and for each patient and even for oneself—though not *just* for oneself. Among those resources is the capacity to sustain a certain distance from the suffering of patients while at the same time remaining attentive and engaged in the way Reich describes. As Gregory puts it, the physician must, as part of integrity in the face of suffering, maintain "composure and firmness of mind."

INTEGRITY AND LEGITIMATE SELF-INTEREST. Of the four virtues, integrity alone seems not to have limits. Indeed, it is also a bedrock form of legitimate self-interest, as will become clear throughout the course of this book, because of integrity's self-renewing character and its sustaining synergy with self-effacement, self-sacrifice, and compassion.

The Four Fundamental Virtues as the Basis for Bioethics in the Clinical Setting

Even though self-effacement, self-sacrifice, and compassion are properly limited in their implications, together with integrity they constitute the basis of the ethical principles of beneficence and respect for autonomy. When these virtues are made real in the moral lives of physicians, when they are the individually necessary material conditions for the physician-patient relationship and when together they constitute the sufficient material conditions for that relationship, self-effacement, self-sacrifice, compassion, and integrity constitute the material basis for beneficence and respect for autonomy because these fundamental virtues regulate and discipline the physician. The physician's mere and legitimate self-interests are justifiably blunted so that the physician focuses on and acts in a sustained way to protect and promote the interests of the patient. The physician-patient relationship is thus created and sustained as a moral relationship by the physician's commitment to these virtues.

The patient also has obligations to the physician, to respect the physician's legitimate self-interests, and the patient has an interest in the physician's commitment to the four fundamental virtues. As we shall see in this book, the patient also has an obligation to respect the physician's autonomy. Here we want to emphasize that a moral relationship with patients does not require that patients acknowledge or carry out their obligations to the physician. A moral relationship is created by the physician's commitment to the four fundamental virtues. Thus, the creation of the moral relationship between physicians and patients is asymmetrical.[64] The patient's acknowledgment and fulfillment of obligations to the physician helps to sustain this moral relationship.

These four fundamental virtues, then, create and sustain the obligation of the physician to protect and promote the interests of the patient. That obligation becomes fully concrete and particular when the patient is presented to the physician (a matter taken up later in this section). The virtues provide the initial concreteness and particularity of that obligation. The ethical principles of beneficence and respect for autonomy provide further particularization of that obligation. First, they provide the framework for articulating in a reliable fashion the concrete scope and the particular implications of this obligation. Second, ethical principles shape the relative significance of beneficence-based and autonomy-based interpretations of this obligation. Before showing how and why this is the case, however, the concept of the "interests of the patient" must be elucidated, an important task to which we now turn.

The Concepts of the "Interests of the Patient" and "In the Patient's Interest"

The language of the patient's "interest" and "interests," including "best interest" and "best interests," enjoys widespread use in the literature of bioethics, as does the language "in the patient's interest." However, insufficient attention has been given to the concept of an interest and to the connections between that concept and the ethical principles of beneficence and respect for autonomy.[65]

Interests Generally

Feinberg's analysis of the concept of "interests" provides a useful reference point. Feinberg links interests to "stakes" that people may have.

> All interests are in this way types of risks: the word "stake" has its primary or literal use to refer to "the amount risked by a party to a wager, or match, or gamble, a thing whose existence, or safety, or ownership depends on

> some issue." In general, a person has a stake in X (where X may be a company, a career, or some kind of "issue" of events) when he stands to gain or lose depending on the condition of X.[66]

Feinberg then goes on to provide a further distinction, between "interest" and "interests."

> One's interests, then, taken as a miscellaneous collection, consist of all things in which one has a stake, whereas one's interest in the singular, one's personal interest or self-interest, consists in the harmonious advancement of all of one's interests in the plural.[67]

On what basis could an individual be said reliably to have an interest, that is, a stake in something? One way to answer this question is from a perspective that is, as it were, "external" to the particular point of view of an individual whose interests we seek to identify. A second way to answer this question is to take an "internal" point of view, the point of view of the individual in question. There are two main variants on each of these responses. Of these four possible viewpoints on an individual's interests, only three—social role, subjective, and deliberative interests—we shall argue, are appropriate for bioethics (See Fig. 1–1.)

Needs-Based Interests

The first of the two "external" bases for defining an individual's interests is needs. Patients may be thought to have a stake in health care because they are thought to need its "issue," the preservation or restoration of health. Need can be understood as the absence of something that would normally be expected to characterize an individual, and that is important for that individual's existence or quality of life. Satisfying an individual's needs has to do with satisfying the necessary and jointly sufficient conditions for that individual's existence or quality of life. Satisfying needs allows that individual to live a full human life or as Pellegrino and Thomasma put it, to achieve "ultimate good."[68] This ultimate good, on such an account, defines when something is in an individual's interest, because, obviously, realizing *ultimate* good for someone means, by definition, that one's needs are met and thus that "all of one's interests in the plural" are harmoniously advanced.[69]

This way of defining a patient's interest must assume that there is a philosophically accepted, final, noncontestable account of human nature and the good for humans. On such an account each patient needs, and

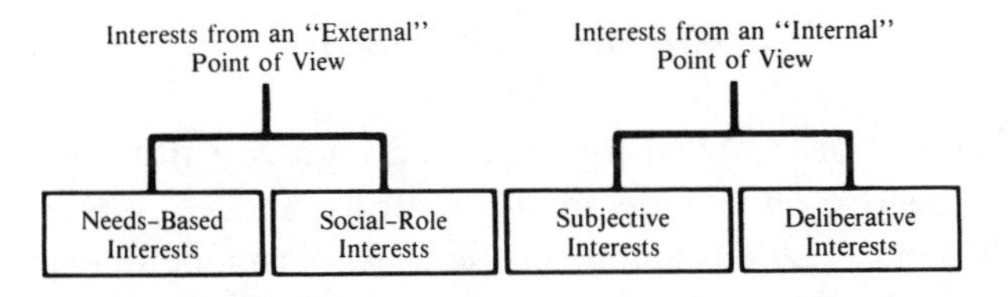

Figure 1-1 A taxonomy of interests.

therefore has an interest in, achieving the good for humans. Health needs can thus be understood as primary social goods, on the basis of the concept developed by Rawls.[70] Health needs, as Kleinig puts it, are "things which it is supposed a rational man wants, whatever he wants."[71] Such a view requires a settled, irrefutable account of what the good for humans is, "that which it is supposed a rational man wants." This, in turn, requires a settled, irrefutable philosophical account of human nature. The latter task falls to the subspecialty of philosophy known as philosophical anthropology.

The history of philosophical anthropology is marked by competing accounts of what human nature is, for example, primarily rational, primarily experiential, primarily aesthetic, or primarily religious.[72] These competing accounts are just what we should expect to find, if we take human biology seriously. Variation is the defining feature of biological life forms and human life forms are no exception. Human nature involves a bundle of traits that can be variously expressed in various environments. In short, biology teaches us that there is no unitary, stable, fixed human nature. Hence there is no one characteristic to be taken to be *the* defining characteristic of human nature. If human nature itself is inherently variable, then there is no single good for humans—there are many, variable goods, with a cluster of goods appropriate to each variant on human nature. This fundamental feature of human nature is illustrated nicely by the competing accounts of human nature that have emerged in the history of philosophical anthropology and the competing accounts of human goods that have emerged, as well, in the history of philosophical ethics. These deeply conflicting results of a 2,500-year intellectual history should chasten us and make us deeply skeptical of any claim to the finality and irrefutable truth of some account of the good, or "ultimate good," for humans. Even if such an account were possible, it is not required to make sense of the principle of beneficence in bioethics for the clinical setting, as we will show.

Social-Role Interests

General theories of the good for humans do not constitute the sole "external" perspective on an individual's interests. Indeed, it is a mistake to think so. There is a less assuming but serviceable enough "external" perspective, namely, that which defines an individual's interests in terms of the "issue" of various social roles that an individual plays. Thus, for example, teachers occupy a social role, one "issue" of which is that their students learn and develop intellectually. Parents occupy a social role, one "issue" of which is that their children mature into independent adults. Military officers occupy a social role, one "issue" of which is that their subordinates carry out the combat mission of destroying an enemy's capacity and will to fight with a minimum of casualties. Teachers, parents, and military officers can reasonably be said, therefore, to have among their interests interests that are solely a function of their social roles. No appeal to some final, irrefutable account of the good for humans is required. Indeed, such accounts are irrelevant for understanding the interests that structure social roles.

Social roles count properly as "external" perspectives because they are not a function of the particular outlook of any particular individual, but constructs precisely meant to embrace many individuals with all of their different concrete values and preferences. Consider, for example, the social role of citizenship in a modern democracy. It confers on all citizens alike and equally a variety of interests, including the protection and fostering of liberty, the establishment of representative forms of self-government, the benefits of the rule of law, and checks on abuses of the exercise of power by the government. Because the concept of a social role does not require, as a matter of logical necessity, an appeal to a settled theory of the good for humans, it provides an "external" account of interests that is separate, and therefore also immune, from the criticisms of the type that Engelhardt advances against accounts that define the interests of patients in terms of human needs and the good for humans.[73]

The social role of being a patient, then, provides an external perspective on the interests of patients.[74] The basis for this social role does not involve something as grand and lofty as an account of *the* good for humans, but something more modest: an account of "issues" or outcomes (1) that are among those historically taken to be among human goods across cultures but are not therefore or necessarily equivalent to *the* human good and (2) that medicine as a social institution is competent to seek on our behalf when we are presented for care. The competence of medicine involves the accumulated scientific knowledge, as well as accumulated clinical skills and experience, of physicians. These, in turn, should be understood as an objective basis for the competence of the health care professions, where "objective" means satisfying some rigorous intersubjective epistemological test.

As noted above, this understanding of an external account of the interests of patients does not logically require any reference to accounts of *the* good for humans. Thus, it is immune to Engelhardt's critique of such accounts' failure as part and parcel of the failure of "the Enlightenment hope . . . that reason alone (through philosophy) could disclose the character of the good life and the general canons of moral probity."[75] It is crucial for all that follows to recognize that this basis for an account of the interests of patients lacks the intellectual and therefore moral authority of a settled account of the human good, were such an account possible. Instead, a social-role-based account is more modest and stringently limited in its scope, because it cannot logically claim to be *the* single external perspective from whose viewpoint all human goods could be finally, uncontestably identified.

The social-role-based account of patients' interests is limited in its perspective by the limited competencies of medicine. Medicine cannot achieve all, not even most, human goods, only some, namely, health-related goods. These goods are of enduring significance and even prominence across cultures.

Such an account is also limited by the modest epistemological claims of the health care professions—not to objective "truth" but to intersubjectively validated modes of clinical judgment and intervention. Indeed, the latter are variable phenomena with important implications for the variability of the moral authority of beneficence-based clinical judgment, as we shall see in the next section.

It is of significant historical and philosophical interest that John Gregory, mentioned earlier, did not rely in his medical ethics on a theory or account of the human good. Instead, he appeals to an understanding of the human goods that medicine can be expected to seek on behalf of patients: ". . . the *practice of medicine,* by which I understand, the art of preserving health, of prolonging life, and of curing diseases."[76] This is a prudent, cautious basis for understanding the competencies of medicine, a feature of Gregory's medical ethics that has not been sufficiently appreciated in contemporary bioethics. Gregory's medical ethics demonstrates philosophically that there is no logical requirement that bioethics adopt some account of *the* human good as the basis for an external perspective on the interests of patients.

Gregory's perspective is also philosophically important because, while it makes powerful claims for the competencies of medicine, it does not make extravagant claims. This more modest understanding of the competencies of medicine, we believe, was abandoned for the majority of this century, during which time the competencies of medicine were thought to be limitless. This social experiment medicine and society found to be a failure, leading to a return to the historical view.

Subjective Interests

There are two varieties of internal perspectives from whose vantage point the interests of patients can be understood. The first appeals to the values and beliefs of a particular individual, on the basis of which that person chooses to have a stake in an "issue" or outcome of events. We call this first perspective the "subjective interests" account. We note here three important features of this first internal perspective on the interests of patients.

First, there is no constraint on the type or variety of the values and beliefs that a particular individual might appeal to in defining her interest. Each of us is free to range widely. The scope of interests can thus be, and usually is, far wider than that afforded by the limited competencies of medicine. Moreover, because medicine is not competent to evaluate the worth of nonhealth-related human goods, it must be silent on the subject. That is, patients bring to their care many health-related and nonhealth-related values and beliefs. For example, the Jehovah's Witness patient holds a health-related value, getting well and preventing unnecessary death. She also holds a nonhealth-related, specifically religious value, obeying the commands of God as set out in Holy Scripture. Physicians have *no* theological competencies and so cannot with intellectual integrity claim to be able to judge the worth or value of such a religious belief—which is a staple of all the world's religions. Indeed, intellectual integrity prohibits such judgments.

Second, there need be no intersubjective or other epistemological test on the values and beliefs to which a particular individual happens to appeal as the basis for identifying her interests, nor on the judgments and decisions that issue from this process. A particular patient, therefore, may have a quite personal and subjective (in the sense of "not subjected to intellectual rigor") understanding of her interests.

Third, this perspective on the interests of patients is limited, in two ways. No particular individual values all human goods, only some of them. Thus, this first internal perspective on patients' interests need not provide an account of *the* human good. This perspective is also limited by its subjective nature, as this term is defined just above. The lack of intellectual rigor gives this perspective an inherently unstable dimension. After all, we often find that we were poorly informed or even mistaken about what our interests were subjectively, when we determine those interests more reflectively, deliberately.

Deliberative Interests

This brings us to the second internal perspective or vantage point from which the interests of patients can be understood. This vantage point results from a particular individual applying intellectual discipline and rigor to the process of identifying her interests. By analogy to accounts of rational desires[77] that result from a process of deliberation, we call this perspective the "deliberative interests" account. Deliberative interests are determined on the basis of careful reflection and deliberation, given adequate information about our present situation and prospects.[78] We note here the significant features of this account.

First, again by analogy to rational desire theories, deliberative interests are those that a particular individual identifies after a process of gathering, considering, and attempting to understand information. The latter, in our view, involves both cognitive understanding,[79] namely, a determination of probable consequences of different choices or events, and evaluative understanding,[80] a careful estimation of the worth of those probable consequences in terms of an individuals' more stable, settled values and beliefs, including values and beliefs about one's ethical obligations to others. Second, this perspective is necessarily limited in the scope of human goods it considers, as a direct result of the intellectual discipline essential to it. This is because this discipline imposes constraints on the values and beliefs thought to be relevant and requires evaluative understanding.

Third, there is a modest but significant epistemological test for this perspective, namely, being able to give to oneself or others an account of the results of applying intellectual discipline in the process of identifying one's interests. This is less demanding than the intersubjectivity test of the social-role account but more demanding than the subjective-interests account. Satisfying this modest epistemological test gives greater stability to deliberative interests than the stability (often, lack of same) of subjective interests.

The social-role account, the subjective interests account, and the deliberative interests account are each limited in their intellectual and therefore moral authority in significant ways, as noted above. The scope of the second and third can overlap with the first, but none has a scope completely or fully in common with either of the others. (See Table 1–1.)

None of these three perspectives on the interests of patients can claim to be exhaustive of the patient's interests as a whole. Each perspective is partial, though authoritative within that partial scope. This will be crucial later for our reading of beneficence and respect for autonomy as prima facie principles.

Interests Generally: A More Precise Account

On the basis of the preceding discussion, we rephrase Feinberg and offer the following, more precise account of the concept of the interests of patients:

> One's interests as a patient, taken as a miscellaneous collection, consist of all things in which one has a stake on the basis of either the social role interests account, the subjective interests account, or the deliberative interests account. One's personal interest or self-interest comprises the harmonious advancement of all of one's interests, in the plural, i.e., interests determined on the basis of one or more of the three accounts.

In One's Interest

Feinberg's analysis of the concept of what is "in one's interest" also provides a useful reference point for our analysis of this important concept.

> Here [i.e., in "the analysis of another common idiom, namely, 'X' is in Jones's interest."] we should distinguish initially between two interpretations: (1) "X promotes some one particular interest of Jones," e.g., his interest in pecuniary accumulation or in artistic achievement, and (2) "X promotes Jones's self-interests," i.e., all of his interests as a group.[81]

Table 1-1 Types of Interests and Their Scopes

Social-Role Interests	Those things in which one has a stake in virtue of occupying social role.
Subjective Interests	Those things in which one has a stake because they happen, perhaps unreflectively, to be valued by one.
Deliberative Interests	Those things in which one has a stake because they are valued in a settled way, after adequate information is obtained and carefully considered.

Feinberg further analyzes the latter in the following terms:

> The analysis of (2) "X is in Jones's self-interest" is more complicated . . . As a start, we can say that this means that X somehow promotes Jones's interests (the things he has a stake in) as a group. We have already suggested that this means that X contributes to the harmonious advancement of Jones's interests. . . . What sort of conditions count as "harmonious advancement?" Three kinds of cases should be distinguished. In the first . . . X advances Jones's interests "harmoniously" by promoting *all of them,* either equally or unequally. In the second, X promotes a particular interest Y of Jones's, or a set of such interests, without impairing any of his other interests. In the third case, X promotes some of Jones's interests and impairs others, but the ones promoted are superior in some relevant way to those that are impaired, so that the result is a net gain for Jones as a whole.[82]

Feinberg's analysis cannot, we believe, be taken whole into bioethics; it can, however, be adapted with modifications of each of his three senses of "in Jones's interests." First, medicine can only rarely advance *all* of the patient's interests. There is almost always some health-related risk or "downside" associated with any medical intervention. One important exception, as we shall see in Chapters 3 and 6, concerns obstetric interventions of documented benefit for the fetal patient, for example, cesarean delivery for well-defined fetal indications. By contrast, gynecologic and obstetric interventions all involve some increment of risk for the (pregnant) woman and so should not be understood as advancing unequivocally all of her social-role interests, much less all of her subjective or deliberative interests.

Second, some medical interventions can advance some social-role interests without impairing others. Relatively safe over-the-counter medications, such as alcohol-free cough medicines, treat morbidity, pain, and suffering, without incremental increased risk of mortality, injury, or handicap. More controversially, some have argued that there are "routine" situations in medicine, that is, those in which the nonhealth-related values and beliefs of the patient are not at stake.[83] Put more precisely, routine medical care advances health-related interests without impairing subjective or deliberative interests, because these interests in fact coincide with social-role interests. This is the case, for example, with encouraging patients to undertake breast self-examination or in the prescribing or recommending medication for a simple vaginal yeast infection.

Third, medical care typically involves the advancement of some interests at the expense of impairing others, for example, hysterectomy for protracted, postpartum hemorrhage. Hysterectomy in this case promotes a woman's health-related interest in avoiding unnecessary mortality, but at the price of impaired social-role interests, loss of a major anatomical system and its functions, and perhaps impaired subjective or deliberative interests, depending on her assessment of the sequelae of hysterectomy in terms of her health-related and other values and beliefs.

A central task of a framework for bioethics is to address the issue of when one or more interests, of whatever of the three sorts, should be regarded as "superior" to others. Buchanan and Brock accurately describe this task when they write, about the "best interests principle:"

> The qualifier "best" [in what they term the "best interests principle"] . . . signals the complex and comparative nature of the judgment: Some interests (such as the interest in avoiding death or chronic pain) are generally more important than others in that advancing them makes a greater contribution to the individual's good, and a particular decision can advance some of the individual's interests while thwarting others. Thus the best interest principle instructs us to determine the *net* benefit for the patient of each option, assigning different weights to the options to reflect the relative importance of the various interests they further or thwart, then subtracting costs or "disbenefits" from the benefits, for each option. The course of action to be followed, then, is the one with the greatest net benefit to the patient. The mere fact that a treatment would benefit the patient is not sufficient to show that it would be in the individual's best interests, since other options may have greater net benefits, or the costs of the option to the patient—in suffering and disability—may exceed the benefit.[84]

It is sometimes the case in clinical practice that one management plan carries a clearly greater *net* benefit—*all* interests considered—than others. In such cases, the language of "best interests" can be used as suggested by Brock and Buchanan, with the following crucial modification: from which one or more of the three perspectives on patients' interests that intervention is "best" must be specified. In addition, because there could be competing accounts of which intervention has the greatest net benefit, the superiority of one account over the others must be reliably established.

Increasingly in health care, the trade-offs between advanced and impaired interests differ qualitatively, not just quantitatively, as a function of the different scopes of each of the three types of patient's interest. The differences among those scopes are qualitatively different. Thus, it will often be difficult to say with final authority which one intervention is best because none of the accounts of patients' interests can, we believe, claim such authority. Indeed, qualitative diversity constitutes a further reason to doubt final authority, because no one of the three accounts possesses sufficient scope (See Table 1–1) to negotiate different estimations of net benefit resulting from each of the three accounts of interests. The implication that is important here is that reliable clinical judgment, that is, that which takes into account what is in the patient's interest from all three perspectives, frequently results in the identification of a range or continuum of management plans that are in the patient's interest. Such judgment also identifies what is *not* in a patient's social-role interest, that is, what lies outside the continuum of alternatives expected to produce net benefit, construed from the perspective of the social-role account, and plans that are not in the patient's deliberative interests. This will be crucial later, particularly in our discussion of justified limits on patients' refusal of interventions. (See Chapter 7.)

Finally, we will adopt, with two slight qualifications, Feinberg's understanding of what it means to advance or not to advance someone's interest. An interest is advanced when it is satisfied or realized to some degree. An interest can also be impaired. An interest is impaired when it is "set back," "defeated," "thwarted," "impeded," or "doomed."

> To *set back* an interest is to reverse its course, turn it away, put it back toward the point from which it started. To *defeat* an interest is to put it to utter rout, to conclusively and irrevocably set it back by destroying the conditions that are necessary for its advancement or fulfillment, as death can set back some interests once and for all. . . . To *thwart* (or block, or frustrate) an interest is to stop its progress without necessarily putting it in reverse. . . . To *impede* an interest is to slow its advancement without necessarily stopping or reversing it, to hinder or delay.[85] A final way of harming a person is to *doom* one of his interests, to foreordain its defeat.[86]

The first qualification that we add concerns the concept of "protecting" a patient's interests. This occurs when interests are protected from impairment, that is, neither impaired nor advanced. That is, in clinical practice there is a middle ground between impaired and advanced interests, namely, when impairment of interests is prevented and when those interests remain unchanged in their degree of satisfaction or realization. The second qualification is that when interests are advanced we shall say they are promoted.

The Virtues of Self-Effacement, Self-Sacrifice, Compassion, and Integrity as the Basis for Bioethics in the Clinical Setting Restated

We are now in a position to flesh out further the account in the previous section of the virtues of self-effacement, self-sacrifice, compassion, and integrity as the basis for the ethical principles of beneficence and respect for autonomy. These virtues blunt mere self-interest and legitimate self-interest in favor of protecting and promoting the interests of the patient. Mere self-interest comprises those subjective interests of the physician that come to the fore in response to social and other differences between the physician and the patient. Legitimate self-interest, by contrast, comprises deliberative interests of the physician that are identified when, on reflective and careful consideration, the physician takes account of both the physician's obligations to patients and to others in the physician's life and those settled, stable values and beliefs in the enrichment of which the physician finds deep and abiding satisfaction. The four fundamental virtues provide the basis for the obligation to protect and promote the patient's interests by creating and sustaining that obligation. The protection and promotion of the patient's interests requires that the three accounts on those interests—the social-role account, the subjective interest account, and the deliberative interest account—be accommodated and their differences negotiated in clinical ethical judgment. Integrity requires this. The ethical principles of beneficence and respect for autonomy structure this interpretive process. We thus turn to a consideration of their meaning, scope, and relative significance in terms of the different ways, and extent to which, they translate the three accounts of patients' interests into clinical practice.

The Principle of Beneficence

The Meaning of the Principle

The principle of beneficence has an ancient pedigree in the history of bioethics. It is arguably the core ethical principle of the Hippocratic Oath: "I will apply dietetic measures for the benefit of the sick according to my ability and judgment; I will keep them from harm and injustice."[87]

The appeal is to the competency of the physician, to undertake what we would now call nutritional interventions, as the basis for the benefits that are to be sought on the patient's behalf. Thus, the benefits of surgery are not to be sought by the Hippocratic physician, the tasks of surgery being left to those suited and competent to undertake them.

In the texts that accompany the Oath, there is a more general formulation of the principle: "Declare the past, diagnose the present, foretell the future; practice these acts. As to diseases, make a habit of two things—to help, or at least to do no harm."[88]

One wants to know, however, in just what ways the physician is to help. Such a general formulation of the principle, because of its abstractness, is impossible to apply to a particular patient in the clinical setting. It is, as Clouser and Gert put it, a "chapter heading for discussion" and not a concrete guide to behavior.

This way of presenting the principle of beneficence persists in the literature to this day. The ethical principle of beneficence is typically understood to require the physician to act in such a way that the consequences of the physician's behavior for the patient are reliably expected to produce a greater balance of goods over harms for the patient. This formulation of the principle, just as its predecessor in *Epidemics,* is very abstract. To be made concrete, beneficence needs to be connected to its basis.

Recall that this basis comprises the four fundamental virtues that together blunt the mere and legitimate self-interests of the physician and move the physician to protect and promote the interests of the patient. We saw in the previous section that there are two perspectives from which those interests can be understood, an external and an internal perspective. On the basis of the external perspective, the social-role account of the patient's interests, the goods and harms that give meaning or content to the principle of beneficence in the clinical setting can be reliably specified. That is, medicine is competent to identify the social-role interests of any patient. Put in the language of the preceding section, *the ethical principle of beneficence obligates the physician to protect and promote the social-role interests of the patient.* These interests are defined, in turn, on the basis of the competencies of medicine to seek limited, but important, human goods on the basis of accumulated scientific and clinical knowledge, skill, and experience.

The social-role interests that medicine is competent to seek on behalf of patients, in our view, comprise the following: the prevention of premature or unnecessary death *and* the prevention, cure, or at least management of disease, injury, handicap, and unnecessary pain and suffering. These are the goods that the social institution of medicine is competent to pursue on behalf of patients and in which individuals who are patients have a stake by virtue of the social role of being a patient. Together these goods provide the concrete meaning for the principle of beneficence.

This formulation is quite compressed and requires further elaboration, if the meaning of the principle of beneficence is to be clear. First, this rendering of the meaning of the principle of beneficence is antivitalist, where "vitalist" means that the good that should be sought for patients is the preservation of life without qualification, that is, preservation of biological life at all costs. On a vitalist view of beneficence, preventing death is the good to be sought for patients. This, of course, sets an impossible goal for medicine, one that it is simply not competent to seek on behalf of patients. Medicine is competent, however, to seek the more modest goal of preventing premature or unnecessary death.

Second, the terms "premature" and "unnecessary" require some amplification. "Premature" death, we believe, means as a rule that the death of the patient will occur before life expectancy, adjusted for the health status of the patient. The death of an otherwise healthy woman from uncontrollable hemorrhage postpartum or from cervical cancer at, say, 29 years of age would count as a premature death, a death every reasonable effort should be made to prevent. "Unnecessary" death, we believe, means that the death of the patient could have been prevented at a reasonable cost vis-à-vis iatrogenic morbidity where "morbidity" should be read to include disease, injury, handicap, and unnecessary pain and suffering. The death of an otherwise healthy woman postpartum from total exsanguination when administration of blood products would have been an effective preventive measure is unnecessary in this sense. The death of a patient in a persistent vegetative state or of a patient with an incurable, very advanced, terminal gynecologic cancer, by contrast, would not count as an unnecessary death. The death of such patients would therefore not constitute a harm to such patients in the sense that an unnecessary death occurred. Killing a patient whose death is either premature or unnecessary contradicts the goods that medicine is competent to seek for patients. Thus, there is a very strong beneficence-based prohibition against the killing of the patient.[89]

Third, "necessary" pain and suffering, we believe, means pain and suffering that are themselves unavoidable means to reasonable attempts to achieve the other goods of beneficence in health care. "Unnecessary" pain and suffering, by contrast, produce no good for the patient; they are only harmful. "Pain" we understand to mean a report in the central nervous system of tissue damage or threat of tissue damage. "Suffering" we understand to mean the experience of thwarted goals, plans, intentions, desires, preferences, and so on. A patient can be in pain without suffering and can suffer without being in pain, although pain of significant degree usually is accompanied by suffering. Since almost all medical interventions involve some increment of pain or suffering, the determination of whether that pain or suffering is necessary or unnecessary is a crucial dimension of beneficence-based clinical judgment.

Fourth, the emphasis on "and" in our formulation of the goods medicine is competent to pursue for patients is deliberate, for the simple reason—already noted in the previous section on the interests of patients—that medical interventions almost always involve some "downside" in the form of iatrogenic disease, injury, handicap, or unnecessary pain and suffering. In other words, medical interventions usually do not promote all of the patient's social-role interests, but rather some at the expense of others.

The Scope of the Principle

The scope of the principle of beneficence in bioethics is limited by the competencies of medicine to those goods in which patients can have a stake in virtue of those competencies. The social-role interests of patients are certainly not equivalent to *the* good for humans, on whatever account of that good the reader might prefer. Moreover, the social-role interests of patients do not encompass all of the *goods* that humans value, only some of them. There are goods that humans value as much as, perhaps more than, the goods that medicine is competent to seek on our behalf, a consideration that will be important for the relative significance of the principle of beneficence vis-à-vis the principle of respect for autonomy. In short, while the competencies of medicine are increasingly powerful, their scope and thus the scope of the principle of beneficence are limited to what scientifically trained and clinically experienced physicians can reasonably aim to achieve on our behalf when we are patients.

Beneficence-Based Clinical Judgment about What Is in the Patient's Interest

Beneficence-based clinical medical interventions, that is, disease prevention and health management strategies, can be in the patient's interest in one of three ways. First, some interventions can promote all of the patient's social-role interests, that is, with no impairment of those interests whatsoever. This will rarely be the case, however. In the discussion above of the concept "in the patient's interest" we said that cesarean delivery for well-defined fetal indications promotes all of the fetus' interests. (The present discussion assumes that the fetus is sometimes a patient, the argument for which appears in Chapter 3.) For example, cesarean delivery for prolonged, severe fetal distress at term is reasonably understood to prevent a premature death (the death of any at-term fetus without a lethal anomaly is a premature death by definition) and to prevent further morbidity. Cesarean delivery for well-documented, complete placenta previa clearly prevents death and morbidity; the alternative, vaginal delivery, is likely to produce stillbirth or short-term survival with severe morbidity.

Second, some interventions promote some social-role interests without impairing others. Delivery of high-risk pregnancies in a tertiary hospital, for example, promotes the social-role interests of both the pregnant woman and the fetus, without impairing others. At best, the risks of both mortality and morbidity are reduced or, at least, the risks of mortality are reduced without the risks of morbidity being increased—vis-a-vis delivery in a community hospital.

By their very nature these first two beneficence-based senses of "in the patient's interest" involve no trade-offs among the goods that together constitute the social-role interests of the patient. As a consequence, these two forms of beneficence-based clinical judgment about what is in a patient's interest are inherently noncontroversial.

This is not the case for the third sense of beneficence-based clinical judgments about what is in a patient's interest, namely, those that do involve trade-offs between social-role interests that are expected to be promoted and social-role interests that are expected to be impaired. Cesarean delivery for maternal complications, for example, well-documented, complete placenta previa, greatly reduces the risks of mortality to the pregnant woman because the risk of mortality from not having a cesarean delivery exceed those of cesarean delivery by a factor of more than 50. To be sure, there is some risk of intraoperative and postoperative morbidity from cesarean delivery. However, the small incidence of these risks pales in comparison quantitatively with those of mortality should labor proceed and vaginal delivery ensue. Negotiating these clear-cut trade-offs in beneficence-based clinical judgment seems to be a straightforward matter.

Matters, however, are not always so straightforward. Consider, for example, the administration of tocolytic agents in the attempt to arrest premature labor. On the one hand, such an intervention, if successful, will reduce the risk of fetal and neonatal mortality and morbidity. On the other hand, there are significant risks of mortality and morbidity—more so the latter than the former—for the pregnant woman. How should the trade-offs here be negotiated?

As a rule, preventing premature or unnecessary death takes priority among the social-role interests of the patient because, if such death occurs, none of the other social-role interests of the patient can be achieved.

Death simply forecloses once and for all the opportunity to do so and thus dooms all of the other social-role interests. On this basis, the beneficence-based justification for administration of certain tocolytic agents relies on the fact that in the short run the risks of mortality to the pregnant woman are small and manageable, whereas those to the fetus/neonate are considerably greater. At some point, of course, it can and does happen that the risks of mortality or grave morbidity to the pregnant woman equal or exceed those to the fetus/neonate. For the latter at this point there is the alternative of delivery followed by aggressive neonatal management, whereas the alternative for the pregnant woman of continuing tocolytic therapy is relatively greater risk of grave morbidity and even mortality. In such circumstances, because of the risks to both the pregnant woman and the fetus, beneficence-based clinical judgment supports stopping the tocolytic therapy and initiating aggressive neonatal management, if there is a live birth.

So far these examples show how negotiating among the social-role interests when trade-offs are involved can be mainly a matter of quantitative judgment. There can also be qualitative judgments about trade-offs among the social-role interests of the patient. Qualitative judgment, we believe, is frequently a feature of beneficence-based clinical judgment, a feature of such judgment that has been insufficiently appreciated. Consider, for example, whether cesarean delivery for fetal distress should be undertaken when the pregnancy involves the already diagnosed, by karyotype, fetal anomaly of trisomy 13. Such a diagnosis, which can be achieved with certainty, involves a prognosis of over 95 percent mortality by age two and in virtually all cases severe, irreversible loss of developmental potential secondary to severe central nervous system anomalies. Infants with trisomy 13, as it were, simply exist at a level of biological function that itself is in chronic, irreversible failure, resulting in the eventual death of almost all affected children before the end of 2 years.

A qualitative judgment about such matters could reasonably conclude that the death of such a child is not unnecessary and that, therefore, no harm in the form of an unnecessary death comes to such a child from death. This conclusion is supported by the observation that aggressive neonatal management may involve significant risks of disease, injury, or unnecessary pain and suffering. That is, the risks of morbidity from aggressive obstetric management followed by aggressive neonatal management may be significant. It follows from this consideration of qualitative judgment about the management of trade-offs among social-role interests that nonaggressive obstetric management of fetal distress in such a pregnancy is justified. By this we mean that nonaggressive management is not plainly inconsistent with reasonable beneficence-based clinical judgment and that such judgment, on qualitative grounds, provides a rationale for nonaggressive management. At the same time, aggressive management is not decisively ruled out. It, too, is justified, although the qualitative beneficence-based judgment just described would conclude that there is only a minimal beneficence-based obligation to provide aggressive obstetric management. Hence, both aggressive and nonaggressive obstetric management are reasonable alternatives for the intrapartum management of a pregnancy complicated by trisomy 13, as far as beneficence-based clinical judgment is concerned. (See Chapter 6 for a more extended discussion of the management of pregnancies complicated by fetal anomalies.)

There is a further justification for this conclusion. We noted earlier that in qualitative judgment about trade-offs among social-role interests it will often be difficult to say with final authority which trade-off is clearly the better. Hence, both alternatives win a place in beneficence-based clinical judgment as being in the patient's interest. Interestingly, when quantitative judgments are "close," that is, when the increment of risks are nearly equal, final authority will also be difficult to achieve. The latter consideration explains why there continues to be controversy, for example, about where to set thresholds for aggressive obstetric management of fetal distress that is not yet either prolonged or severe.

Variability and Uncertainty in Beneficence-Based Clinical Judgment

It follows directly from these considerations that there can be both variability and uncertainty in beneficence-based clinical judgment, both quantitative and qualitative. These are not inherently problematic or disabling features of such judgment, unless one takes the view—as some seem to do—that the epistemology of clinical judgment should be understood in terms of the two-valued logic of truth and falsehood. For example, some have reasoned—a line of reasoning that seems to have wide currency—that clinical judgment about the expected outcomes of cesarean delivery for complete placenta previa is subject to disabling uncertainty because there have been some exceptions to the grim neonatal and maternal prognosis in some celebrated court cases.[90]

This line of reasoning mistakenly holds clinical judgment to a standard that it can never satisfy: clinical judgment is to be trusted only when it turns out that it is never false in an individual case. Of course, on this standard of truth, all clinical prognostic judgments must be judged possibly false and therefore disabled by uncertainty. The problem with such an epistemological standard is that it ignores the inherent variability of quantitative and qualitative beneficence-based clinical judgment described just above. Given such inherent variability, certain knowledge of outcomes is not available in advance. Hence, those who adopt his line of reasoning espouse an epistemological standard that has little or nothing to do with the clinical reality of matters, namely, the inherent variability of beneficence-based clinical judgment. The appropriate epistemological test for inherently variable clinical judgment focuses on its reliability.[91]

Determination of the reliability of clinical judgment rests on two factors: (1) the process of reaching a particular clinical judgment; and (2) the data upon which that clinical judgment is based. As to the first factor, a clinical judgment is reliable when that judgment would with high probability be replicated by a second, equally informed, rigorous judger. No other test makes sense, especially for qualitative beneficence-based clinical judgment and for quantitative judgment when the trade-offs are "close." As to the second factor, a clinical judgment is reliable when the data upon which it is based do not vary and are not expected to vary. This is an especially important consideration, again, for qualitative and quantitative beneficence-based clinical judgments.

Determining the reliability of both qualitative and quantitative beneficence-based clinical judgments entails four main considerations. First, the physician must rigorously assess the probability of self-limitation or spontaneous resolution of the patient's condition. This assessment should be based on accumulated clinical experience—not just one physician's—regarding the variability of data concerning these matters. In addition, the expected outcomes of alternative management strategies need to be specified as precisely as possible. This will enable the physician to identify with confidence when qualitative and close-call quantitative trade-offs among social-role interests must be taken into account in evaluating alternative management strategies.

Second, the physician must appreciate that prognostic clinical judgment is not about individual cases, but concerns the natural history of particular diseases under different management strategies. Prognostic judgment is not about what will or will not occur but about different probabilities of the different outcomes of different management strategies. That a highly improbable outcome of a management strategy later occurs in fact does not at all mean that the prior prognostic judgment and expectation that the most common outcome was expected to occur was "wrong."

Third, to insist nonetheless that physicians can be and frequently are "wrong" in their clinical prognostic judgments makes sense only if one is so fortunate to have at hand what medical students and residents fondly and somewhat ruefully dub the "retrospectoscope." This clinical tool possesses one endearing feature: it always affords a crystal clear picture of what was really going on. Unfortunately, its drawback is that this finding always comes too late to be of any use when it is really needed. Our point in using this metaphor is not to entertain. Instead, we use it to underscore the epistemological status of prognostic clinical judgment: that status is not captured by the two-valued logic of truth and falsehood about individual cases.

Fourth, in addition to these epistemological factors, qualitative and close-call quantitative judgments introduce variability and uncertainty. Consider qualitative judgments about when preventing the severity and chronicity of some forms of morbidity should be the primary beneficence-based consideration, rather than preventing premature death, for example, Stage IV ovarian cancer. Clearly, when it is no longer possible to achieve the latter good, the former properly becomes the primary beneficence-based consideration. Matters are less clear when attempting to prevent premature death is futile or virtually futile.[92] This is also the case when a judgment is reached that because of very severe, irreversible morbidity and very high probability of eventual mortality in the near term, the death of the patient is not unnecessary and so it is not a harm to that patient. Reasonable people, starting from the same set of data, will reach different judgments in such matters. Clinical judgment will thus be variable and resultant uncertainty will not be eliminable.

This is not, however, a disabling feature of beneficence-based clinical judgment, unless one thinks that beneficence-based clinical judgment must always yield the one, true, uncontestable account of what is in the patient's social-role interest, an account that excludes as false or unreasonable all other accounts. But this again is to set an impossible standard. Instead, the way to manage the inherent variability and resultant uncertainty of qualitative and close-call quantitative beneficence-based clinical judgment is to recognize that *the proper outcome of beneficence-based clinical judgment is often the determination of the range or continuum of reasonable assessments of what is in the patient's social-role interest.* None of these can rationally be construed to exclude the others as false or unreasonable, because no assessment can hope to claim the final epistemological authority for doing so. However, the range or continuum, considered as a whole, does serve as the basis for excluding all other available alternatives as unreasonable *in beneficence-based clinical judgment*. This will be important later when we consider the relative significance of the principles of beneficence and respect for autonomy.

Beneficence-Based Objections to Paternalism

No discussion of the principle of beneficence is possible without at least initial consideration of the problem of paternalism, which, following Beauchamp and Childress, we understand "as the overriding of a person's wishes or intentional actions for beneficent reasons."[93] This formulation indicates the line of argument that usually follows: because it is (sometimes or at all times) an unjustified offense to the autonomy of persons, paternalism is not acceptable in clinical practice. That is, the usual way of thinking about paternalism in the literature focuses on autonomy-based objections to paternalism. We will consider these when we consider the principle of respect for autonomy. Here we want to examine a topic that has been largely neglected, as far as we can tell: *beneficence-based* objections to paternalism.

On the basis of the preceding analysis there are only three possible types of beneficence-based clinical judgment that count as clear-cut:

1. a reliable judgment that all of the patient's interests will be promoted by a management strategy and that there is only one such strategy;
2. a reliable judgment that some of the patient's interests will be promoted but none impaired, that there is only one such strategy, and that no judgment of the first type is possible; and
3. a reliable quantitative judgment that a strategy is expected to prevent premature or unnecessary death, that there is only one such strategy, and that no judgment of the first two types is possible.

In all other cases of reliable beneficence-based judgments, those judgments will be variable, because there will be competing reasonable, beneficence-based judgments about what is in the patient's social-role interest.

The three types of clear-cut beneficence-based clinical judgment exclude all other available management alternatives as unreasonable and therefore not acceptable, but *only* on beneficence-based grounds. To think that such grounds should function alone as the basis for determining what is in the patient's interest *as a whole* involves a form of hubris: that the social-role interests of the patient are the *sole* interests of the patient. This is simply false. Our first beneficence-based objection to paternalism therefore is that for these types of clinical judgment it is simply a mistake to hold that their results should be implemented *all things having been considered,* that is, when the subjective and deliberative interests of the patient have also been taken into account. It only follows that the results of such clinical judgment should be implemented *the social-role interests of the patient having been taken into account.* To think otherwise is to think that beneficence-based clinical judgment is about *the* good for patients. This, it should now be abundantly clear, is a fundamental conceptual error. Determination of *the* good for patients must be made, if it can be made at all, in public policy.

Our second objection concerns the conclusion that one of a variable set of beneficence-based judgments about what is in the patient's interest should be implemented, as if it were the "best" in the sense that it excludes all others as unreasonable. The mistake here is to fail to appreciate that variable beneficence-based clinical judgment means that reliable clinical judgment identifies a range or continuum of alternatives, any one of which is properly regarded to be in the patient's interest. To assume that any one of these is *the* alternative that is *alone* in the interest of the patient is therefore a patently false assumption. To go on, further, to assume that this one alternative should be carried out *all things having been taken into account* does not follow because, *the social-role interests of the patient having been considered, there are reasonable alternatives.* This is our second beneficence-based objection to paternalism.

If the physician makes the further assumption that the range or continuum of reasonable alternatives entails that a patient's preference for an alternative not within that range or continuum should not be implemented *all things having been considered* is to make the same mistake noted above about paternalism based on clear-cut beneficence-based clinical judgments. The subjective and deliberative interests of the patient must also be taken into account. The only thing that therefore follows is that, *the social-role interests of the patient having been taken into account, no alternative outside the range or continuum of reasonable alternatives should be implemented.*

In short, one can advance beneficence-based objections to paternalism of two kinds: (1) some forms of paternalism mistakenly assume that the scope of beneficence-based judgments includes all relevant interests of the patient and thus can speak to *the* good for patients, a form of hubris regarding the competencies of the health care professions; or (2) some forms of paternalism deny the inherent variability and uncertainty of beneficence-based clinical judgment.

What to Make of Primum non Nocere or "First, Do No Harm"

Primum non nocere or "First, Do no harm" enjoys a prominent status in the thinking of many physicians and some currency in the literature of bioethics.[94] Curiously, this is a maxim without a history. It does not occur in the Hippocratic Oath or accompanying texts, for example. Moreover, it involves several confusions, the principal one of which is the assumption that the maxim can always be carried into effect in clinical practice. This assumption is false.

The dictates of the maxim are consistent with clear-cut beneficence-based judgments of the first two types discussed above—(1) a reliable judgment that all of the patient's interests will be promoted by a management strategy and that there is only one such strategy and (2) a reliable judgment that some of the patient's interests will be promoted but none impaired and that there is only one such strategy and that no judgment of the first type can be sustained. For virtually all other beneficence-based clinical judgments their results involve some downside, some impairment of the patient's interests. That is, they are not unequivocally in the patient's interest but judged on balance to be so. *Primum non nocere* would seem to exclude these as unreasonable clinical judgments. In short, *primum non nocere* eliminates as unjustified the implementation of most beneficence-based clinical judgments. Indeed, it is hard to know when in the history of medicine *primum non nocere* would not have had this effect.

"First, Do no harm" does apply in beneficence-based clinical judgment that is variable and uncertain, because the range or continuum, as such, of reasonable alternatives does exclude as unreasonable on beneficence-based grounds all other alternatives. This is because these other alternatives involve only impairment of and not protection of the social-role interests of the patient. As a consequence, they cannot be understood in beneficence-based clinical judgment to be in the patient's interest. To implement any one of them would only do harm. Thus, "First, Do no harm" is a corollary of the principle of beneficence but only when it is reinterpreted to mean: no management strategy that is judged only to do harm to the patient's social-role interests is justified in beneficence-based clinical judgment. This is also, in our view, the appropriate understanding of the principle of nonmaleficence: it is a corollary of the principle of beneficence, not an independent principle. For example, a beneficence-based prohibition against killing a patient is no less strong than a nonmaleficence-based prohibition.

Table 1-2 Beneficence-Based Action Guides

1. Management strategies based on clear-cut beneficence-based clinical judgments ought to be implemented *the social role interests of the patient having been taken into account.*
2. Any one of the range or continuum of management strategies based on variable and uncertain beneficence-based clinical judgments may properly be implemented *the social role interests of the patient having been taken into account.*
3. Management strategies that lie outside the range or continuum of those based on variable and uncertain but reliable beneficence-based clinical judgments ought not to be implemented *the social role interests of the patient having been taken into account.*

The Principle of Beneficence as a Set of Concrete Guides to Action

Considered by itself, the principle of beneficence on the account that we have given constitutes more than a "checklist" of items to be considered. It provides concrete guides—more than one of them because of the heterogeneity of beneficence-based clinical judgment. Those guides appear in Table 1–2.

These action guides are obviously not absolute, the final story for bioethics in the clinical setting. Their limited character in this respect is a direct function of several factors:

1. the limited scope of interests that the health care professions are competent to address, namely, the social-role interests of patients;
2. the heterogeneity of reliable beneficence-based clinical judgment from the clear-cut to the variable and uncertain; and
3. the fact that most reliable beneficence-based clinical judgments are variable and uncertain because of the persistent downside to most clinical management strategies.

For these reasons, the above three action guides are *prima facie* in that they must be considered together with the action guides that issue from clinical judgments that take account of the subjective and deliberative interests of patients. The latter are structured by the principle of respect for autonomy, to which we now turn.

The Principle of Respect for Autonomy

The Meaning of the Principle

Unlike the principle of beneficence, the principle of respect for autonomy in bioethics is entirely a creature of our own century, although the roots of the principle go back several centuries in the history of Western political philosophy. Also, unlike the principle of beneficence, which was developed within medicine in response to cultural resources available to it, the principle of respect for autonomy has been developed outside medicine, in the law and in political philosophy. This historical feature of the principle of respect for autonomy is crucial for understanding its meaning in bioethics.[95]

Beneficence-based clinical judgment was the whole of bioethics before our century. Even when the language of rights does appear, for example, in the history of medical ethics, those rights are derivative from the beneficence-based obligations of the physician.[96] The rights of patients, properly understood as self-originated, have their origin in some morally important feature or characteristic of the patient that is independent of all other considerations. The law provides an important reference point for understanding this, because American common law gave expression to such independent moral status of the patient and the origin of rights in that status. The law understands respect for autonomy in terms of the nature and implications of the legal principle of respect for self-determination.

AUTONOMY AS LEGAL SELF-DETERMINATION. An important, precedent-setting case was *Schloendorff* v. *Society of New York Hospital*. The decision in this case dates from 1914 in New York state. In 1908, Ms. Schloendorff was admitted to the New York Hospital, at a charge of $7.00 per week, with "some disorder of the stomach." After some time as an "inmate" of the hospital, one Dr. Bartlett "discovered a lump, which proved to be a fibroid tumor." The consulting physician, Dr. Stimson, advised an operation. The patient consented to an "ether examination" to determine the "character of the lump," "but notified Dr. Bartlett, as she says, that there must be no operation." Ether was administered, a physical examination of her abdomen was performed, and while Ms. Schloendorff was unconscious, "a fibroid tumor was removed." "Her testimony is that this was done without her consent or knowledge." This approach makes perfectly good sense in beneficence-based clinical judgment of the time, because removing the tumor upon its discovery after the ether examination prevents the avoidable morbidity and mortality risks of a second anesthesia, after the "ether examination," that is, physical examination of an abdomen made nonrigid by anesthesia.[97]

Judge Cardozo apparently did not agree that such a beneficence-based account was the whole of the legal story, however. He introduced a contrapuntal theme to beneficence-based clinical judgment. His language rings out in a distinctively American cadence: "Every human being of adult years and sound mind has the right to determine what shall be done with his body; and a surgeon who performs an operation without his patient's consent commits an assault, for which he is liable in damages."[98]

Apparently recognizing that such a rule might be too rigid, Cardozo admits one—and only one—exception for the legal authority to act on beneficence-based clinical judgment: "This is true except in cases of emergency, where the patient is unconscious, and where it is necessary to operate before consent can be obtained."[99]

Three important implications follow from this early version of autonomy as legal self-determination:

1. The physician retains authority and power to make beneficence-based clinical judgments because Cardozo's principle leaves their integrity as such intact.
2. The physician no longer possesses authority and power to act on such judgments, a significant change from the exclusively beneficence-based approach of the preceding millennia.
3. The authority and power to authorize acting on beneficence-based clinical judgment is vested in the adult, competent patient.

The legal principle of self-determination has undergone historical development in the common law of the United States. A key case in this respect is *Canterbury* v. *Spence,* from the United States Court of Appeals for the District of Columbia from 1972.[100] In 1958 Mr. Canterbury, then an employee of the Federal Bureau of Investigation, underwent—with his consent—a laminectomy procedure to repair a " 'filling defect' in the region of the fourth thoracic vertebra." Postoperatively, Mr. Canterbury was permitted to leave his bed for the purpose of voiding, experienced an unattended fall during one such episode, and experienced paralysis from the waist down. In an attempt to correct this paralysis a second surgery was performed, again with Mr. Canterbury's consent, and Mr. Canterbury subsequently "required crutches to walk, still suffered from urinal incontinence and paralysis of the bowels, and wore a penile clamp." Mr. Canterbury, in the process of consenting to the first surgery, was not informed about the risk of paralysis from unguarded falls.[101]

On the basis of cases from state courts, Judge Robinson and the Court's majority went beyond the *Schloendorff* concept of simple consent—the patient's agreement to or refusal of an intervention—to what the court termed "true consent." Interestingly, "true consent" turns out to be a function of disclosure by physicians of information to patients. Two key passages from *Canterbury* are worth citing:

> True consent to what happens to oneself is the informed exercise of a choice, and that entails an opportunity to evaluate knowledgeably the options available and the risks attendant upon each.[102] . . . the physician discharges the duty when he makes a reasonable effort to convey sufficient information although the patient, without the fault of the physician, may not fully grasp it.[103]

The *Canterbury* court was quick to point out the limited nature of the disclosure required. In doing so the *Canterbury* court anticipated and rejected a common—but uninformed—objection of physicians:

> The discussion need not be a disquisition, and surely the physician is not compelled to give his patient a short medical education; the disclosure role summons the physician only to a reasonable explanation. This means generally informing the patient in nontechnical terms as to what is at stake: the therapy alternatives open to him, the goals expectably to be achieved, and the risks that may ensue from particular treatment and no treatment. So informing the patient hardly taxes the physician and it must be the exceptional patient who cannot comprehend such an explanation in at least a rough way.[104]

On this approach to legal self-determination, respect for autonomy involves the "opportunity" for the patient to evaluate alternatives and to make choices among them. On the basis of this (slightly) enriched legal principle of self-determination the following is the case:

1. The physician retains authority and power to make beneficence-based clinical judgments, as with *Schloendorff,*
2. the physician has a new obligation to explain those judgments, in terms of the benefits and risks of available alternatives, to the patient at a level that the patient can understand,
3. The adult, competent patient possesses sole power to authorize the physician to act on beneficence-based clinical judgment, even when
4. the competent, adult patient does not "fully grasp" the physician's explanation.

On the basis of this brief legal history, four important clinical implications of autonomy as legal self-determination can be identified.[105] First, it is clear who possesses the power to make authoritative decisions governing interventions undertaken by physicians: the competent, adult patient—and no one else; in particular, not the physician, not the patient's family, not hospitals, not payers, not institutions of self-government, and not society.

Second, the power to make authoritative decisions can be exercised by the competent, adult patient in advance, via a living will,[106] via durable power of attorney,[107] or via prior relevant statements, provided that there is legally satisfactory evidence for their having, in fact, been made. In the United States, this last form of "advance directive" is valid only in some states. (See Chapter 5.)

Third, the power to make authoritative decisions can be exercised by others on behalf of minor children and the never competent patient, subject to tests of reasonableness and prudence.

Fourth, this power of the patient does not leave the physician powerless—the common belief of many physicians to the contrary notwithstanding. The physician can, and bears the responsibility to, form his or her will in beneficence-based clinical judgments. That is, legal self-determination challenges only the power to *act* on beneficence-based clinical judgments; it does not challenge the intellectual integrity or ethical legitimacy of such judgments themselves.

While the law in these respects provides a useful reference point for understanding the principle of respect for autonomy, the legal concept of self-determination must be subjected to critical scrutiny, if we are to understand respect for autonomy as an ethical principle. As we read these and other cases in which the principle of self-determination is developed, legal self-determination is a "thin" concept of autonomy because it makes no reference to the particularities of the individual patient, especially to whether the exercise of legal self-determination is a function of the patient's subjective or deliberative interests. Legal self-determination refers only in an abstract way to the distribution and exercise of power in the patient-professional relationship. By "power" we mean the ability to form and to effect one's will. Even if the patient does not "fully grasp" information, his or her power to authorize intervention remains intact. This is conceptually and, therefore, clinically at least curious.

AUTONOMY AS MORAL AUTONOMY. Autonomy as legal self-determination is not adequate for understanding the concept of individual autonomy and the ethical principle of respect for individual autonomy, given the abstract nature of legal self-determination. To remedy this problem, we need to attend to the concept of autonomy as moral autonomy. This sense of autonomy is not entirely independent from the legal sense, but is distinct from it in an important fashion: it accents the moral particularities of each individual. That is, moral autonomy acknowledges that each of us is, in some important sense, a unique configuration and history of particular values and beliefs that form the basis for our determination of our own subjective and deliberative interests.

The values and beliefs that form the basis of each individual's interests are rarely *de novo*. Instead, they derive or are adapted from such factors as personal experience, family upbringing and traditions, and religious belief and faith communities, to name only some of the cultural resources each draws upon in shaping one's values and beliefs. One important implication of this is that, while each individual's perspective on one's interests and on what is in one's interest is unique—none of us are altogether alike in this respect—the resources upon which we draw as we develop our unique perspective can often be common to many. This is especially the case with religious beliefs and traditions, which usually are sustained and given life in a community of belief. Thus, while each individual's perspective on one's interests is unique and, therefore, is particular to that individual, the source of all of those interests need not be unique or idiosyncratic.

By emphasizing respect for the concrete, actual values and beliefs of each individual as, ultimately, an independent basis for one's moral status, respect for moral autonomy avoids the abstract character of respect for legal self-determination. By doing so, it adds an important dimension to the meaning of respect for autonomy: respect for the integrity and meaning of the patient's values and beliefs and the subjective and deliberative interests to which they give rise, even and especially when those interests do not coincide with the physician's beneficence-based judgment concerning the patient's social-role interests. That is, to the power to control decision making and outcomes—contributed by autonomy as legal self-determination—moral autonomy adds respect for the particular, concrete *basis* in the patient's life, her values and beliefs, for decision making and outcomes. Moral autonomy, not legal self-determination, makes for autonomy-based clinical judgment about an *individual* patient.

The most important implication of this feature of moral autonomy is that, in setting out its meaning, no concrete content can be given in advance without reference to the particular individual whose interests are at stake. In this way, respect for autonomy differs sharply from beneficence and, in doing so, highlights the peculiar nature of beneficence-based judgments: they are based on a determination of the patient's social-role interests, which, in turn, are a function of the competencies of medicine, which, in turn, can be determined independently of any particular patient's values and beliefs. That is, social-role interests are not a function of the values and beliefs of a particular patient, while subjective and deliberative interests of a particular patient can have no content apart from her actual values and beliefs, a second major dimension of autonomy as moral autonomy.

The Scope of the Principle

The scope of the principle of respect for autonomy is limited, but not for the same reason that the scope of beneficence is limited, namely, the competencies of medicine to seek goods on our behalf. The scope of respect for autonomy is limited in two ways.

First, no individual appeals to all possible values and beliefs in forming her own unique configuration of values and beliefs. There is not time and world enough for mortal beings to undertake such a task. Moreover, each of us is limited by the particular sources of morality into whose history we are born and raised at a particular time. For example, the importance in bioethics of the right of informed consent, the right to make decisions by a patient about his or her future—so prominent in the last several decades—is in considerable measure a function of the historical impact of the civil rights and consumer movements in the United States. Forty years ago in the United States, and today in other countries, things were and are different.

Second, each individual's values and beliefs give rise to different sorts of interests: subjective interests and deliberative interests. Subjective interests can be a function of whim as well as preference, a function of lifelong, settled—even if inchoately expressed—values and beliefs or values and beliefs that one is trying out, experimenting with in one's life. Subjective interests are thus inherently at risk for being unstable.[108] As far as some senses of respect for autonomy in the literature go, for example, respect for autonomy as a side constraint,[109] or respect for autonomy as a lexically ordered first principle,[110] such considerations are irrelevant. Autonomous refusal of health care interventions must be respected, that is, not overridden. This implication makes sense, though, only if one puts aside the issue of the potential instability of subjective interests. In effect, these senses of respect for autonomy do precisely that because they abstract from the particular values and beliefs of the patient to the conceptual category of persons as such, in a manner directly analogous to and derivative from respect for legal self-determination.

Deliberative interests are more stable, to the extent that they are a function of the patient determining her interests on the basis of adequate information and both cognitive and evaluative understanding of that information.[111] Respect for autonomy as respect for deliberative interests is not abstract, but concrete: respect for the integrity of a particular individual's values and beliefs that the process of forming deliberative interests itself produces. Respect for autonomy in this sense is limited in scope, as well, because an inevitable feature of deliberative interests is that they are formed on the basis of assigning some, however rough, but serviceable priority to one's values and beliefs, a process that necessarily cannot be all-encompassing of one's actual values and beliefs, much less all possible values and beliefs in one's culture.

Autonomy-Based Clinical Judgment about What Is in the Patient's Interest

Autonomy-based clinical judgment medical interventions, that is, prevention and management strategies, are in the patient's interest when those interventions are consistent with either the individual patient's subjective or deliberative interests. This occurs when the autonomous patient gives actual expression to those interests or when others undertake on the behalf of the formerly but now no longer autonomous patient a determination of those interests, which is usually called "substituted judgment" in the bioethics literature.[112] Thus, for example, whether the utilization of an assisted fertilization technique, such as in vitro fertilization or gamete intrafallopian transfer, is in an infertile woman's interest is a function of her determination of either her subjective or deliberative interests, and whether discontinuation of life supports for a patient with a terminal gynecologic cancer is justified is a function of either her subjective or, probably more appropriately, deliberative interests.

It is important here for us to underscore the fact that we are *not* claiming that respect for autonomy is invalid if it is based only on respect for the patient's subjective interests. We *are* claiming, however, that respect for autonomy has two distinct senses, depending on which interests the patient utilizes as the basis of her decisions. Those two senses will become important later, especially in Part II, on the clinical strategies of preventive ethics, and in Part III, on the strategies for managing ethical crises in gynecologic and obstetric practice.

Variability and Uncertainty in Autonomy-Based Clinical Judgment

There can obviously be variability in autonomy-based clinical judgment and in a variety of ways. First, by definition, autonomy-based clinical judgment about one individual cannot be presumed to apply to another individual. Across individuals—especially when those individuals appeal to quite different values and beliefs—there will be considerable, unpredictable variability of autonomy-based clinical judgment.

Second, over time for any given patient, there can be—though not necessarily need be—variability in autonomy-based clinical judgment based on the subjective interests of that patient. There can also be uncertainty in those cases where the patient merely expresses acceptance or refusal and provides little or no indication of her underlying values and beliefs.

Third, by their very nature, the subjective and deliberative interests of an individual patient may vary, because deliberative interests result from reflection upon, and thus regulation and correction of, subjective interests. As patients gather more information and assess it, they sometimes "change their minds." Perhaps this is not the most accurate description. It could also be the case that they are shifting from a subjective-interests basis for their decision making to a deliberative-interests basis. Something very much like this process goes on, we believe, when a pregnant woman is surprised to learn that her pregnancy is complicated by a fetal anomaly or that an asymptomatic patient is informed that her PAP smear has been diagnosed as Stage I cervical cancer. Decision making about the subsequent disposition of the pregnancy or about management of newly diagnosed cervical cancer can often be best understood as a process in which the patient's subjective interests are challenged by unexpected information with the result that the patient's interests must be more carefully determined. The result often is that the woman makes subsequent decisions on the basis of increasingly well-formed deliberative interests.

Autonomy-Based Objections to Paternalism

The previous discussion of beneficence-based objections to paternalism already indicates the general nature of autonomy-based objections to paternalism: beneficence-based clinical judgment, because of its limited scope, does not take account of subjective and deliberative interests of the patient. In failing to do so, it sets up the unwitting physician—that is, the physician who acts as if beneficence-based clinical judgment were the whole story of bioethics in the clinical setting—for failing to respect the integrity of the values and beliefs of the patient. That those values and beliefs are the patient's, that they constitute in a fundamental way her identity as a unique individual, and that the integrity of those values and beliefs is not necessarily undermined by morbidity or the threat of mortality—all of these are offended by paternalism. From this point of view, obviously, paternalism bears the burden of proof, at the very least, and is probably almost always unjustified, at most.

Table 1-3 Autonomy-Based Action Guides

1. The physician is ethically obligated in all cases to acknowledge and respect the integrity of the values and beliefs of the patient, even and especially when those values and beliefs lead to the expression of subjective or deliberative interests that are inconsistent with the patient's social-role interests or the physician's subjective or deliberative interests.
2. The physician is obligated to elicit the patient's subjective-interests-based or deliberative-interests-based preferences, as appropriate, about her health care.
3. Management strategies consistent with the subjective interests of the patient ought to be implemented.
4. Management strategies consistent with the deliberative interests of the patient ought to be implemented.
5. Management strategies inconsistent with the subjective interests of the patient ought not to be implemented, because they involve unjustified paternalistic interference with autonomy as self-determination.
6. Management strategies inconsistent with deliberative interests ought not to be implemented, because they involve unjustified paternalistic interference with autonomy as moral autonomy.

The Principle of Respect for Autonomy as a Set of Concrete Guides to Action

Considered by itself, the principle of respect for autonomy on the account that we have given constitutes more than a "checklist" of items to be considered. It provides concrete action guides—more than one of them because of the heterogeneity of autonomy-based clinical judgment. Those guides appear in Table 1–3.

These action guides are obviously not absolute, the final story for bioethics in the clinical setting. Their limited character in this respect is a direct function of several factors: (1) the limited scope of values and beliefs that serve as the basis for both subjective and deliberative interests, with the scope of the latter narrower than the former; (2) the inherently unstable nature of subjective interests; and (3) the variability for any individual patient of subjective interests over time or between subjective and deliberative interests over time.

The Relative Significance of the Principles of Beneficence and Respect for Autonomy in Clinical Judgment

Most often the principles of beneficence and respect for autonomy work in a synergistic fashion in clinical judgment. Sometimes, however, the action guides generated by beneficence and those generated by respect for autonomy may not be consistent in a particular case or set of circumstances. That is, because clinical ethical judgment—if it is to be comprehensive—must take into account social-role, subjective, and deliberative interests of the patient, the potential for ethical conflict within clinical judgment is a built-in feature of clinical judgment. When, as is the case sometimes in obstetrics, there are two patients whose interests are at stake, the potential for ethical conflict is heightened.

Sometimes, as we noted at the beginning of this chapter, action guides of beneficence and respect for autonomy conflict such that there is a crisis. Either the physician must act unreasonably in beneficence-based clinical judgment, that is, the physician must violate beneficence-based action guide #3 (See Table 1–2) in order to respect the patient's autonomy, or the physician must act unreasonably in autonomy-based clinical judgment, that is, the physician must violate both autonomy-based action guides #5 and #6 (See Table 1–3) in order to respect beneficence-based clinical judgment. All other conflicts among the remaining action guides are merely conflicts.

In a case of ethical conflict, the relative significance of the principles of beneficence and respect for autonomy cannot be settled in advance, by some decisive, theoretical rank-ordering of the two principles. This is because the limited scope and inherent variability and uncertainty of the ethical principles of beneficence and respect for autonomy denies each the status of a lexically ordered first principle that would always override the other in clinical judgment. Instead, the two principles are on theoretically equal, limited footing, with differences worked out in the clinical setting. The two are prima facie principles. The clinical strategies for working out the differences between the principles are those of preventive ethics, because all ethical conflicts that are not crises are resolvable within the physician-patient relationship. (See Part II.)

Ethical crises can only be resolved outside the physician-patient relationship. This is because ethical crises involve disputes about power, the power to determine which action guide will be violated and which honored. (See Part III.)

When Is a Human Being a Patient?

This question must be asked, because it will be crucial in the third and subsequent chapters on obstetrics. The preceding discussion of the relative significance of the principles of beneficence and respect for autonomy provides an adequate basis for a reliable answer.

It should, we trust, be clear by now that our fundamental theoretical commitment regarding bioethics—a commitment we believe we have corroborated in this chapter—is that clinical judgment is inescapably and disablingly defective if it does not take account of all of the interests of the patient: social-role, subjective, and deliberative interests alike. Any attempt to answer the question just posed that does not take account of all three types of interests is just as inescapably and disablingly defective. Thus, a human being is not a patient just when that individual consents to be a patient—a solely autonomy-based answer—or just when that individual is physically presented to a health care professional—a solely beneficence-based answer.

An answer that takes into account all three types of interest, we believe, is the following:[113]

> An individual human being is a patient when he or she (a) is presented to a physician (b) for the purpose of applying clinical interventions that are reliably expected to protect and promote the interests of that individual—construed as social-role, subjective, or deliberative interests as it is justified to do so—and thus to some reasonable degree are in that individual's interest.

On the basis of this answer, not all individuals need be autonomous in order to be patients. The never autonomous, which includes the profoundly and severely mentally retarded and—as we shall argue in the next chapter—some fetuses, are patients when they are presented to a physician whose competencies can protect and promote the social-role interests of those individuals. The autonomous or formerly autonomous are patients when they are presented to a physician whose competencies can protect and promote their social-role interests, as well as their subjective and deliberative interests.

This answer to the question, "When is a human being a patient?," is required to distinguish patients from research subjects and human beings undergoing innovate therapy, that is, upon whom a medical experiment is being performed without the benefit and protection of a research protocol. Research subjects are presented to the physician, but not for the purpose of applying clinical interventions that are reliably expected to protect and promote the interests of that individual and thus to some reasonable degree are in that individual's interest. This is certainly the case for subjects in the experimental arm of a randomized clinical trial. It is, interestingly, also the case for all subjects in a randomized trial, because randomization eliminates any *reliable expectation* that the individual patient's social role interests will be protected and promoted in the most effective way. It is precisely because randomization places this expectation at risk that the role of the physician is so ethically different from that of the clinical investigator.

Patients as Strangers: A Malignant Concept

The preceding discussion of beneficence and respect for autonomy has important implications for the concept of the patient as "stranger." This language has come to prominence recently.[114] To say that the patient is a stranger to the physician has a benign sense, namely, that the physician and patient have no prior social acquaintance. There is a malignant sense of the patient as "stranger," however. This sense implies something more, that the physician lives in a world so removed from that of patients that the physician possesses no ethically reliable access to an understanding of the patient's interests.[115] This concept of the patient as a moral stranger is malignant because it is destructive of the physician-patient relationship as a moral relationship and has no reliable conceptual foundation. On the account that we have given of social role interests of patients and of beneficence, the physician does reliably have access to an understanding—with all of the limitations noted above—of the social role interests of any patient. Thus, no patient can be a stranger to any physician in the second sense of the term. Moreover, it is reasonable to assume that for a patient who presents herself to a physician, health-related concerns may shape, to some degree, her subjective interests. Such concerns necessarily shape deliberative interests. Thus, no patient can be a stranger in the second sense of the term. To insist otherwise is either to adopt a concept of beneficence utterly disconnected from the interests of patients (which could not meaningfully then be termed "beneficence" at all) or to adopt a theory of the privacy of values and beliefs of patients that would render those values and beliefs species of a private language, a view that encounters formidable, disabling philosophical opposition.[116] In a minimalist legal relationship, described earlier, patients are indeed moral strangers. But this cannot be the case for a moral relationship with patients. To think otherwise is to equate the moral to the minimalist legal physician-patient relationship, which, it should now be clear, is a mistake.

Obligations to Third and Fourth Parties to the Physician-Patient Relationship

The physician-patient relationship is now situated within the context of third and fourth parties to that relationship. Third parties include individuals and institutions whose interests can be affected, for better or worse, by what occurs within the physician-patient relationship. These third parties include family members of the patient, the patient's larger community—especially religious community, if there is one—and the institutions that own or manage the resources consumed in the care of patients. The latter include employers of patients or patients' spouses or parents, individual and group practices from the solo fee-for-service practitioner through the large, fee-for-service group practice to health maintenance organizations, large-scale delivery systems such as the U.S. Department of Veterans Affairs and military health care, hospitals, and private and public payers. Fourth parties include those entities retained by payers to retrospectively or prospectively manage the expenditure of money in the care of patients, for example, through the use of various case management strategies and required prior authorization for hospital admission.

Family as a Third Party

In this book, we do not understand "patient" to include the spouse, children, other family members, or "significant others" of the individual patient. In particular, the spouse, partner, or parent of the female or pregnant patient is not a patient, but a third party to the physician-patient relationship. Obviously, the social role subjective, or deliberative interests of such a third party can be promoted or impaired as a consequence of what occurs within the physician-patient relationship.

Third and Fourth Parties That Own or Manage Resources Consumed in the Care of Patients

Third and fourth parties that own or manage resources consumed in the care of patients loom larger and larger in clinical practice. The ethical dimensions of and justification for their influence on or even involvement in clinical decision making must be carefully identified. The following considerations are essential, in our view.

It is crucial, at the outset of consideration of this topic, that physicians and patients, especially the former, understand that most of the resources consumed in the care of patients are no longer solely owned by patients and physicians, as was once the case in the now distant past. Some of these resources are owned by private entities—mainly the employers of patients, patients' spouses, or patients' parents and the insurance companies with which they may contract to provide health care "benefits." Some of these resources are owned publicly—by local, state, and federal governments. The managers of health care resources include both private entities—for example, private hospitals and fourth party companies in the health care management business on behalf of private and public owners of resources—and public entities, including public hospitals and delivery systems such as the Veterans Affairs or the various branches of military health care. The managers of health care also finance health care of patients.

Because these resources are owned by others, neither the physician nor the patient has an overriding positive right to their use. Moreover, the nature and extent of the obligation of owners and managers of health care resources to expend them in the care of patients is an unsettled matter, for example, the obligations of a private hospital to uninsured patients. These two considerations, obviously, have within and between them the makings of considerable ethical conflict between the obligations of the physician to third and fourth parties and the beneficence-based and autonomy-based obligations of the physician to the patient. These conflicts have to do with the fair or just allocation of health care resources.

Conflicts with third parties should be prevented. Indeed, increased efforts must be expended toward this important goal, lest those ethical conflicts unnecessarily evolve into ethical crises. The principle of justice is the basis of preventive ethics strategies for scarce resources. (See Parts II and III.)

How This Framework for Bioethics Differs from Others

The framework that we have set out and defended in this chapter is based methodologically in both philosophy and medicine. Other approaches to bioethics exist in the literature. The framework for bioethics in the clinical setting that we set out and defended in the previous section differs in important ways from others in the literature. We therefore want to outline how they differ from our own.

Bioethics and the Law

The law has been employed prominently as a methodological basis of bioethics. This is not surprising, given the high frequency of malpractice suits in medical care. There is thus a natural tendency on the part of many physicians in gynecologic and obstetric practice to equate ethical conduct, right behavior, with what the law permits and unethical conduct, wrong behavior, with what the law prohibits. In the literature, there has been a strong association between bioethics and the law. Annas, for example, argues on the basis of court opinions and holds that all of obstetric ethics can be summarized in a single legal rule: respect for the liberty and rights of the pregnant woman.[117]

The problems with taking the law as the basis of gynecologic and obstetric ethics are several. First, the law, especially the common law, is primarily reactive. That is, the law—both the common law, written by courts, and statutory law, enacted by legislatures—responds to civil complaints or issues that attract significant public attention. The law addresses those complaints and issues, with a view to resolving them and to some extent discouraging their recurrence. This preventive dimension of the law is mainly negative in character, that is, providing incentives to avoid legally culpable action. This preventive dimension of law has led to considerable emphasis on "defensive" medical practice. Such practice increasingly focuses the concern of the physician on protecting him or herself, rather than protecting the interests of patients. A truly preventive posture would focus primarily on the latter, thus emphasizing the prevention of ethical conflict in gynecologic and obstetric practice as a primary clinical consideration. As we shall argue in Part II, the clinical strategies of preventive ethics are essential to gynecologic and obstetric practice.

Second, the law is incomplete in that there are many areas of gynecologic and obstetric concern that the law does not, and probably will not, address. For example, some state courts have issued court orders for cesarean delivery for fetal distress or placenta previa.[118] However, no court has addressed, or is likely to address, a pregnant woman's disinclination to maintain an *excellent* record of conduct during her pregnancy, but only to maintain an *adequate* record.

Third, the law is largely silent on the virtues that physicians in gynecologic and obstetric practice ought to cultivate. Yet, attention to virtues such as self-effacement, self-sacrifice, compassion, and integrity is critical for any adequate response to society's concerns about the dehumanization of gynecologic and obstetric practice. Indeed, as we argued above, four virtues—self-effacement, self-sacrifice, compassion, and integrity—are individually necessary and jointly sufficient conditions for creating and sustaining a moral relationship with the patient.

Fourth, the law is subject to internal conflict. On the one hand, statutory and regulatory law governing publicly funded health care seems to obligate physicians to do less for their patients. On the other hand, the common law of malpractice seems to obligate physicians to do more.

In summary, making the law the methodological basis of bioethics imposes serious limitations, because it burdens bioethics unnecessarily by putting it at risk for being reactive, as well as negative or defensive in its preventive dimensions rather than positive. The law is also incomplete, and inconsistent. These are obviously serious shortcomings.

Nevertheless, there are some areas in which the law is settled, for example, informed consent for invasive procedures on competent patients. Well-established law commands respect ethically in a democratic society. To think, therefore, that gynecologic or obstetric ethics is intellectually autonomous from matters of settled law involves serious misconception in gynecologic and obstetric ethics. For example, to articulate ethical principles or "conditions" for ethically justified invasive clinical research in normal pregnant women without situating those principles within the considerable and settled body of statutory and regulatory law protecting human research subjects, as some have done,[119] involves this misconception.

Despite the shortcomings noted here, the law does provide two valuable reference points for bioethics. First, in the discussion above of the principle of respect for autonomy, we saw that the law is crucial for understanding one dimension of the ethical principle of respect for autonomy, namely, autonomy as legal self-determination.

Second, in the law the physician-patient relationship is understood to be a fiduciary relationship, not simply contractual. Such a relationship presupposes, we have argued, the virtues of self-effacement, self-sacrifice, compassion, and integrity. The law cannot, however, provide an ethical account of those virtues and so the law must be supplemented crucially by philosophy. In the absence of those virtues, the physician-patient relationship is merely contractual, to which sort of relationship the law is just barely adequate, because the legal relationship in a contract is minimal, lacking the fuller legal dimensions of a fiduciary relationship. Indeed, in the absence of the fundamental virtues of self-effacement, self-sacrifice, compassion, and integrity, the physician-patient relationship is reduced to a solely commercial, nonfiduciary relationship.

Bioethics and Religious Beliefs and Traditions

In subtle, and sometimes not so subtle ways, religious belief has been employed as the methodological basis of bioethics. Consider, for example, the "right to life" position on the morality of abortion.[120] Advocates of this position typically assert that the fetus is an unborn child and has a right to life, which is violated by abortion in all—or almost all—cases and is, therefore, murder in those cases.

Such a view holds, in effect, that the fetus independently possesses the right to life on grounds that everyone should accept. In particular the fetus is thought to possess such a right independently of at least four parties: the woman in whose uterus it is gestating; fathers; health care professionals; and society at large. On closer examination, however, it is plain that there are serious problems with this view.

First, the philosophical grounds for independent rights of the fetus are in hot and endless dispute, as are theological grounds.[121] Second, in the Judeo-Christian tradition, with its emphasis on stewardship over life as a gift from God, there is no independent right to life on the part of human beings, a right that they generate in and of themselves. In this tradition, the moral status of a human being is generated from the relationship between God as creator and that human being as God's creature. Any rights that creatures may have do not originate in themselves but in God.

By attending to these problems, we are in a position to see that advocates of the right to life position must either claim grounds for the independent rights of the fetus that are beyond dispute or acknowledge that the Judeo-Christian tradition would frame matters in very different ways, namely, in terms of our dependence on God, the fetus' theologically dependent moral status. The first alternative is ruled out as an intellectual impossibility because no such grounds can be conclusively established either philosophically or theologically. The second alternative is frankly theological and therefore is not something with which everyone should be expected to agree in a pluralistic society.[122]

There is yet a further problem: "right to life" does not refer to a single right but, in our view, to at least three. These are (1) the right not to be killed unjustly, (2) the right not to have technological, biological, social, and other basic life supports discontinued unjustly, and (3) the right to have all such basic life supports continued for as long as it is reasonable to do so. These rights, however, make different demands upon the pregnant woman. For example, the first version seems limited by very few exceptions, whereas the third version must admit of many exceptions because no human being has an overriding positive right to the property or body of another human being. The right to life movement thus suffers from a fundamental lack of clarity about the concept of a right to life and its clinical, ethical, and legal implications.

Another problem with basing bioethics on religious or theological grounds worth noting here is the use of theological concepts as if they are secular philosophical concepts. This problem is illustrated in the work of Evans and Fletcher, who appeal, for example, to a "graded" moral status of the fetus as the basis for their evaluation of selective termination of multifetal pregnancies.[123] The source for this concept, as is plain from their reliance on a key reference,[124] is the history of Christian theology. Evans and Fletcher do not appeal to secular philosophical foundations for independent moral status of the fetus, perhaps because all such proposed foundations are in dispute. In any case, the point of our criticism is that gynecologic and obstetric ethics that relies crucially on theological bases should be clearly defined as such and its limited applicability in a pluralistic society recognized. McNaughton, for example, is notable in that he undertakes to do so.[125]

In summary, making religious beliefs the methodological basis of gynecologic and obstetric ethics imposes serious limitations on bioethics, because of an appeal to foundations that cannot be expected to be accepted by everyone in a pluralistic society. This is because bioethics based on religious belief requires all to accept (1) the existence of a deity or some equivalent transcendent reality and (2) a particular interpretation within a particular faith community of what the deity or equivalent transcendent reality deems to be the ultimate good of human beings. But no reasonable person should expect these two conditions to be satisfied in a pluralistic society. Even if this were not a problem, key theological concepts that are employed in debates about ethical issues in obstetrics, such as the right to life, are equivocal. Approaches to bioethics that rely on theological foundations without acknowledging this fact cannot escape these criticisms.

Despite the shortcomings noted here, religious beliefs and traditions provide an important reference point for bioethics. Religious beliefs can, obviously, be a major source of influence on the values and beliefs of physicians and patients. The role of religious beliefs in the formation of what we term the physician's "private conscience" will be crucial for our discussion of abortion, in Chapters 5 and 6. The importance of religious beliefs for the values and beliefs of patients, especially when those values and beliefs differ from those of the physician, and thus for the patient's subjective and deliberative interests cannot be emphasized enough. The obligation of the physician to respect the integrity of the patient's religious values and beliefs, an integrity that makes those values and beliefs immune to criticism from a clinical point of view, helps to underscore the concrete meaning and application of the ethical principle of respect for autonomy. The crucial role of religious beliefs in clinical practice and for institutional policy has only recently received attention in bioethics.[126]

Bioethics and Professional Education and Training

Professional education and training have undoubted influence on the morality of physicians, if for no other reason than the length and intensity of that education and training. Hence, it comes as no surprise that there are appeals to education and training as the basis for bioethics, for example, in ubiquitous appeals in the bioethics literature to professional codes or oaths. Codes and oaths, however, are inadequate because their basis is either disputed—appeals to divinity as the sanction for an oath—or is unclear—as in the case of many codes of ethics. To be sure, students and trainees model themselves on role models of right behavior and good character, but this process is often unreflective and intuitive at best and inchoate at worst. Accounts of what morality in health care ought to be should be based on more self-conscious and thus more stable grounds than these, if they are to possess intellectual and moral authority.[127]

Despite these shortcomings, professional education and training provide an important reference point for bioethics. Education and training still emphasize the patient and the care of the patient. At their best, education and training still emphasize the moral life of professionalism, a life in service to others. Powerful role models and codes of professionalism are vital to sustaining the moral life of medicine. Making sense of the moral life of professionalism in terms of both virtues and ethical principles is another way to understand the main task we have aimed to carry out in this chapter.

Bioethics and Personal Experience

Personal experience is another powerful source of morality in medical practice for the simple intuitive reason that what worked well in the past should work well now. This rule of thumb is disabled by a serious problem, because, when applied to personal experience, the rule of thumb can take on a highly variable meaning. What worked for one physician didn't work for another and further appeals to personal experience quickly founder because there is no possibility that a third individual's personal experience can adjudicate disputes authoritatively. In short, personal experience is a highly idiosyncratic basis for bioethics and thus an inadequate basis for the management of ethical conflict in gynecologic and obstetric practice. That idiosyncracy must be tested and corrected from the broader perspective afforded by ethical analysis and argument. Thus, personal experience is ruled out as an endpoint. Still, it remains an obvious reference point for many of us. The point for bioethics is that personal experience must be subjected to critical scrutiny. Part I of this book is designed to provide each reader with frameworks for doing so in her gynecologic and/or obstetric practice.

Bioethics and Professional Consensus

Consensus has a natural appeal as a source of morality for medicine, since well-formed consensus commands intellectual respect in scientific and clinical reasoning. Appeals to consensus are thus very powerful in clinical medicine, especially when that consensus can be documented empirically, or even more when it has been derived from a rigorous process and reliable database.

Consensus in bioethics can be documented by empirical studies. Such studies are surely important for descriptive ethics, the study of what people actually believe morality to be. Whether consensus is important for normative ethics, the study of what morality ought to be, is problematic. An important example of consensus that has been documented in bioethics, not just on correct behavior but also on underlying ethical principles, has been claimed in gynecologic and obstetric ethics on the basis of accepted social science methodology and has resulted in descriptive ethics.

The most prominent example is the investigation of practices and allegiance to ethical principles in genetic counseling internationally.[128] To be sure, Fletcher and Wertz,[129] and Fletcher separately,[130] acknowledge the limits of their methodology but at the same time they interpret the data as providing strong support for the centrality of such ethical principles as respect for autonomy. They claim that approaches to or theories of ethics should be tested and corrected against this consensus. In effect, and subtly, they offer empirical validation for a normative ethical principle.

There are serious methodological problems with using consensus as the methodological basis of bioethics. Consensus in scientific and clinical judgment occurs when there is a sufficient body of data about a particular medical intervention, a body of data with clear, statistically significant trends, and when there is a high probability that there will be a lack of variance in future data regarding that medical intervention. That is, consensus can be achieved in scientific and clinical judgment when there is well-established, highly reliable information about present and expected data and about the replicability of judgments based on those data.

Such reliability cannot be established in empirical studies of ethical opinion. In bioethics it is more important to know *why* individuals regard an ethical virtue or principle as guiding than it is to know *that* they believe that it is guiding. Once this distinction is recognized the marked variance among possible reasons for holding respect for autonomy as a basic principle of genetic counseling, a key finding for Wertz and Fletcher, must also be recognized. These would include such heterogeneous considerations as the legal principles of self-determination and privacy, fear of malpractice, religious beliefs, political ideologies, professional education, or simple custom or habit of a professional group.[131] Because of this variance, the meaning in bioethics and the clinical implications of respect for autonomy will vary widely, perhaps incoherently. That is, the reasons why the principle of respect for autonomy is important to respondents of a survey do not necessarily fit into a connected, well-reasoned pattern. The fact that there is consensus provides no antidote to this potential incoherence, because the weight of numbers does not amount to a rigorous philosophical account of an ethical principle. Such an account would indeed provide an antidote to incoherence. It is even possible for a small minority to have the only well-reasoned accounts of a principle, a possibility that social science survey methodology cannot rule out.

In summary, consensus as the methodological basis of bioethics involves the serious shortcoming of taking widespread agreement on behavior, virtues, or principles to be intellectually authoritative despite the potential variability, even incoherence, of the reasons that lead to such agreement. Consensus misses the point that quality of argument, not quantity of opinions, is crucial. Opinions should be tested against well-made arguments, not vice versa. Critical analysis and argument, not data, constitute the materials and methods of bioethics as normative ethics, which concerns what morality ought to be in health care. Descriptive ethics, the only result of consensus methodologies in bioethics, provides a useful reference point: data on the actual opinions of physicians or patients. But this reference point must be subjected to the sustained critical scrutiny provided by normative ethics, so that the social wisdom that may exist in evolved social practices can be identified and critically evaluated. The goal of doing so is to identify and critically evaluate the moral wisdom that may exist in evolved social practices.

Bioethics and Inappropriate Appeals to Authority

Inappropriate appeals to authority play a surprisingly prominent role in bioethics. In the literature of gynecologic and obstetric ethics this usually takes the form of appeals to the conclusions of experts, or prominent individuals, or groups, as if the conclusions of such individuals or groups were authoritative in the sense of being immune to well-founded criticism because they have achieved closure on the subject, for example, ubiquitous appeals to the work of the President's Commission on Ethical Issues in Medicine and in Biomedical and Behavioral Research.[132] The problem is that the intellectual authority of any expert view in bioethics depends on the quality of the analysis and argument that supports the view and not on the prestige of an individual, an academic institution, professional association, or government commission or agency. These individuals or institutions may well have produced a well-reasoned account, which can then serve usefully as the springboard for further inquiry. The methodological mistake of inappropriate uses of authorities is to overlook the need to critically evaluate that account and thus avoid the pitfalls of premature closure.[133] There are often competing, well-argued accounts on particular issues in gynecologic and obstetric ethics just as there are often controversies in medical practice.

Some individuals may respond to reasonable competing accounts as if they were a problem. The response often takes the form in medical controversies of dogmatically asserting a solution. Inappropriate uses of authorities in gynecologic and obstetric ethics, in effect, do the same thing. Dogmatic responses to well-reasoned, competing accounts are never acceptable in bioethics, although they may be necessary as a *temporary* administrative last resort to establish clear policies in the clinical setting. Inappropriate uses of authorities also fail to appreciate the principal virtue of accepting controversy. Accepting controversy maximizes the possibility of respecting both the autonomy of the pregnant woman and the integrity of clinical judgment. A central tenet of this book is that well-reasoned diversity is not the problem in gynecologic and obstetric ethics; arbitrary closure is. The latter is a serious shortcoming of inappropriate uses of authorities.

In the lay media, this problem takes the form of provocative printed quotations or electronic "sound bites" from individuals who, on the basis of their scholarly accomplishments, may or may not be experts in gynecologic and obstetric ethics. Even when they are from individuals with good scholarly credentials, however, isolated quotations and "sound bites" are simply incapable of constituting thoughtful analysis and argument.

Apart from these serious procedural objections, there are substantive objections to this sort of inappropriate use of authorities, because frequently the expert statement cannot be supported by philosophical arguments.[134] For example, some recent statements of ethics experts concerning the initiation of a pregnancy for the purpose of producing an infant bone marrow donor for a sibling with cancer appealed to positions on the proper moral purpose for conceiving children.[135] There is, to be blunt, no accepted philosophical basis of any kind for making such a claim. Such a claim is nothing more than an expression of the subjective opinion of the authority figure who made the claim. Socrates pointed out 2.5 millennia ago that, however strongly held, subjective opinions cannot count as philosophical arguments. They are, as Socrates would say, "mere opinions," because they cannot be sustained by philosophical argument.

In summary, inappropriate uses of authorities as the methodological basis of gynecologic and obstetric ethics involve the misconception of locating that authority in such irrelevant factors as the prestige of an expert or that person's facility of producing sound bites on demand. The intellectual authority that gynecologic and obstetric ethics can hope to possess rests on careful analyses and arguments and the quality of thinking that goes into them and nowhere else. Given the seriousness of their shortcomings, inappropriate appeals to authority do not even serve as useful reference points for bioethics.

Bioethics and Institutional Policies and Practices

Institutional policies and practices possess considerable, though little appreciated, influence on the perceptions of physicians about what morality in medical care ought to be. Thus, if a physician's criteria for repeat cesarean delivery or disclosure practices regarding the need for a hysterectomy conform to those of the gynecologic or obstetric service, the physician may tend to assume that those criteria are therefore justified. If this or any other institutional policy is the result of consensus, however, all of the shortcomings of consensus discussed above apply. Worse, some institutional policies and practices originate from the dicta of powerful institutional figures, for example, department or service chairpersons or committees. Such *ex cathedra* dicta, at best, emanate from one or more of the above methodological bases for bioethics and so are subject to their shortcomings. Sometimes institutional policies and practices have obscure or unknown origins and have not been critically examined in many years. Their intellectual authority is therefore minimal. Indeed, such policies and practices are more often the source of ethical conflict than a basis for reliably managing ethical conflict.[136] They do not serve, therefore, as useful reference points for bioethics.

Conclusion

In this chapter we have set out the basis for the identification of ethical conflict in clinical practice generally, as a prelude to the next two chapters, in which we shall set out frameworks for the identification of ethical conflict in gynecologic practice and for the identification of ethical con-

Table 1-4 The Identification of Ethical Conflict in Clinical Practice

Areas of No Conflict

1. The physician is ethically obligated in all cases to acknowledge and respect the integrity of the values and beliefs of the patient, even and especially when those values and beliefs lead to the expression of subjective or deliberative interests that are inconsistent with the patient's social-role interests or the physician's subjective or deliberative interests. (Autonomy-based action guide #1).
2. The physician is obligated to elicit the patient's subjective-interests-based or deliberative-interests-based preferences, as appropriate, about her health care.

Ethical Conflict

2. Implementation of management strategies based on clear-cut beneficence-based clinical judgment (beneficence-based action guide #1) vs. implementation of management strategies based on the subjective interests of the patient (autonomy-based action guide #3).
3. Implementation of management strategies based on clear-cut beneficence-based clinical judgment (beneficence-based action guide #1) vs. implementation of management strategies based on deliberative interests of the patient (autonomy-based action guide #4).
4. Implementation of any one of the continuum of beneficence-based management strategies (beneficence-based action guide #2) vs. implementation of management strategies based on subjective interests of the patient (autonomy-based action guide #3).
5. Implementation of any one of the continuum of beneficence-based management strategies (beneficence-based action guide #2) vs. implementation of management strategies based on deliberative interests of the patient (autonomy-based action guide #4).
6. Beneficence-based management plans (beneficence-based action guides #1 or 2) vs. interests of third parties.
7. Autonomy-based management plans (autonomy-based action guides #3 or 4) vs. interests of third parties.

Ethical Crisis

8. Implementation of a management strategy outside the continuum of beneficence-based clinical judgment (in violation of beneficence-based action guide #3) vs. implementation of a management strategy inconsistent with either the subjective interests of the patient (in violation of autonomy-based action guide #5) or the deliberative interests of the patient (in violation of autonomy-based action guide #6).
9. Implementation of a management strategy outside the continuum of beneficence-based clinical judgment (in violation of beneficence-based action guide #3), or implementation of a management strategy inconsistent with the subjective interests of the patient (in violation of autonomy-based action guide #5), or implementation of a management strategy inconsistent with the deliberative interests of the patient (in violation of autonomy-based action guide #6) vs. interests of third parties.

Table 1-5 Topical Areas of Gynecologic and Obstetric Ethics

Gynecologic Ethics	*Obstetric Ethics*
Contraception and family planning	Assisted reproduction
Ectopic pregnancy	Directive vs. non-directive counseling for fetal benefit
Abortion before viability	Routine offering of antenatal diagnosis
Gynecologic diseases	Fetal anomalies
Critical care of female patients	Prematurity
The terminally ill patient	Critical care of the pregnant patient

flicts and crises in obstetric practice. The identification of ethical conflicts and crises in clinical practice can be summarized conveniently, based on the preceding discussion. (See Table 1–4.)

A framework for gynecologic ethics concerns the physician's beneficence-based and autonomy-based obligations to the female patient, either when there is no fetus present or when the fetus is not a patient. A framework for obstetric ethics concerns the physician's beneficence-based and autonomy-based obligations to the pregnant woman and beneficence-based obligations to the fetus, when the fetus is a patient. This ethical distinction between gynecology and obstetrics can be simply stated: gynecology concerns the management of one patient, the female patient, and obstetrics concerns the management of two patients, the pregnant patient and the fetal patient. On this basis, we present a classification of topics for both gynecologic and obstetric ethics. (See Table 1–5.)

This classificatory scheme does not necessarily conform to present gynecologic and obstetric practice, hence, it must be subjected to critical scrutiny. We will justify this classificatory scheme by setting out and defending frameworks for gynecologic and obstetric ethics, a task to which we turn in the next two chapters. Doing so will complete the task of Part I of this book, providing the readers with the cognitive and practical clinical tools for identifying ethical conflict and crisis in gynecologic and obstetric practice.

NOTES

1. By "well-documented, complete placenta previa" we mean the following: (1) Transabdominal or transvaginal ultrasound examination is performed by individuals competent in the technique and interpretation of its results; (2) the placenta is clearly visualized on ultrasound examination to cover the cervical os completely; (3) to maximize reliability, ultrasound examination should be performed shortly before delivery. The reliability of the examination varies inversely with the time remaining before expected date of delivery, because of increased variability of data regarding outcome the earlier the examination is performed. Satisfaction of these three criteria makes a false

positive diagnosis of complete placenta previa highly unlikely. See William J. Ott, "Placenta Previa," in Frank A. Chervenak, Stuart Campbell, and Glenn Isaacson (eds.)., *Textbook of Ultrasound in Obstetrics and Gynecology* (Boston: Little Brown, 1993) pp. 1493–1502; and D. Farine, H.E. Fox, and I.E. Timor-Tritsch, "Placenta Previa: Transvaginal Approach," in *Textbook of Ultrasound in Medicine,* pp. 1503–8.

2. Warren T. Reich, "Introduction," in Warren T. Reich (ed.), *Encyclopedia of Bioethics* (New York: Macmillan, 1978), pp. xv–xxiii.

3. We use "institution" deliberately broadly, to cover everything from the solo, fee-for-service physician in private practice, through group practices and hospitals, to large-scale private delivery (e.g., Kaiser Permanente) and private payment (e.g., private insurance) and public delivery (U.S. Department of Veterans Affairs) and payment (e.g., Medicare and Medicaid) schemes.

4. We do not attribute virtues to institutions, because this matter is not relevant to the questions addressed in this book. For a useful discussion, see Stephen Wear, "The Moral Significance of Institutional Integrity," *Journal of Medicine and Philosophy* 16 (1991):225–30.

5. Martin Benjamin, "Lay obligations in Professional Relations," *Journal of Medicine and Philosophy* 10 (1985):85–103.

6. See, for example, Mark Siegler, Edmund Pellegrino, and Peter Singer, "Clinical Medical Ethics," *The Journal of Clinical Ethics* 1 (1990):5–9; "Research in Clinical Ethics," *The Journal of Clinical Ethics* 1 (1990):95–99; "Teaching Clinical Ethics," *The Journal of Clinical Ethics* 1 (1990):175–180; "Ethics Committees and Consultants," *The Journal of Clinical Ethics* 1 (1990):263–67.

7. This is how we read H. Tristram Engelhardt, Jr., *The Foundations of Bioethics* (New York: Oxford University Press, 1986).

8. A notable exception is Howard Brody, *The Healer's Power* (New Haven, CT: Yale University Press, 1992).

9. See H. Tristram Engelhardt, Jr., *The Foundations of Bioethics,* Chapter 1. A sufficient condition is that, if it occurs, that for which it is the sufficient condition then occurs. A necessary condition is that, if it does not occur, that for which it is the necessary condition does not occur. In logic a sufficient condition is the antecedent of a hypothetical proposition (If a, then b), while a necessary condition is the consequent, b.

10. Others have taken a similar starting point for bioethics, notably Edmund Pellegrino and David Thomasma. See their *A Philosophical Basis for Medical Practice* (New York: Oxford University Press, 1981) and *For the Patient's Good: The Restoration of Beneficence in Health Care* (New York: Oxford University Press, 1988). We disagree with their concept of the patient's "wounded humanity," because not all patients have illnesses when they have diseases. Moreover, not all patients have diseases, notably pregnant patients. In addition, the phenomenological approach of Pellegrino and Thomasma does not show that disease *by itself* "wounds" the humanity of the patient, for they take no account of the contribution to this "wounding" by the authoritarian physician and bureaucratic structures.

11. Baruch A. Brody, "The Quality of Scholarship in Bioethics," *Journal of Medicine and Philosophy* 15 (1990):161–78.

12. K. Danner Clouser, "Bioethics," in Warren T. Reich (ed.), *Encyclopedia of Bioethics* (New York: Macmillan, 1978), pp. 115–27.

13. Arthur Caplan, "Ethical Engineers Need Not Apply: The State of Applied Ethics Today," *Science, Technology and Human Values* 6 (1980):24–32; "Applying Morality to Advances in Biomedicine: Can and Should This be Done?," in William Bondeson, H. Tristram Engelhardt, Jr., Stuart F. Spicker, and Joseph M. White (eds.), *New Knowledge in the Biomedical Sciences* (Dordrecht, The Netherlands: D. Reidel Publishing Co., 1981), pp. 155–68.

14. ibid., and Laurence B. McCullough, "Biomedicine, Health Care Policy, and the Adequacy of Ethical Theory," in William Bondeson, H. Tristram Engelhardt, Jr., Stuart F. Spicker, and Joseph M. White (eds.), *New Knowledge in the Biomedical Sciences*, pp. 167–75.

15. This can fairly be said of Tom L. Beauchamp and James F. Childress, *Principles of Biomedical Ethics*, 3rd ed., (New York: Oxford University Press, 1990).

16. This can fairly be said of Pellegrino and Thomasma, *For the Patient's Good* and Solomon Pepper, *Doing Right: Everyday Medical Ethics* (Boston: Little, Brown and Company, 1983).

17. See, for example, Ronald A. Christie and C. Barry Hoffmaster, *Ethical Issues in Family Medicine* (New York: Oxford University Press, 1986).

18. K. Danner Clouser and Bernard Gert, "A Critique of Principlism," *Journal of Medicine and Philosophy* 15 (1990):221.

19. ibid., 222.

20. ibid., 227.

21. See Albert R. Jonsen and Stephen Toulmin, *The Abuse of Casuistry: A History of Moral Reasoning* (Berkeley: University of California Press, 1988) and Albert R. Jonsen, Mark Siegler, and William Winslade, *Clinical Ethics: A Practical Approach to Ethical Decisions in Clinical Medicine,* 3rd. ed. (New York: Macmillan, 1992). For a useful critique of this methodology in bioethics, see John Arras, "Getting Down to Cases: The Revival of Casuistry in Bioethics," *The Journal of Medicine and Philosophy* 16 (1991):29–51.

22. Albert R. Jonsen and Stephen Toulmin, *The Abuse of Casuistry*.

23. See Baruch A. Brody, *Death and Dying Decision Making* (New York: Oxford University Press, 1988).

24. We take these criteria from Baruch A. Brody, "The Quality of Scholarship in Bioethics;" K. Danner Clouser and Bernard Gert, "A Critique of Principlism;" and Ronald M. Green, "Method in Bioethics: A Troubled Assessment," *Journal of Medicine and Philosophy* 15 (1990):179–98. Some readers may notice that we make no mention of "deontology", "consequentialism," or other such terms. We omit them because we believe that ethics generally and bioethics in the clinical setting in particular are too complex to be captured by such simple labels. For the reader who nonetheless insists on such labels, our approach is a mixed but disciplined one.

25. This list owes a debt to Alfred North Whitehead, *Process and Reality: An Essay in Cosmology* (New York: The Free Press, 1969).

26. See H. Tristram Engelhardt, Jr., *The Foundations of Bioethics*.

27. See, for example, Hilary Putnam, *The Many Faces of Realism* (LaSalle, Ill.: Open Court, 1987).

28. For a discussion of plausibility as a test of ethical theory, see Shelly Kagan, *The Limits of Morality* (New York: Oxford University Press, 1990).

29. We adopt this wonderful and apt phrase from John Stone, "He Makes a House Call," in his book of poetry, *In All This Rain* (Baton Rouge, La.: Louisiana State University Press, 1980), p. 5. See also his "The Long House Call," in his *In the Country of Hearts: Journeys in the Art of Medicine* (New York: Delacorte Press, 1990), p. 35.

30. See, for example, Robert M. Veatch, *A Theory of Medical Ethics* (New York: Basic Books, 1981).

31. See, for example, Pellegrino and Thomasma on beneficence in *For the Patient's Good*. They seem ultimately to collapse beneficence into respect for autonomy.

32. Tom L. Beauchamp and James F. Childress, *The Principles of Biomedical Ethics*, p. 195.

33. ibid., p. 196.

34. For a more general version of this argument, namely, that we are embedded in and

constituted by our relationships to each other, as Leibniz correctly taught, see Edmund L. Pincoffs, *Quandaries and Virtues: Against Reductionism in Ethics* (Lawrence, Kans.: University Press of Kansas, 1986). Medicine, because of its peculiar moral character as a life in service to patients, requires as mandatory virtues that Pincoffs treats as non-mandatory. Pence argues for the virtues on the basis that "contractualism is not the ideal," because "patients really want to be treated by physicians who practice the virtues." Gregory E. Pence, *Ethical Options in Medicine* (Oradell, N.J.: Medical Economics Company, Book Division, 1980), p. 199. This approach leads him to an account of virtues that shares with ours the virtue of compassion. Our argument is not based on some appeal, empirical or intuitive, of what patients "really want," that is, need. Instead, we examine the virtues from the physician's perspective, that is, what must be the case about the character of physicians such that they are routinely moved to create and are bound by the obligation to protect and promote the interests of each particular patient. For a very useful, concise introduction to virtue theory in ethics, see Greg Pence, "Virtue Theory," in Peter Singer (ed.), *A Comparison to Ethics* (Oxford: Basil Blackwell, Inc., 1991), pp. 249–58.

35. We do not deny that some physicians and some patients will find a minimalist, contractual relationship adequate. We do deny that this account can provide a basis for the physician's obligation to attend to the distinctive interests of each patient, so that each patient is treated as an individual person. Moreover, we believe that a minimalist, contractual relationship will be experienced by some patients as dehumanizing. We also wonder whether physicians will, in fact, find this approach to patient care to be satisfactory over time.

36. Keith S. Fineberg, J. Douglas Peters, J. Robert Willson, and Donald A. Kroll, *Obstetrics/Gynecology and the Law* (Ann Arbor, Mich.: Health Administration Press, 1984), Chapter I, especially p. 13.

37. Henry Campbell Black, *Black's Law Dictionary* (St. Paul, Minn.: West Publishing Co., 1979), p. 563.

38. Immanuel Kant, *Foundations of the Metaphysics of Morals*, trans. L.W. Beck (Indianapolis: Library of Liberal Arts, 1959).

39. This view of informed consent has been criticized for its ritualistic nature. See Stephen Wear, *Informed Consent: Patient Autonomy and Physician Beneficence Within Clinical Medicine* (Dordrecht, The Netherlands: Kluwer Academic Publishers, 1992).

40. This would seem to follow from Engelhardt's *The Foundations of Bioethics*.

41. John Gregory, *Lectures on the Duties and Qualifications of a Physician* (London: W. Strahan, 1772), p. 18.

42. Thomas Percival, *Percival's Medical Ethics*, Chauncey D. Leake, ed. (Baltimore: Williams and Wilkins, 1927).

43. See Baruch A. Brody, *Life and Death Decision Making*, on courage, *passim*.

44. See Laurence B. McCullough, "Historical Perspectives on the Ethical Dimensions of the Patient-Physician Relationship: The Medical Ethics of Dr. John Gregory," *Ethics in Science and Medicine* 5 (1978):47–53.

45. John Gregory, *Lectures on the Duties and Qualifications of a Physician*, pp. 19–20.

46. Warren T. Reich, "Speaking of Suffering: A Moral Account of Compassion," *Soundings* 72 (1991):83–108. See also his "The Case: Denny's Story" and "Commentary: Caring as Extraordinary Means," *Second Opinion* 17 (1991):41–56.

47. Reich, "Speaking of Suffering," p. 86.

48. ibid., 93.

49. ibid., 88.

50. ibid., 94.

51. ibid., 91.

52. ibid., 98. This need not involve feeling what the patient feels, but feeling that the

patient feels and experiencing one's own suffering of the patient's suffering. An interesting account of suffering is also provided by Eric Cassell. See his "The Nature of Suffering and the Goals of Medicine," *New England Journal of Medicine* 306 (1982):639–645 and his *The Nature of Suffering and the Goals of Medicine* (New York: Oxford University Press, 1991).

53. Cf. Baruch Brody, *Life and Death Decision Making,* pp. 35–37.

54. Edmund D. Pellegrino, "Altruism, Self-Interest, and Medical Ethics," *Journal of the American Medical Association* 258 (1987):1939–40.

55. See, for example, ibid.

56. ibid.

57. In effect, Pellegrino advocates a false heroism.

58. For example, Colonel William B. Travis defied General Sam Houston's orders to abandon the Alamo as a hopeless cause. General Lord Cornwallis found himself with his back to the York River and cut off by the French Fleet from reinforcements. Rather than sacrifice his troops in a lost cause, he did the correct thing as an officer—he surrendered.

59. To date, in our judgment, no obstetric or gynecologic procedure has been demonstrated to satisfy these three criteria.

60. This now involves state legislatures, the federal legislature, the federal executive branch, and several professional associations.

61. For more on informed consent, see Chapter 4, Ruth R. Faden, and Tom L. Beauchamp, *A History and Theory of Informed Consent* (New York: Oxford University Press, 1986), and Stephen Wear, *Informed Consent.*

62. It is important to recall that the practice of medicine is a privilege, not a right. Hence, no right to practice on the part of the physician is at stake.

63. John Gregory, *Lectures on the Duties and Qualifications of a Physician,* p. 20.

64. Medicine is not unique in this respect. The same argument could be made about the other traditional professions—namely, the law, the ministry, and the military (officer corps).

65. An important, recent exception is Bonnie Steinbock, *Life Before Birth: The Moral and Legal Status of Embryos and Fetuses* (New York: Oxford University Press, 1992). Steinbock approaches the moral status of the fetus in terms of interests the fetus may be said reliably to have. Steinbock takes the view that consciousness is a necessary condition for the possession of interests, a concept that she sees as tightly connected with having welfare of one's own. In short, only those entities that *generate* interests can reliably be said to have interests. As will become clear in this section, we take the view that one can have interests in virtue of being in a social role constituted by those interests, even though one may generate neither the social role nor the interests that constitute it.

66. Joel Feinberg, *Harm to Others* (New York: Oxford University Press, 1984), pp. 33–34.

67. ibid., p. 34.

68. Edmund Pellegrino and David Thomasma, *For the Patient's Good,* pp. 77–83.

69. Alan Goldman emphasizes the importance of needs in his interpretation of the basic norm of medicine, what he (mistakenly) calls the "Hippocratic Principle" of "do no harm:" "Notice that this norm appeals to the patients' health/needs, rather than to his desires or rights." See his *The Moral Foundation of Professional Ethics* (Totowa, N.J.: Rowman and Littlefield, 1980), p. 157.

70. John Rawls, *A Theory of Justice* (Cambridge: Harvard University Press, 1971).

71. John Kleinig, *Paternalism* (Totowa, N.J.: Rowman and Littlefield, 1983), p. 119.

72. Irwin C. Lieb, *The Four Faces of Man: A Philosophical Study of Practice, Reason, Art and Religion* (Philadelphia: University of Pennsylvania Press, 1971).

73. See H. Tristram Engelhardt, Jr., *The Foundations of Bioethics, passim.*

74. This is *not* the same concept as Engelhardt's person in the social sense, in his

Foundations of Bioethics, passim. The social-role interests of patients are conceptually independent from whether or not the patient is a person, in Engelhardt's sense. The social-role interests of patients are, instead, a function of the competencies of the health care professions.

75. H. Tristram Engelhardt, Jr., *The Foundations of Bioethics,* p. 3.

76. John Gregory, *Lectures on the Duties and Qualifications of a Physician,* p. 2.

77. James Griffin, *Well-Being: Its Meaning, Measurement, and Moral Importance* (Oxford: Oxford University Press, 1989).

78. Deliberative interests involve actually having additional information about one-self. They thus do not involve the more hypothetical nature of rational desires, what one would desire if one had more information. The concept of deliberative interests thus provides a concrete, actual example of rational desire. This becomes important later, in Chapter 4.

79. Becky C. White, *Competence to Consent* (Dordrecht, The Netherlands: Kluwer Academic Publishers, 1994).

80. ibid.

81. Joel Feinberg, *Harm to Others,* p. 38.

82. ibid., p. 39, emphasis original.

83. See Laurence B. McCullough and Stephen Wear, "Respect for Autonomy and Medical Paternalism Reconsidered," *Theoretical Medicine* 6 (1985):295–308.

84. Daniel Brock and Allen Buchanan, *Deciding for Others* (Cambridge: Cambridge University Press, 1991), pp. 122–23, emphasis original.

85. Joel Feinberg, *Harms to Others,* p. 53, emphasis original.

86. ibid, p. 54, emphasis original.

87. Hippocrates, *Oath of Hippocrates,* Ludwig Edelstein (trans.), in Owsei Temkin and C. Lilian Temkin (eds.), *Ancient Medicine: Selected Papers of Ludwig Edelstein* (Baltimore: John Hopkins University Press, 1967), p. 6.

88. Hippocrates, *Epidemics,* in W.H.S. Jones (trans.), *Hippocrates,* 4 vols. (Cambridge, Mass.: Harvard University Press, 1923), vol. 1, p. 165.

89. Carson Strong has claimed that our approach to obstetric ethics did not include a strong prohibition against killing. We think his criticism was mistaken, though it was useful in pointing us to the need to be clear on this point. See Carson Strong, "Delivering Hydrocephalic Fetuses," *Bioethics* 5 (1991):1–22.

90. See, for example, George Annas, "Protecting the Liberty of Pregnant Patients," *New England Journal of Medicine* 316 (1988):1213–14.

91. Our account of reliability can be placed in the larger context of recent literature on the epistemology of reliabilism. See, for example, Alvin I. Goldman, *Epistemology and Cognition* (Cambridge, Mass.: Harvard University Press, 1986) and his *Liaisons: Philosophy Meets the Cognitive and Social Sciences* (Cambridge, Mass.: The MIT Press, A Bradford Book, 1991). Our approach to reliability combines indicator (the nature of the clinical information on which prognostic clinical judgment is based) and process (the replicability of the prognostic clinical judgment by a rigorous judger) accounts. See Thomas D. Senor, "Ecumenical Reliabilism and the Demon World," *Proceedings and Addresses of the American Philosophical Association* 66 (1993): 109 (abstract).

92. By "futile" we mean that there is no or very low (<3%) probability of an intended effect occurring. For a discussion of futility, see Leslie J. Blackhall, "Must We Always Use CPR?," *New England Journal of Medicine* 317 (1987):1281–85; Tom Tomlinson and Howard Brody, "Ethics and Communication in Do-Not-Resuscitate Orders," *New England Journal of Medicine* 318 (1988):43–46; Tom Tomlinson and Howard Brody, "Futility and the Ethics of Resuscitation," *Journal of the American Medical Association* 264 (1990):1276–80; John D. Lantos, Peter A. Singer, Robert M. Walker, et al., "The Illusion of Futility in Clinical Practice," *The American Journal of Medicine* 87 (1989):81–84; and Lawrence J. Schneiderman, Nancy S. Jecker, and Albert R. Jonsen, "Medical Futility: Its Meaning and Ethical Implications," *Annals of Internal Medicine* 112 (1990):949–54.

93. Tom L. Beauchamp and James F. Childress, *Principles of Biomedical Ethics*, p. 214.

94. See, for example, Carson Strong, "Court-Ordered Treatment in Obstetrics: The Ethical Views and Legal Framework," *Obstetrics and Gynecology* 78 (1991):861–68.

95. See Ruth Faden and Tom L. Beauchamp, *A History and Theory of Informed Consent, passim.*

96. See Laurence B. McCullough, "Medical Ethics, History of: Britain and the United States in the Eighteenth Century," in Warren T. Reich (ed.), *Encyclopedia of Bioethics*, pp. 957–63.

97. *Schloendorff* v. *Society of New York Hospital*, 211 N.Y. 125, 126, 105 N.E. 92, 93 (1914). The quoted material is from the edited version of the case in Judith Areen, Patricia A. King, Steven Goldberg, and Alexander Morgan Capron (eds.), *Law, Science and Medicine* (Mineola, N.Y.: The Foundation Press, 1984), pp. 353–56.

98. ibid. It is interesting that Cardozo wrote his opinion during the very time in the history of the United States when our legislatures were significantly restricting self-determination when it came to the use of drugs. Thus, if one tempered the common law with statutory law, one would not reach the view that legal self-determination is absolute, contra Cardozo and the legal tradition and commentary that flows from this case.

99. ibid.

100. *Canterbury* v. *Spence*, 464 f. 2d 772, 785 (D.C. Cir. 1972). The quoted material is taken from the edited version of the case in Judith Areen, et al. (eds.), *Law, Science and Medicine*, pp. 372–85.

101. ibid.

102. ibid.

103. ibid.

104. ibid.

105. For a fuller, excellent account of this history, see Ruth Faden and Tom L. Beauchamp, *A History and Theory of Informed Consent.*

106. A "Living Will" is a legal document in which one refuses life-prolonging medical intervention in advance of a time in which one is terminally ill and incompetent. See Chapter 5.

107. "Durable Power of Attorney" is a document in which one assigns to another the power to make medical care decisions in advance of a time at which one is unable to do so for oneself. See Chapter 5.

108. Subjective interests thus are not, or at least need not be "authentic" in Miller's sense of the term. See Bruce Miller, "Autonomy and the Refusal of Life Saving Treatment," *Hastings Center Report* 11 (1981):22–28.

109. See H. Tristram Engelhardt, Jr., *The Foundations of Bioethics.*

110. See Robert M. Veatch, *A Theory of Medical Ethics.*

111. Deliberative interests may, but need not always, be authentic in Miller's sense of the term. See Bruce Miller, "Autonomy and the Refusal of Life Saving Treatment." Nor need they be "deeply sedemented," as John Arras suggests in his "The Severely Demented, Minimally Functional Patient: An Ethical Analysis," *Journal of the American Geriatrics Society* 36 (1988):938–44.

112. In a substituted judgment, one individual (for example, a family member) substitutes his or her judgment and decision for another (for example, the patient).

113. This account of when a human is a patient differs from that offered by Mathieu, who simply asserts, but nowhere argues, that "[t]he ability to treat a fetus as a patient has no bearing whatsoever on its status as a person, nor does it reflect any light on what our obligations to the fetus should be." Deborah Mathieu, *Preventing Prenatal Harm: Should the State Intervene?* (Dordrecht, The Netherlands: Kluwer Academic Publishers, 1991), p. 17. What we say here and argue in Chapter 3 can be read as a decisive refutation of the second part of Mathieu's claim. The first part of her claim is irrelevant to whether the fetus is a patient. (See Chapter 3.)

114. See, for example, David J. Rothman, *Strangers at the Bedside: A History of How Law and Bioethics Transformed Medical Decision Making* (New York: Basic Books, 1991).

115. This is the import of Engelhardt's account: "I use the term 'moral strangers' to signal the relationship people have to one another when they are involved in moral controversies and do not share a concrete moral vision that provides the basis for the resolution of controversy, but instead regard one another as acting out of fundamentally divergent moral commitments. When one meets another as a moral stranger, one meets in circumstances where there is no community of moral commitment that could in principle resolve the difference and allow the disputants to regard cooperation in the matter at issue as warranted in terms of content-full moral principles." H. Tristram Engelhardt, Jr., *Bioethics and Secular Humanism: The Search for a Common Morality* (Philadelphia: Trinity Press International, 1991), pp. xiii–xiv.

116. See Ludwig Wittgenstein, *Philosophical Investigations,* trans. G.E.M. Anscombe (Oxford: Basil Blackwell, 1963).

117. George J. Annas, "Protecting the Liberty of Pregnant Patients;" Sherman Elias and George J. Annas, *Reproductive Genetics and the Law* (Chicago: Year Book Medical Publishers, 1987), pp. 253–62; Sherman Elias and George J. Annas, "Perspectives on Fetal Surgery," *American Journal of Obstetrics and Gynecology* 145 (1987):807–12; George J. Annas, "Pregnant Women as Fetal Containers," *Hastings Center Report* 16 (1986):13–14; and George J. Annas, "Forced Cesareans: The Most Unkindest Cut of All," *Hastings Center Report* 12 (1982):16–17, 45.

118. See, for example, *Jefferson* v. *Griffin Spalding County Hospital Authority,* 274 Ga. 86, 274 S.E. 2d 457 (1981); *In Re Baby Jeffries,* No. 14004 (Jackson Country, Mich. P. Ct. May 24, 1982). For a useful, concise discussion of current legal trends, see Lawrence J. Nelson, "Legal Dimensions of Maternal-Fetal Conflict," *Clinical Obstetrics and Gynecology,* 35 (1992):738–48. For a detailed review, see Deborah Mathieu, *Preventing Prenatal Harm, passim.*

119. Richard L. Berkowitz, "Invasive Studies During Normal Pregnancy," *Obstetrics and Gynecology* 75 (1990):1041–42.

120. James Bopp (ed.), *Restoring the Right to Life: The Human Life Amendment* (Provo, Utah: Brigham Young University Press, 1984).

121. See Charles E. Curran, "Abortion: Contemporary Debate in Philosophical and Religious Ethics," in Warren T. Reich (ed.), *Encyclopedia of Bioethics,* pp. 17–26; John R. Noonan (ed.), *The Morality of Abortion* (Cambridge: Harvard University Press, 1970); and Andre E. Hellegers, "Fetal Development," *Theological Studies* 31 (1970): 3–9.

122. For a discussion of the limits of theologically based ethics, see H. Tristram Engelhardt, Jr., *The Foundations of Bioethics* and *Secular Humanism: The Search for a Common Morality.*

123. M.I. Evans, John C. Fletcher, and I.E. Zador, "Selective First-Trimester Termination in Octuplet and Quadruplet Pregnancies: Clinical and Ethical Issues." *Obstetrics and Gynecology* 71 (1988):289–96. For further discussion of selective termination of multifetal pregnancies, see Chapter 6, pp. 181–185.

124. G. R. Dunstan, "The Moral Status of the Human Embryo: A Tradition Recalled," *Journal of Medical Ethics* 1 (1984):38–42. In subsequent discussions, curiously, Evans and Fletcher drop this reference, but retain the concept of graded moral status. See Mark I. Evans, John C. Fletcher, and Charles Rodeck, "Ethical Problems in Multiple Gestations: Selective Termination," in Mark I. Evans, John C. Fletcher, Alan O. Dixler, and Joseph Schulman (eds.), *Fetal Diagnosis and Therapy: Science, Ethics, and the Law* (Philadelphia, Pa.: J.B. Lippincott Company, 1989), pp. 266–76.

125. M. McNaughton, "Ethics and Reproduction," *American Journal of Obstetrics and Gynecology* 162 (1990):879–82.

126. Frank A. Chervenak and Laurence B. McCullough, "Does Obstetric Ethics Have Any Role in the Obstetrician's Response to the Abortion Controversy?," *American Journal of Obstetrics and Gynecology* 163 (1990):1425–29.

127. For an interesting discussion of the adequacy of codes of ethics, see Ronald S. Gass, "Introduction: Codes of the Health Care Profession," in Warren T. Reich (ed.), *Encyclopedia of Bioethics,* pp. 1725–30. A very useful source on the development of medical ethics in the eighteenth century is Robert Baker, Roy Parker, and Dorothy Park (eds.), *Codification of Medical Morality, Volume I: The Eighteenth Century* (Dordrecht, The Netherlands: Kluwer Academic Publishers, 1993).

128. Dorothy C. Wertz and John C. Fletcher (eds.), *Ethics and Human Genetics: A Cross-Cultural Approach* (New York: Springer-Verlag, 1989). Similar work has been done regarding abortion, sex selection, and selective termination of multifetal pregnancies. See Mark I. Evans, Arie Drugan, Sidney F. Bottoms, et al., "Attitudes on the Ethics of Abortion, Sex Selection, and Selective Pregnancy Termination Among Health Care Professionals, Ethicists, and Clergy Likely to Encounter Such Situations," *American Journal of Obstetrics and Gynecology* 164 (1991):1072–99.

129. John C. Fletcher and Dorothy C. Wertz, *Ethics and Human Genetics, passim.*

130. John C. Fletcher, "Ethical and Human Genetics: A Cross-Cultural Perspective," in Dorothy C. Wertz and John C. Fletcher (eds.), *Ethics and Human Genetics,* pp. 457–90.

131. Jonathan Moreno, "Ethics by Committee: The Moral Authority of Consensus," *Journal of Medicine and Philosophy* 14 (1988):411–32 and "What Means This Consensus?: Ethics Committees and Philosophic Traditions," *The Journal of Clinical Ethics* 1 (1990):38–43. For a more extended discussion of the role of consensus in bioethics, see Robert M. Veatch and Jonathan Moreno (eds.), *Journal of Medicine and Philosophy* 16 (1991):371–463, issue on "Consensus Panels and Committees: Conceptual and Ethical Issues."

132. This commission was established under President Carter and completed its work under President Reagan. It produced volumes from 1981 to 1983. For a critique of such public ethics, see Baruch A. Brody (ed.), *The Journal of Medicine and Philosophy* 15 (1990):345–48, issue on "The Role of Philosophy in Public Policy," and Laurence B. McCullough, "Methodological Concerns in Bioethics," *The Journal of Medicine and Philosophy* 11 (1986):17–37.

133. For an example of the failure to do so, see Kenneth J. Ryan, "Ethics in Obstetrics and Gynecology," *American Journal of Obstetrics and Gynecology* 151 (1985): 840–43.

134. James Rachels, "When Philosophers Shoot from the Hip," *Bioethics* 5 (1991): 67–71.

135. Associated Press, "Baby is Conceived to Save Daughter," *New York Times,* February 17, 1990. The expert quoted as holding this view is Alexander Morgan Capron, a law and medical professor at the University of Southern California. See also Robin D. Clark, John Fletcher, and Gloria Peterson, "Conceiving a Fetus for Bone Morrow Donation: An Ethical Problem in Prenatal Diagnosis," *Prenatal Diagnosis* 9 (1989):329–34.

136. Edmund Erde, private communication. That unexamined institutional practices and policies are frequently a cause of ethical conflict in the clinical setting we dub the "Erde Rule."

2 | A Framework for Gynecologic Ethics in the Clinical Setting

In the previous chapter we set out and defended a framework for bioethics in the clinical setting. We argued that such a framework must start with the individually necessary and jointly sufficient material conditions for the physician-patient relationship as a moral relationship. These conditions are provided by the virtues of self-effacement, self-sacrifice, compassion, and integrity, because these virtues create and sustain the physician-patient relationship as one in which the physician acts primarily to protect and promote the interests of the patient. The obligation to protect and promote the patient's interests is made clinically applicable by the ethical principles of beneficence and respect for autonomy, respectively. We also noted that the physician-patient relationship exists in the context of third parties and fourth parties. The physician has obligations to protect and promote the legitimate interests of these third and fourth parties, as well as obligations to the patient. This framework for bioethics in the clinical setting, we showed, permits the physician to identify ethical conflicts and crises between beneficence-based and autonomy-based obligations owed to the patient and conflicts and crises between obligations owed to the patient and obligations owed to third and fourth parties. In this chapter we shall adapt this framework to gynecologic practice. Our goal is to develop a framework for gynecologic ethics in the clinical setting that permits the identification of ethical conflict and crises in gynecologic practice.

Gynecological practice deals with one patient, the female patient. This stands in sharp contrast to obstetric ethics, which deals with two patients.

(See Chapter 3.) A framework for gynecologic ethics, therefore, simply adapts the framework for bioethics from Chapter 1 to the setting of gynecologic practice. This can be done concisely; hence, the relatively compact length of the present chapter.

Four Basic Virtues: Self-Effacement, Self-Sacrifice, Compassion, and Integrity

What we said in Chapter 1 about self-effacement, self-sacrifice, compassion, and integrity as together forming the basis for the ethical principles of beneficence and respect for autonomy applies completely here. The commitment by the physician to these virtues creates and sustains the physician-patient relationship by making a reality the obligation to protect and promote the patient's interests. This obligation, in turn, is interpreted in clinical practice by the principles of beneficence and respect for autonomy. Before discussing the two principles, we comment on a particular dimension of self-sacrifice, namely, its ethical implications for the physician's response to changes in the economics of medical care and for self-aggrandizement. (These comments also apply to obstetric practice.)

The Importance of Self-Sacrifice in the Present Economics of Medical Care

In the present economic environment of medical practice, there are, we believe, powerful incentives for the physician to give personal monetary concerns high priority, and even primary consideration. This is morally problematic.

Adequate remuneration is certainly among the legitimate interests of the physician, simply because remuneration is among the legitimate interests of everyone who works for a living. Other factors affect this legitimate interest. Four are especially worthy of note. First, physicians experience a delay of entry into the work force and so their years of earning power are reduced vis-à-vis the average. Second, American society, along with others, places a high value on physician services and, as a consequence, physicians enjoy a very high average income. Third, persistent efforts by payors to control the growth of the cost of medical care have created many constraints on and incentives to the ability of physicians to increase their income. Fourth, physicians entering the profession in the last decade or so, like their peers in other ways of life, may find themselves living at a lower economic standard than physicians of earlier times or their own parents. Fifth, this last factor is compounded by the sometimes significant levels of debt that physicians may carry into practice from undergraduate college or medical school.

These five factors make for a volatile mix, with the effect that developing and sustaining a clear and reasonable understanding of one's legitimate economic interests presents an ongoing moral challenge to the physician in gynecologic practice. (The same is true of obstetric practice, which is certainly not unique in this respect.) A careful consideration of the nature of self-sacrifice provides the physician with powerful tools for fashioning an ethically justifiable response to these five factors, as well as to any other factor that can distort the legitimate economic interests of the physician.

Monetary reward, of a higher-than-average level (vis-à-vis other occupations), constitutes a reasonable expectation for physicians, provided that it is understood to be an effect or result of a commitment to excellence in clinical practice. Another result of this commitment is quality care of patients. We are aware of no evidence to support a belief that these two effects will not continue to follow from a commitment to practice medicine well, with excellence. Economic changes in medical care have, so far, not disrupted the cause-effect relationship between a commitment to excellence and remuneration. They have only diminished the size of the effect. But compression of earnings, even real reduction in earnings, is *not* unique to medicine; it is a broadly based phenomenon in our economy in recent years.

On this understanding of the remuneration of physicians, the quality of patient care remains the primary consideration with financial reward an independent effect of the commitment to excellence. By this we mean that reasonable financial reward is not sought as an end, with the care of patients the means to that end. The care of patients and reasonable financial reward are *both* ends, with neither a means to the other. That is, the commitment to excellence in patient care has a "double effect,"[1] or two effects of which it is the cause: (1) quality care of patients, and (2) remuneration. Quality care of patients and remuneration, on this understanding of them, are causally independent: neither is, nor therefore need be, the means to the other.

The virtue of self-sacrifice has an important ethical implication here, because it requires that this arrangement be preserved. The moral demands of the virtue of self-sacrifice are violated when patient care becomes the means to monetary reward. By making patient care the *means* to monetary reward, rather than an independent end or goal, patient care is relegated to secondary status in a systematic way. The physician's pecuniary interests thus take first place and, in the process, threaten to eclipse the interests of patients. This is because patients can be subjected to management strategies that, in reasonable beneficence-based judgment, benefit patients only to a slight degree or cannot be thought to benefit patients at all, but which do increase compensation. Given the persistent "downside" of medical interventions discussed in Chapter 1, patients can also be subjected to systematic risk of harm as the means to the physician's remuneration.

It is not too extreme to say that physicians who fail to abide by the moral and economic logic of the virtue of self-sacrifice become economic predators on their patients. This is, obviously, a powerful vice. Indeed, it is a corrosive force that could destroy the moral underpinnings of medicine generally, not just a particular physician-patient relationship.

Thus, the virtue of self-sacrifice requires physicians to sacrifice making patient care a means to remuneration. Not doing so would eliminate one of the necessary conditions for the physician-patient relationship as a moral relationship. By appreciating this aspect of self-sacrifice, the physician keeps monetary reward an end or goal that is casually independent of quality patient care, which is preserved as itself an end or goal in the physician's moral life.

Self-Aggrandizement

Self-aggrandizement, the seeking after of reputation and power for their own sake, also constitutes a vice vis-à-vis self-sacrifice, especially in the academic setting. The distinction between self-aggrandizement and a legitimate interest in one's reputation is made along the same lines as above. The repute of colleagues and patients will follow in its own course from the commitment to excellence in patient care. Such repute is a happy side effect of quality patient care, and, so long as it is nothing more, is among the physician's legitimate interests. If self-aggrandizement becomes the physician's goal, the interests of patients are subordinated to that goal, and reputation and power must be regarded as forms of mere self-interest and therefore, self-aggrandizement. This is because self-aggrandizement does not serve the interests of patients, but rather uses patients in a predatory fashion.

Self-aggrandizement can be a major problem for academic physicians. Reputation and power in the academic medical setting tend to accrue to those who produce revenues or publications. The inclination to pursue these as goals is particularly strong in the academic setting, because they are rewarded with promotion and tenure. It is one of the ironies—if not contradictions—of academic medicine that it rewards the pursuit of self-interest on the part of physicians in their role as faculty members but still expects them to be role-models of professionalism, the moral life in service to others. The assumption seems to be that students, residents, and patients benefit from rewarding the faculty's pursuit of self-interest.

There are dangers here. In the academic medical setting, its rhetoric to the contrary notwithstanding,[2] teaching is decreasingly valued as a goal. In good teaching the student comes first. It is our observation that in the present milieu of academic medicine—as in research universities generally—faculty committed to good teaching undertake that goal without genuine institutional support. Good teaching amounts to a "private" moral commitment, sustained only by like-minded colleagues. This basis for the moral life of the physician-teacher strikes us as inherently unstable. It needs to be stabilized by genuine institutional commitments to good teaching.

Publication requires research and, in research with human subjects, there can be no reliable expectation that the interests of the patient will be protected and promoted as a matter of course, as explained in Chapter 1. Those interests must be promoted by design. A physician interested in collecting cases of advanced cervical cancer for the purposes of a randomized trial of experimental management of that cancer can protect and promote the interests of patients by providing safeguards, such as insistence on a meaningful informed consent process and stopping rules based on both safety and statistical considerations. A physician gathering cases to develop and master a new procedure, for example, minimal site surgery, must be much more careful, given the direct and powerful economic incentives that are inevitably involved and the absence of legally mandated oversight. Such activity must be stringently reviewed, to protect patients from becoming merely a means to the economic advantage of the physician. The fact that the physician's academic department stands also to gain adds the confounding factor of conflict of interest. Institution-wide policies seem necessary to manage this conflict of interest with integrity.

The problem of self-aggrandizement is compounded still further in the private practice setting. The profession, perhaps through the American College of Obstetricians and Gynecologists, needs to develop mechanisms that will promote ethical integrity and thus protect and promote the interests of patients.

The Virtues as the Basis for Gynecologic Ethics in the Clinical Setting

The virtue of self-effacement erases the mere self-interests of the physician, but not always the physician's legitimate self-interests. The virtue of self-sacrifice blunts mere self-interest, particularly in remuneration or self-aggrandizement that are detached from the commitment to excellence in patient care. Self-sacrifice thus crucially defines a dimension of legitimate self-interest. As argued in Chapter 1, self-sacrifice does not always blunt other forms of legitimate self-interest. Self-effacement and self-sacrifice create the physician-patient relationship as a moral relationship. The virtues of compassion and integrity sustain that moral relationship. In doing so, these four virtues serve as the individually necessary conditions for the physician-patient relationship in gynecologic practice. Together these four virtues provide the sufficient condition for the physician-patient relationship as a moral relationship, because they have the effect in practice of focusing the concern of the physician, and moving the physician to act, on the protection and promotion of the interests of the patient. Insofar as they are relevant, the social-role, subjective, and deliberative interests of the patient shape the interests of the patient. How such shaping occurs can be interpreted clinically in terms of the ethical principles of beneficence and respect for autonomy. We thus turn to a consideration of these principles in gynecologic practice, along the lines of which they were considered in Chapter 1.

The Principle of Beneficence

The principle of beneficence shapes the physician's understanding of the interests of the female patient in terms of the social-role interests of the patient.

Beneficence-Based Obligations to the Female Patient

The ethical principle of beneficence obligates the physician in gynecologic practice to protect and promote the patient's social-role interests. These comprise the prevention of premature or unnecessary death *and* the prevention, cure, or at least amelioration of disease, injury, handicap, and unnecessary pain and suffering. As a rule, beneficence-based obligations to the female patient will give priority to preventing her premature or unnecessary death, because a premature or unnecessary death makes impossible or dooms the realization of her other social-role interests. It will sometimes be the case that gynecologic management of nonlife-threatening problems will either promote all of the female patient's social-role interests or promote some of those interests without impairing others. That is, sometimes beneficence-based gynecologic clinical judgment is clear-cut. It is also true that both quantitative and qualitative trade-offs will be involved, as discussed in Chapter 1. As a consequence, beneficence-based clinical judgment in gynecology will typically be subject to uncertainty and variability. In response to this moral fact, beneficence-based clinical judgment typically will aim to identify the range or continuum of gynecologic interventions that are in the female patient's social-role interest. As a whole, this continuum sets the boundaries on both what is reasonable in beneficence-based clinical judgment—all alternatives within the continuum—and what is unreasonable in beneficence-based clinical judgment—all alternatives outside the continuum. The latter are not in the female patient's social-role interest, that is, insofar as beneficence-based clinical judgment is concerned. This approach provides beneficence-based grounds to oppose paternalism, as explained in Chapter 1.

The Principle of Beneficence as a Set of Concrete Guides to Action in the Gynecologic Management of the Female Patient

Considered by itself, the principle of beneficence on the account that we have provided constitutes more than a mere "checklist" of items to be considered in gynecologic practice. It provides concrete action guides for the physician in gynecologic practice—more than one of them, because of the heterogeneity of beneficence-based clinical judgment, as explained in Chapter 1. Those guides are summarized in Table 2–1.

It is important to emphasize that these beneficence-based action guides cannot be regarded as absolute, that is, always controlling of the physician's behavior. The limited character of these guides is a direct function of several factors: (1) the limited scope of interests of female patients taken into account by beneficence-based clinical judgment; (2) the heterogeneity of reliable beneficence-based clinical judgment from the clear-cut to the variable and uncertain; and (3) the fact that most reliable beneficence-based clinical judgments are variable and uncertain because of the persistent downside to most clinical management strategies in gynecology.

Table 2-1 Beneficence-Based Action Guides for Gynecologic Practice

1. Management strategies based on clear-cut, beneficence-based clinical judgments about what is in the female patient's interest ought to be implemented, *the social-role interests of the female patient having been taken into account.*
2. Any one of the range or continuum of management strategies based on variable and uncertain beneficence-based clinical judgments about the interests of the female patient may properly be implemented, *the social-role interests of the female patient having been taken into account.*
3. Management strategies that lie outside the range or continuum of those based on variable and uncertain but reliable beneficence-based clinical judgments about the interests of the female patient ought not to be implemented, *the social-role interests of the female patient having been taken into account.*

The Principle of Respect for Autonomy

The principle of respect for autonomy shapes the physician's understanding of the interests of the female patient in terms of the subjective and deliberative interests of the patient.

Autonomy-Based Obligations to the Female Patient

In gynecologic practice the female patient possesses subjective interests and is capable of forming deliberative interests. Any assumption to the contrary is unwarranted.[3] Hence, the physician in gynecologic practice owes autonomy-based obligations to the female patient.

Unlike the principle of beneficence, no content can be provided a priori, that is, without conferring with the female patient, or reliable surrogates of female patients who irreversibly lack the capacity for autonomous decision making, for the subjective and deliberative interests that give substance and meaning to autonomy-based clinical judgment. That content can only be provided by the female patient or, when that patient is unable to do so, by those reliably thought to represent her subjective and deliberative interests. Autonomy-based clinical judgment about what is in the female patient's interest concerns her judgment about which gynecologic interventions protect and promote her subjective and deliberative interests.

The subject matter of gynecology is especially rich in subjective and deliberative interests, because it involves such human concerns as sexuality and reproduction. It is important to note that there is nothing in the concepts of either subjective or deliberative interests, as we have developed them here, that excludes the possibility that they may include the female patient's concerns, hopes, plans for, and sense of obligation to others, family members in particular. That is, subjective interests need not be exclusively self-regarding, although they can be. Deliberative interests in gynecologic ethics may be more likely to be both self-regarding and other-regarding for some patients. This is not, however, a matter of cognitive or moral necessity. How the female patient negotiates trade-offs between self-regarding and other-regarding concerns in forming her deliberative interests is a matter for her to decide alone.

In addition, the deliberative interests of the female patient will be formed in response to a consideration of her own social-role interests and the physician's beneficence-based judgment about what is in her social-role interest. Thus, the physician's beneficence-based clinical judgments play a vital role in the formation of the female patient's deliberative interests.

As we shall see in Parts II and III of this book, the formation by the female patient of her deliberative interests plays a crucial role in the strategies for both preventing and managing ethical conflict and crises in gynecologic practice. Rather than get ahead of ourselves at this point, we return to the task of identifying autonomy-based obligations of the physician to the female patient.

Chief among these will be to avoid paternalism. In terms of the previous chapter we can say that paternalism involves the imposition of beneficence-based clinical judgment about what is in the female patient's social-role interest on the autonomous female patient without her consent. When the female patient, by refusing intervention, in effect refuses any longer to be a patient, there is no cognitive or moral authority to any beneficence-based judgment regarding her social-role interests that she is obligated to remain a patient. Because of the limited scope of beneficence-based clinical judgments, they possess no authority to mandate that someone become or remain a patient. This is a matter for public policy, courts, and legislatures to decide. (See Chapter 7.) To think otherwise is to misunderstand in a fundamental fashion the limited nature of the principle of beneficence in bioethics. When the female patient remains a patient but refuses all reasonable (in beneficence-based clinical judgment) interventions in favor of an unreasonable course, then ethical conflict becomes ethical crisis, as explained in Chapter 1. In response to this situation the strategies for preventing ethical conflict and crisis in gynecologic practice (Chapter 5) and managing ethical crisis in gynecologic practice (Chapter 7) should be implemented.

The Principle of Respect for Autonomy as a Set of Concrete Guides to Action in the Gynecologic Management of the Female Patient

Considered by itself, the ethical principle of respect for autonomy on the account that we have provided for it here constitutes more than a "checklist" of items to be considered. It does provide action guides to the physician in gynecologic practice—more than one of them because of the heterogeneity of autonomy-based clinical judgment, as explained in Chapter 1. Those guides are summarized in Table 2–2.

The Relative Significance of the Principles of Beneficence and Respect for Autonomy in Gynecologic Clinical Judgment

The relative significance of the ethical principles of beneficence and respect for autonomy in gynecologic ethics concerns how the conflicts between guides to action based on these two principles should be addressed in clinical practice. This topic will be taken up in detail in Parts II and III of this book.

Our approach will be distinctive in that we shall emphasize the importance for the physician and female patient alike of the expression of her deliberative, not just subjective, interests. This is especially the case for

Table 2-2 Autonomy-Based Action Guides for Gynecologic Ethics

1. The physician in gynecologic practice is obligated in all cases to acknowledge and respect the integrity of the values and beliefs of the female patient, even and especially when those values and beliefs lead to the expression of subjective or deliberative interests that are inconsistent with the female patient's social-role interests or the physician's subjective or deliberative interests.
2. The physician in gynecologic practice is obligated to elicit the female patient's subjective-interests-based or deliberative-interests-based preferences, as appropriate, about her health care.
3. Gynecologic management strategies consistent with the subjective interests of the female patient ought to be implemented.
4. Gynecologic management strategies consistent with the deliberative interests of the female patient ought to be implemented.
5. Gynecologic management strategies inconsistent with the subjective interests of the female patient, when these are the only interests expressed, ought not to be implemented, because they involve unjustified paternalistic interference with autonomy as self-determination.
6. Gynecologic management strategies inconsistent with the deliberative interests of the female patient ought not to be implemented, because they involve unjustified paternalistic interference with autonomy as moral autonomy.

nonroutine matters, that is, when the social-role interests of the female patient are vitally at stake. This occurs when the patient's health status is a risk for serious, far-reaching, and irreversible change. Health status is valued, in part, because it is a necessary condition for the pursuit of anyone's subjective or deliberative interests. The setting back of the social-role interests of a patient can therefore set back her subjective and deliberative interests. Serious risks to health status involve anatomic or physiologic changes that greatly set back interests. Such risks are far-reaching when several such changes may occur. Such risks are irreversible when the setback to interests that those risks might cause cannot reliably be expected to be reversed. The serious, far-reaching, and irreversible setting back of any patient's social-role interests almost always threatens to set back her subjective and deliberative interests.[4] Thus, for example, the female patient's decisions about the management of such conditions as uterine cancer or infertility are serious matters. Granted, they are not always entered into in a reflective fashion. However, to permit them to be entered into or, worse, continued in an unreflective fashion or to fail to take the opportunity to encourage reflective decisions—that is, to elicit expression of the woman's deliberative interests—sets up the physician-patient relationship for preventable, serious, even unmanageable (in some cases) ethical crises.

Moreover, to do so is to show a profound disrespect for the female patient, treating lightly in her life what she should not, without reflection, consider to be light matters, as one might, if—in the language of Chapter 1—one equated respect for autonomy with respect for legal self-determination. Doing so is one of the most dehumanizing things the physician could do to a female patient, because it paternalistically treats the female patient as less than an adult.

Obligations to Third and Fourth Parties to the Physician-Patient Relationship

In general, the obligations of the physician in gynecologic practice to third and fourth parties to the physician-patient relationship are the same as they are in clinical practice generally, although the spouse of the female patient poses some special considerations as a third party.

This is because the spouse or partner of the gynecologic patient may have a vital stake in the patient's decisions about the management of her gynecologic disease. After all, the spouse or partner may be a contributing factor to the etiology of such disease. In addition, the spouse or partner can be a crucial contributor to management of disease, especially

Table 2-3 The Identification of Ethical Conflict in Gynecologic Practice

Areas of No Conflict

1. The physician in gynecologic practice is ethically obligated in all cases to acknowledge and respect the integrity of the values and beliefs of the female patient, even and especially when those values and beliefs lead to the expression of subjective or deliberative interests that are inconsistent with the female patient's social-role interests or the physician's subjective or deliberative interests. (Autonomy-based action guide #1).
2. The physician in gynecologic practice is obligated to elicit the female patient's subjective-interests-based or deliberative-interests-based preferences, as appropriate, about her health care.

Ethical Conflict

3. Implementation of management strategies based on clear-cut beneficence-based clinical judgment (beneficence-based action guide #1) vs. implementation of management strategies based on the subjective interests of the female patient (autonomy-based action guide #3).
4. Implementation of management strategies based on clear-cut beneficence-based clinical judgment (beneficence-based action guide #1) vs. implementation of management strategies based on deliberative interests of the female patient (autonomy-based action guide #4).
5. Implementation of any one of the continuum of beneficence-based management strategies (beneficence-based action guide #2) vs. implementation of management strategies based on subjective interests of the female patient (autonomy-based action guide #3).
6. Implementation of any one of the continuum of beneficence-based management strategies (beneficence-based action guide #2) vs. implementation of management strategies based on deliberative interests of the female patient (autonomy-based action guide #4).
7. Beneficence-based management plans (beneficence-based action guides #1 or 2) vs. interests of third parties.
8. Autonomy-based management plans (autonomy-based action guides #3 or 4) vs. interests of third parties.

Ethical Crisis

9. Implementation of a management strategy outside the continuum of beneficence-based clinical judgment (in violation of beneficence-based action guide #3) vs. implementation of a management strategy inconsistent with either the subjective interests of the female patient (in violation of autonomy-based action guide #5) or the deliberative interests of the female patient (in violation of autonomy-based action guide #6).
10. Implementation of a management strategy outside the continuum of beneficence-based clinical judgment (in violation of beneficence-based action guide #3), or implementation of a management strategy inconsistent with the subjective interests of the female patient (in violation of autonomy-based action guide #5), or implementation of a management strategy inconsistent with the deliberative interests of the female patient (in violation of autonomy-based action guide #6) vs. interests of third parties.

chronic disease. Controversially, we are willing to say that the gynecologic patient's determination of her deliberative interests regarding the management of her gynecologic disease is incomplete if she does not at least acknowledge the pertinence of her spouse's or partner's deliberative interests in her and in their relationship, his subjective interests being too unstable in our view to merit such consideration. That is, the morally significant relationship in which the gynecologic patient stands to her spouse or partner is not something she is free simply to ignore, unless her spouse or partner consents to being ignored. The role of the physician in this process will be addressed as necessary in subsequent chapters.

In general, then, to the extent that the patient understands herself to be obligated to avoid impairing the interests of her family, she ought to take those interests into account in her decision-making process. To the extent that the physician is bound by general obligations not to impair the interests of the patient's family, the physician should take those interests into account in clinical ethical judgment. Both of these matters, however, are inherently conflictual and there is no settled ethical theory available to manage decisively conflicts that may arise. These conflicts must be managed in practice.

The Identification of Ethical Conflict and Crisis in Gynecologic Practice

Based on the preceding discussion of the elements of a framework for gynecologic ethics, we are now in a position to complete that framework by providing for the identification of ethical conflict and crisis in gynecologic practice in terms of the following taxonomy, which we take to be exhaustive of the extent of such ethical conflict. That is, on the basis of the preceding discussion, the identification of ethical conflict in gynecologic practice can be summarized conveniently. (See Table 2–3.)

Conclusion

Ethical conflicts are usually intellectually provocative and engaging to discuss. Indeed, the gynecologic literature is beginning to include discussion of "four-alarm" cases and issues. However intellectually engaging it may be to consider such cases and issues, their ethically most significant feature for physicians and patients alike in clinical practice should be their prevention. Before turning in Part II to strategies of preventive ethics in gynecologic practice, we first provide in the next chapter a framework for obstetric ethics.

NOTES

1. For a discussion of the principle or doctrine of double effect, see Richard McCormick, *Ambiguity in Moral Choice* (Milwaukee: Marquette University Press, 1973); Richard McCormick and Paul Ramsey (eds.), *Doing Evil to Achieve Good* (Chicago: Loyola University Press, 1978); and Thomas Bole (ed.), *The Journal of Medicine and Philosophy* 16 (1991):465–585, issue on "Double Effect: Theoretical Function and Bioethical Implications."

2. Panel on the General Professional Education of the Physician and College Preparation for Medicine, *Physicians for the Twenty-First Century: The GPEP Report* (Washington, D.C.: Association of American Medical Colleges, 1984).

3. That is, the presumption is that the female patient is autonomous. Any judgment to the contrary carries a considerable burden of proof. The preventive ethics strategies developed in Part II are based on this presumption of autonomy. Indeed, preventive ethics strategies provide the most effective way, in our judgment, to put this presumption into clinical practice.

4. This relationship between serious setbacks to social-role interests and serious setbacks to subjective and deliberative interests seems to be the following. The former seems usually to be a sufficient condition for the latter, but the latter is neither a necessary nor sufficient condition for the former. The reader should note that a serious setback to social-role interests does not imply or entail diminished autonomy. The relationship between serious setbacks to social-role interests and reduced autonomy is highly variable.

3 | A Framework for Obstetric Ethics in the Clinical Setting

In the first chapter we set out and defended a framework for bioethics in the clinical setting. There we argued that such a framework must start with the individually necessary and jointly sufficient material conditions for the physician-patient relationship as a moral relationship. These conditions comprise the virtues of self-effacement, self-sacrifice, compassion, and integrity that blunt the mere self-interests and, though not always, legitimate self-interest of the physician so that he or she can focus primarily on, and act to protect and promote, the interests of the patient. The obligation to protect and promote the interests of the patient is, in turn, interpreted clinically by the ethical principles of beneficence and respect for autonomy. The physician-patient relationship, we also argued, exists in the context of third and fourth parties and the physician has obligations to these parties, as well as to the patient. This framework for bioethics in the clinical setting, we showed, permits the physician to identify ethical conflicts and crises within the physician-patient relationship and conflicts and crises between obligations to the patient and obligations to third parties. In this chapter, we shall adapt this framework to obstetric practice and show how it permits the identification of ethical conflict and crises in obstetric practice.

Obstetrics is unique among all of the health care specialties or fields in that the physician can at times bear responsibility for two patients simultaneously. The pregnant woman is indisputably a patient.[1] When she comes to the physician for antenatal care, she presents herself for the purpose of applying reasonable health care interventions. It is increasingly a commonplace for the fetus to be regarded as a patient.[2] After all, the fetus can be diagnosed throughout a pregnancy and increasingly can be treated. Embryos existing in vitro can be directly presented to and manipulated by the physician. At the same time, the lives of fetuses are terminated by abortion. If all fetuses were patients, abortion would therefore involve the direct killing of a patient—something that, as a rule, violates beneficence-based obligations to patients. Indeed, as we showed in Chapter 1, there is a strong beneficence-based prohibition against the killing of patients whose deaths are premature or unnecessary. Fetuses, then, seem ambiguously to be patients, and their status as such needs to be clarified as a preliminary to setting out and defending a framework for obstetric ethics in the clinical setting.

Accordingly, this chapter is divided into two parts. In the first we address the fundamental question for obstetric ethics: When is the fetus a patient? In the second section, on the basis of what we take to be a defensible answer to this crucial question and on the basis of the framework for bioethics set out and defended in Chapter 1, we set out and defend a framework for obstetric ethics.

When is the Fetus a Patient?

The concept of the fetus as patient has come to prominence in recent years in obstetric literature and practice, largely as a result of developments in fetal diagnosis and management strategies to optimize fetal outcome.[3] This concept, which has become widely accepted and influential in the thinking and behavior of physicians in obstetric practice, possesses considerable ethical significance. When the fetus is a patient, the physician is bound by beneficence-based obligations to protect and promote the social-role interests of the fetus, seemingly on an equal par with the obligations to protect and promote the social-role, subjective, and deliberative interests of the pregnant woman. When the fetus is not a patient, this would not be the case—there would only be obligations to protect and promote the social-role, subjective, and deliberative interests of the pregnant woman.

If one held that the fetus were never a patient, then the only obligations of the physician in obstetric practice would be to the pregnant woman. If one held that the fetus were always a patient, then the potential for conflict between the physician's obligations to the fetus and to the pregnant woman would be ever-present. If, finally, one held that the fetus were sometimes a patient and at other times not a patient, then there would be the potential for conflict between obligations to the fetus and to the pregnant woman, but not an ever-present one. The potential would be present only when the fetus is a patient.

Of these three possibilities, we shall defend the third as the most reasonable response to the question, "When is the fetus a patient?" We shall do so by showing that the first two responses depend on establishing whether or not the fetus has independent moral status, an enterprise doomed to failure. That is, these responses turn on arguments meant to show that some one or more characteristics are required for someone to have independent moral status, that is, independently of any other consideration or individual or society, and on arguments meant to show that the fetus does or does not possess such characteristic or characteristics. We begin, then, our inquiry into the question, "When is the fetus a patient?," with an inquiry to arguments about whether or not the fetus possesses independent moral status.

The Independent Moral Status of the Fetus

A remarkable variety of intrinsic characteristics has been nominated as the basis for arguments about whether or not the fetus possesses independent moral status. These include the moment or time of conception, implantation in the uterine wall, central nervous system development, quickening, or the moment of birth.[4] Given this wide variety of proposed intrinsic characteristics, it should come as no surprise that—in the centuries of debate on this topic—there is considerable variation of views about when the fetus is thought to come to possess independent moral status.

Some think that the fetus possesses independent moral status from the moment or time of conception.[5] At this stage the full genetic complement is present for the gestation of an individual human being and such a potential, it is thought, provides the basis for independent moral status. Others believe that independent moral status comes about by degrees, so that at each point during gestation there is greater and greater increment of independent moral status. This is the view that the fetus possesses "graded"[6] moral status. Still others hold, at least by implication, that the fetus never possesses independent moral status so long as it is in utero.[7] It is only when the fetus is alive and ex utero that it enjoys full moral status and protection.

The debate about these matters stretches over centuries. Indeed, it is one of the oldest ethical debates in Western culture, along with such debates as those concerned with the meaning of citizenship, the proper relationship between humans and the environment, and the nature and limits of political power. Like the debates on these other topics, the debate about the independent moral status of the fetus has never been able to achieve closure on a single account of whether or not—or when, if at all—the fetus possesses independent moral status.

There are powerful and inescapable reasons why this is the case. Debates about the independent moral status of the fetus draw upon all of the sources of morality that can be found in a pluralistic society such as the contemporary United States. Thus, an argument based on any one of them suffers from its methodological limitations, which we attempted to identify at the end of the first chapter. In particular, arguments about the independent moral status based on theological considerations suffer the shortcomings that characterize any argument based on faith and revelation in a pluralistic society: those outside a particular faith community may not accept the conclusions drawn by that particular faith community. There may also be deep disagreement within a faith community.

A compounding factor is that the religious traditions in our world—and they can all be found in well-represented proportions in a large pluralistic society such as that of the United States—have failed to agree on *the* single theological authority for the resolution of differences between religious traditions and faith communities on moral theological questions. This is important because there are quite significant differences on the substantive responses of the world's religions to the issue of the independent moral status of the fetus.[8] In the absence of a universally accepted authority to remove those differences, they will necessarily persist.

The philosophical literature on the subject—which is too vast to cite in detail—suffers from a similar problem.[9] As an intellectual tradition now well into its third millennium in the West, philosophy has developed a wide array of methodologies—as one would expect in any intellectual tradition with such a history and maturity. One result of this methodological pluralism is that philosophy has been unable to settle on a single methodology—the analogy of the long sought-for "unified field theory" in physics—that would settle all methodological disputes in philosophy in a way that any reasonable person would have to accept. Thus, any philosophical argument that the fetus possesses or does not—or cannot—possess independent moral status is methodology-dependent and cannot claim final intellectual authority, despite the persistent fond hopes of many philosophers to the contrary. Moreover, like theologically based responses to the issue of the independent moral status of the fetus, philosophical responses differ substantively, and sometimes very sharply. In the absence of a universally accepted philosophical methodology, those differences will necessarily persist.

Matters become even more complex when one attempts to adjudicate disputes about the independent moral status of the fetus between theological traditions and the secular methodologies of philosophy. There simply is no possibility of closure on a final authority, because theological traditions start with beliefs or principles accepted on the basis of revelation or the experience of a faith community, whereas philosophy starts only with presuppositions, beliefs, or principles that can be supported by rational argument. Philosophy thus must reject what serves as the basis for theological ethics, and theological ethics must regard the skepticism of philosophy about revelation with theology's own skepticism about whether what philosophy proposes to accomplish—to proceed only on the basis of what can be supported by rational argument—can indeed be accomplished with finality. In short, ne'er can, therefore ne'er shall the twain meet.

The alternatives seem plain. One could persist in attempting to establish whether or not the fetus possesses independent moral status. To do so, however, requires that one simply ignore or deny the impossibility of closure in undertaking such a task. Interestingly, the literature on the subject continues to grow. Sooner or later, this way of thinking about the question, "When is the fetus a patient?," falters under the burden of a requirement that, in effect, renders the project ultimately frustrating at best and simply unbelievable at worst. The second alternative is simply to abandon the debate about whether or not the fetus possesses independent moral status and pursue what we shall show is an answerable question: "When does the fetus possess dependent moral status?" It is, we shall argue, possible to answer this question in a reliable fashion, thus making it possible to identify ethically distinct senses of the fetus as patient and their clinical implications. We need to ask not, "Does the fetus possess independent moral status or not?," but, as Warnock usefully puts it, "How ought we to treat the fetus?"[10]

The Dependent Moral Status of the Fetus

All accounts about whether or not the fetus possesses independent moral status commit a common error: they seek to find or reject some time, prior to or at delivery, during which the fetus possesses some intrinsic characteristic that in turn generates independent moral status. This matter is endlessly disputed, because—for the reasons set out above—it is endlessly disputable.

There is no dispute among all of these views, however, that at some time after birth virtually every human being possesses independent moral status. That is, there is some place in the continuum of early human development from conception through childhood at which no reasonable individual could deny that an individual human being possesses independent moral status. One prominent way in which this is put is that at some point every rational individual must agree that virtually every human being is a *person*—a human being who intrinsically generates his or her own moral status independently of every other human being and every social institution.[11] The latest time that has been proposed for the coming to be of persons is in the second year of life.

We take no position on this matter, because our framework for obstetric ethics does not require that we do so. That framework requires only that there is agreement among all the diverse views on the moral status of the fetus about the achievement of independent moral status postpartum, sometime in the second year of life. Before such a time, a human being can be thought to possess *dependent* moral status, so long as reliable links can be established between that earlier time and later achieving independent moral status. We believe that, for the fetus, only two such links can be established: viability and the autonomous decisions of the pregnant woman regarding the previable fetus.

A Note on Fetal Interests

Establishing links between the fetus and later achieving independent moral status involves the following general considerations about fetal interests. Recall from Chapter 1 that an interest exists when an individual has a stake in the issue of events or the activities of an individual or institution. Interests are thus future-oriented by definition: they are concerned with the "issue" of things and an "issue" occurs only in the future. Among the possible issues of human gestation is subsequently achieving independent moral status. There are also other possible issues: death in utero; stillbirth; livebirth followed by death before achieving independent moral status; or livebirth accompanied by central nervous system anomalies—anatomical or physiological—that greatly impair, perhaps even eliminate, the coming to be of independent moral status.

Obviously, achieving independent moral status is among the goods that humans value. When achieving independent moral status is reliably expected to occur as the issue of in utero gestation and subsequent neonatal development, albeit with full technological support, the fetus has a stake in that issue. As a consequence, the fetus reliably linked to later achieving independent moral status has present interests in the individually necessary and jointly sufficient conditions for later achieving independent moral status that medicine as a social institution is competent to address. That is, the fetus that is reliably expected to achieve independent moral status possesses as its interests the social-role interests identified in Chapter 1. The phrase, "reliably expected to achieve independent moral status," is crucial, because it signals that the only moral status appropriate to the fetus is dependent moral status, that is, dependent on reliable links to a future, unambiguously independent moral status. This phrase also points to the nature of the links that establish such status: they must show that the fetus in question is reliably expected to achieve independent moral status. When this is the case, the fetus has an interest in such moral status.

On the account given of subjective interests in Chapter 1, the fetus cannot be thought to possess subjective interests. Because of the immaturity of its central nervous system, the fetus has no values and beliefs that form the basis of such interests. It obviously follows from this that the fetus cannot possess deliberative interests, since these, in turn, are based on subjective interests and reflection on subjective interests. The latter is a task no fetus can accomplish. Hence, there can be no autonomy-based obligations to the fetus. Hence also, there can be no meaningful talk of fetal rights, the fetus' right to life in particular, in the sense that the fetus itself generates rights. Only human beings (or other entities) with subjective or deliberative interests can independently generate rights. In Chapter 1 we showed that the "right to life" is a phrase with three strikingly different meanings. Here we have shown that there is no philosophically meaningful way that any fetus can be thought to generate its own right to life.

Finally, it is worth noting that when the fetus is a patient, it possesses social-role interests in the same way that all patients do. The fetus as patient is not unique in that its interests are future-oriented. *All* medical interventions are future-oriented: they aim to protect and promote patients' interests as their result. A result, by definition, follows from something else; a result will occur in the future. All patients have present interests in the goods of medical care occurring in the future, provided that the individual patient in the present is reliably expected to become the individual patient in the future who will receive or experience those results. We will now identify and defend the links between the fetus and future, independent moral status that satisfy this condition.[12]

The Dependent Moral Status of the Viable Fetus

Viability is the first link between a fetus and later achieving independent moral status. "Viability" means that the fetus can survive ex utero with full technological support, as required to supplement immature or impaired anatomy and physiology, through the neonatal period and into the second year of life during or near the end of which independent moral status comes into existence as a function of some intrinsic characteristic(s) of the infant. Viability is *not* an intrinsic characteristic of the fetus, because viability is a function in all cases of *both* biological capacity—fetal anatomy and physiology—and technological capacity.[13] Both capacities are essential in establishing a link between the fetus and later achieving independent moral status.

Technological capacity to supplement fetal anatomy and physiology varies widely from country to country and even within countries. As a consequence, at the present time there can be no worldwide uniform gestational age to define viability. In the United States, we believe, rigorous, scientifically informed clinical judgment concludes that viability presently occurs at approximately 24 weeks of gestational age.[14]

The ethical significance of viability for the viable fetus is that there are clinical interventions that can reasonably be expected to protect and promote the interests of the fetus by preventing premature death in or ex utero and by preventing, curing, or managing disease, injury, handicap, and unnecessary pain and suffering. In the presence of some fetal anomalies clinical interventions may not be reasonably expected to so clearly protect and promote the interests of the fetus or of the future patient it can become, a matter with important implications for the degree of obligations owed to the viable fetus. This topic will be addressed below, in the section on the principle of beneficence in obstetric ethics.

The viable fetus is not presented to the physician solely as a function of biomedical technology to diagnose, manipulate, or treat it—contrary to what seems to be a widespread belief among physicians.[15] This view is mistaken, because it assumes that the pregnant woman is always obligated to accept whatever morbidity and mortality risks are involved for her in obstetric management thought to protect and promote fetal interests. That is, this view simply assumes that the fetus always comes first and the pregnant woman second. The error here involves a failure to appreciate that the obligation to protect and promote the interests of the patient applies theoretically to all patients equally, even and especially when the physician has more than one patient. Thus, whether the viable fetus is presented to the physician is in part a function of the pregnant woman's autonomous decision to do so.

Recall from Chapter 1 that an individual is a patient when the individual is (1) presented to a physician (2) for the purpose of applying clinical interventions that are reliably expected to protect and promote the interests of that individual. This understanding of the concept of becoming a patient applies in the present context as follows. Viability means that the viable fetus has interests, derived from the biologic-technologic capacity to later achieve independent moral status, that can reliably be expected to be protected and promoted by obstetric interventions. Thus, the second condition is fulfilled. When both conditions are fulfilled the viable fetus is a patient. Both the pregnant woman and her physician therefore have an obligation to protect and promote the fetal patient's interests, including interests in future health.

Obviously, the pregnant woman and her physician must take into account her subjective, deliberative, and social-role interests in her own health. It is certainly among the pregnant woman's legitimate subjective, deliberative, and social-role interests not to be obligated to take unreasonable health risks in the fulfillment of her beneficence-based obligations to the viable fetus. In the latter respect, she can be obligated to the viable fetus only to take those risks reliably thought to be reasonable. Thus, the first condition above is fulfilled when the pregnant woman is reliably thought to be obligated to present the viable fetus for health care. As a rule, this occurs when the interests of the viable fetus will be significantly advanced and when the interests of the pregnant woman will not be significantly impaired. What this means in clinical practice is addressed in Parts II and III.

In summary, when it is obligatory for the pregnant woman to present the viable fetus to the physician for the purpose of applying reasonable interventions, the viable fetus becomes a patient. While the viable fetus possesses this status dependently on the link between viability and later achieving independent moral status, the viable fetus possesses the social-role interests of any patient.

The Dependent Moral Status of the Previable Fetus

The only possible link between the previable fetus and subsequent independent moral status is the pregnant woman's autonomy. This is because technological factors cannot result in the previable fetus later achieving independent moral status. This is, simply, what "previable" means. Recall that, because independent moral status for the fetus cannot be reliably established, the previable fetus has no claim on the pregnant woman or any physician to remain in utero. The previable fetus needs the use of the pregnant woman's body to achieve viability and, later, live birth, but the previable fetus has no independent claim to either. Thus, the previable fetus cannot inherently establish a link to later achieving independent moral status. The link, therefore, between a fetus and subsequent independent moral status, when the fetus is previable, can be established only by the pregnant woman's autonomous decision to confer the status of being a patient on her previable fetus. When she does so in a settled way, the fetus is reliably expected to achieve independent moral status.

Here the earlier discussion about the inherently disputable character of claims for or against the independent moral status of the fetus has direct bearing. There is no compelling reason in bioethics, as a philosophical intellectual undertaking, for the physician, the pregnant woman, or anyone else—the male gamete donor, family members, or the state, in particular—to regard the previable fetus as independently possessing, lacking, or possessing only to some degree, the moral status of being a patient. The ethical implication of this consideration is that the pregnant woman is free to confer, withhold, or, having once conferred, withdraw the moral status of being a patient on or from the previable fetus. Note that she is not obligated to confer, withhold, or withdraw such status except by her own lights. Thus, for example, to think that a pregnant woman who is HIV+ should always have an abortion—which, in effect, is to take the view that she is always obligated to withhold the status of being a patient from her previable fetus—involves a fundamental misunderstanding of the dependent moral status of the previable fetus. Recall, again from Chapter 1, that an individual is a patient when that individual is (1) presented to a physician (2) for the purpose of applying clinical interventions that are reliably expected to protect and promote the interests of that individual. On the basis of the immediately preceding paragraph, it is plain that the pregnant woman is under no ethical obligation to present the previable fetus to the physician. Hence, the first condition can be fulfilled only by her autonomous decision to fulfill it.

Health care interventions cannot reliably be expected to protect and promote the interests of the previable fetus unless it survives subsequent gestation to viability. But whether it is to do so is, again, solely a function of the pregnant woman's autonomy. Hence, the second condition above is fulfilled only as a function of the autonomy of the pregnant woman.

In summary, when the pregnant woman autonomously presents the previable fetus to the physician, that is, when she elects to continue her pregnancy to viability, the previable fetus is a patient. Both the pregnant woman and her physician then, and only then, have an obligation to protect and promote the fetal patient's interests, including interests in future health. While the previable fetus possesses this status dependently on the pregnant woman's autonomy—the only link between the previable fetus and its later achieving independent moral status—the previable fetus, made a patient by the pregnant woman, possesses the social-role interests of any patient. The interests of the previable fetal patient are thus present interests.

Previable fetuses that are what we term near-viable fetuses, that is, those which are 22–24 weeks gestational age, should be regarded as previable fetuses. There are anecdotal reports of survival for fetuses in this group.[16] In our view, aggressive obstetric and neonatal management of such fetuses should be regarded as clinical investigations, that is, as forms of medical experimentation—*not* standard of care. There is no beneficence-based obligation on the part of any pregnant woman to confer the status of being a patient on any near-viable fetus, because the efficacy of aggressive obstetric and neonatal management has yet to be proven.

The Dependent Moral Status of the In Vitro Embryo

A subset of previable fetuses is the in vitro embryos that are created in the process of assisted reproduction techniques. It might at first seem that an in vitro embryo is a patient, because it is directly presented to the physician in the petri dish. However, recall yet again from Chapter 1, that for a human being to be a patient it must also be the case that medical interventions can be applied that are reliably expected to protect and promote that human being's interests. Whether interventions on the in vitro embryo can satisfy this second condition for becoming a patient necessarily depends on whether the in vitro embryo can survive subsequent cell division, transfer, implantation, and gestation to viability. Obviously, the final outcome of this process depends on the decisions of the woman who becomes pregnant via an assisted reproduction technique regarding the dependent moral status of the implanted, previable fetus. Should she deny such status and terminate her pregnancy (including selective termination of some fetuses in a multifetal pregnancy)[17] no benefit of interventions on the in vitro embryo can meaningfully be said to have resulted.

Because the achievement of such benefit only occurs in vivo, the dependent moral status of the in vitro embryo is entirely a function of the woman's decision regarding the status of the fetus as a patient, should an assisted reproduction technique successfully result in the gestation of a previable fetus or fetuses. Whether the in vitro embryo will become a viable fetus and whether interventions on the in vitro embryo will protect and promote the fetus' interests are both functions of the pregnant woman's decision to confer, withhold, or, having once conferred, withdraw the dependent moral status of being a patient on or from the in vitro embryo or subsequent previable fetus. It is therefore justified to regard the in vitro embryo as a previable fetus and not as a patient in and of itself. As a consequence, an in vitro embryo should be regarded as a patient only when the woman into whose reproductive tract that embryo will be transferred confers such status. Just as no woman is obligated to confer, withhold, or withdraw that status for the in vivo previable fetus, so too is she free regarding the determination of the dependent moral status of the in vitro embryo.

The implications for "surrogate" pregnancy are the following: First, the term is a terrible misnomer, and ethically misleading. The woman into whose uterus the embryos are placed is not simply substituting her uterus for another woman's. Instead, that woman is pregnant and, like any other pregnant woman, has sole authority to determine the moral status of the previable fetus(es) as patient(s) or not. Second, no contract requiring invasive antenatal diagnosis or abortion of fetus(es) with detected anomalies is ethically justified, because such a contract denies to the pregnant woman her autonomy regarding the moral status of the previable fetus(es) as patient(s). In short, a so-called "surrogate" pregnancy is just like any other when it comes to the dependent moral status of the fetus. To think otherwise is to be misled by the term "surrogate."

Provisional Dependent Moral Status of the Previable Fetus

For pregnancies in which viability has not yet occurred and in which the pregnant woman is uncertain or unsettled about whether to confer the status of being a patient on the previable fetus, the authors propose that the physician proceed on the assumption that the previable fetus is *provisionally* a patient. Our argument is a variation on Pascal's wager.[18] The advantage of this strategy is that, should the woman subsequently confer on the fetus the status of being a patient, the physician will always have been in a position to attempt to protect and promote the interests of the previable fetus as a patient. Should the woman withhold such status, nothing is lost for the fetus by assuming provisional moral status of the fetus. What this concept means in clinical practice is a very important matter and will be addressed in Part II, for example, concerning directive counseling for fetal benefit.

Dying Fetuses That Are Nonviable

Some fetuses past the statistically normal gestational age for viability suffer from lethal anomalies that can be diagnosed with certainty, for example, anencephaly. Strictly speaking, such fetuses are nonviable because no intervention exists that can reliably be expected to prevent their premature death—either in utero, during the intrapartum period, or early in the postpartum period.[19] In the case of lethal anomalies diagnosed in utero with certainty, preventing imminent, premature death is not a result or "issue" reliably to be expected. Lethal fetal anomalies diagnosed with certainty doom the possible interest of the fetus in later achieving independent moral status, thus making impossible any meaningful talk of a link between such fetuses and later achieving independent moral status.

This does not mean that all social-role interests of such fetuses are necessarily doomed. Instead, such fetuses can meaningfully possess the social-role interests of any dying patient. Some pregnant women may find it important to continue such a pregnancy to term, thus conferring the status of being a dying patient on the fetus, long enough for the fetus at least to become a child, a significant type of dependent moral status, to be sure. In addition, going to term may promote the subjective or deliberative interests of the pregnant woman, for example, to have a chance to see or hold her child as her child dies or to donate organs or tissue for transplantation. In such cases, we believe that it makes philosophical and clinical sense and is humane for the physician to regard the nonviable fetus as an irreversibly dying patient. There is no beneficence-based obligation to irreversibly dying patients to attempt to prevent their death, because it is impossible to do so. No ethical theory—and certainly no ethical frameworks that we set out in this book—obligate the physician to attempt the impossible. When the obligation to prevent death ceases to exist, the other obligations of beneficence move to the fore—to provide comfort and assure the protection of the patient's dignity.

The physician also has obligations to the woman and those she has chosen to involve in her pregnancy, especially the male gamete donor, who may also be her spouse or lover, to see to it that they understand that the situation is impossible and that they have the opportunity to mourn their fetus/child as they see fit as part of the process of creating lifelong stories and memories that will sustain them in their loss. These are part of the autonomy-based obligations of the physician to the pregnant woman as a patient and to those intimately involved third parties to the physician-patient relationship.

"When is the Fetus a Patient?" Answered

On the basis of the foregoing, it is plain that our answer to this question rejects the two extremes of "Always!" and "Never!". Instead, the answer is "sometimes, depending on (1) whether the fetus is gestationally viable and the woman is obligated to present it for care or (2) whether she confers such status on the previable fetus."

There are a number of important ethical implications of this answer. First the moral relationship of the pregnant woman and the viable fetus, and the individual with independent moral status that it will later become, is primarily one of obligation, not freedom. The pregnant woman is the moral fiduciary of the viable fetus. The strength of her beneficence-based obligations to the fetal patient vary, as noted above. Second, the moral relationship of third parties—such as male gamete donors, spouses, parents, and others in the pregnant woman's household—to the viable fetus and also to the pregnant woman is one of obligation, not freedom. These third parties, too, are moral fiduciaries of the viable fetus. The strength of their beneficence-based obligations to the fetal patient vary, with important implications for the ethics of fetal neglect and abuse. (See Chapter 6.) Third, the moral relationship of the pregnant woman to the previable fetus that is a patient, even when she has reached a settled determination of that status, is ambiguous between obligation and freedom, because before viability, the pregnant woman retains the freedom to withdraw the moral status of being a patient from the previable fetus. This ambiguity is crucial for understanding the ethics of antenatal diagnosis. (See Chapter 6.) Fourth, the moral relationship of third parties to the previable fetus that is a patient is primarily one of obligation to the pregnant woman to respect her decision about the moral status of the previable fetus, because their autonomy plays no role in the determination of that status. This too, has important implications for fetal neglect. (See Chapter 6.) Fifth, when the previable or viable fetus is a patient, it possesses the social-role interests of any patient. However, those interests will not be univocal, because fetal complications—for example, fetal anomalies or extreme prematurity—can limit or even defeat the competencies of the health care professions to protect and promote the social-role interests of the fetal patient. Sixth, any beneficence-based obligations of the physician to protect and promote the social-role interests of the fetal patient must be negotiated with the beneficence-based and autonomy-based obligations of the physician to the pregnant woman who is clearly a patient. Seventh, that a pregnant woman has beneficence-based obligations to the fetal patient as its fiduciary does not mean that others, on this basis alone, have the moral authority to enforce that obligation. This is a separate matter entirely and is therefore addressed separately in this book. (See Part III.) Eighth, obligations of the physician to either one or both of these patients must also be negotiated with obligations to third and fourth parties. Addressing these complex matters requires us to develop a framework for obstetric ethics in the clinical setting, in terms of which ethical conflict and crises in gynecologic and obstetric practice can be identified.

A Framework for Obstetric Ethics in the Clinical Setting

A framework for obstetric ethics sets out and defends an account of the ethical principles of beneficence and respect for autonomy in the physician-patient relationship in obstetric practice and an account of the interests of and obligations to third parties to that relationship. The pregnant woman is a patient when she consents or is ordered by a court (See Chapter 7) to be one. The fetus is a patient when the fetus is viable and the pregnant woman is obligated to present it for care or when she confers such status on the previable fetus. A framework for obstetric ethics, as a specialty of the general field of bioethics, finds its basis in the four basic virtues of self-effacement, self-sacrifice, compassion, and integrity.

Four Basic Virtues: Self-Effacement, Self-Sacrifice, Compassion, and Integrity

What we said in Chapter 1 about self-effacement, self-sacrifice, compassion, and integrity as together forming the basis for the ethical principles of beneficence and respect for autonomy applies completely here. We want to add some comments, however, on the special demands of the virtue of self-effacement. Recall from Chapter 1 that this virtue blunts the mere subjective interests of the physician by negating the adverse impact on the physician's attitude and behavior of differences between the physician and the patient in matters of socioeconomic class, education, race, gender, religion, language, manners, hygiene, and, as Gregory put it two centuries ago, the "weakness and bad behavior of patients, and the number of little difficulties and contradictions which every physician must encounter in his practice."[20]

Limits on the Virtues When Self-Effacement Can Become Unjustified Self-Sacrifice

Differences between the physician and the pregnant woman in matters of religion and serious moral convictions can be an especially important consideration in obstetric ethics (and also in gynecologic ethics), because religious beliefs and traditions as well as serious moral convictions constitute important sources of morality for both physicians and patients regarding their views on the independent moral status of the fetus. The implication of the arguments of the preceding section for the physician, as a matter of professional conscience, is that the physician's thinking about the moral status of the fetus must be governed by what secular bioethics can conclude: the moral status of the fetus can only be understood as dependent, not independent, moral status. Obviously, as a "private" individual—that is, in roles other than physician—the physician may subscribe to religious or other serious moral beliefs about whether or not the fetus possesses independent moral status. These are among the subjective and, given their gravity, legitimate interests of the physician. Such beliefs may be very carefully developed and considered and so may also count among the deliberative and therefore legitimate interests of the physician. On either account, the physician has a legitimate interest in protecting the integrity of religious or other serious moral convictions about the independent moral status of the fetus, whether they endorse or reject such status.

In Chapter 1, we treated self-effacement as a virtue that always blunts mere self-interest but that does not always blunt deliberative, legitimate self-interest. Here we want to say more about the latter, because it is not our view that self-effacement always erases or makes irrelevant the legitimate self-interests of the physician, any more than self-sacrifice or compassion do. In some circumstances, self-effacement of religious or other well-founded convictions of the physician about the moral status of the fetus can, in effect, threaten the moral integrity of those convictions. Whether this is indeed the case in particular circumstances should be a matter of careful, prudent judgment on the part of the physician, because such threats are not, we believe, routine. Our point here is that self-effacement of such religious or other serious moral beliefs can sometimes be carried into effect only in the form of sacrificing the moral integrity of those beliefs. The virtue of self-sacrifice would, if it required this sort of personal moral sacrifice, become a tyrannical, self-destructive virtue if it demanded in all cases the sundering of the moral integrity of the private convictions of the physician. A fundamental virtue would then be transformed into a vice.

Thus, we do not hold that self-effacement *always* obligates the physician to ignore and never act on religious or other serious convictions concerning the moral status of the fetus. It follows from this that the patient has an obligation to respect the legitimate interest of the physician in avoiding sundering of his or her moral integrity as a private individual. The physician, therefore, is free to withdraw from the physician-patient relationship when the physician reliably concludes that continuing in that relationship entails a substantial risk of sundering the moral integrity of private convictions, what we term the "private conscience" of the physician. This is especially important for the prerogative of physicians who hold serious "right to life" views on abortion.

In withdrawing, the physician should explain that no judgment is made or implied about the moral integrity of the pregnant woman's beliefs and convictions. Respect for her autonomy, first and foremost, calls for the physician to acknowledge and respect the integrity of the patient's values and beliefs. The physician has no intellectual and therefore no moral warrant among the physician's competencies *as a physician* for reaching any other judgment. As a private individual, the physician does act with justification to protect private conscience, and the pregnant woman has an autonomy-based obligation to respect the prerogative of the physician in this matter. Thus, the virtues reveal a dimension of the ethical obligations of patients to physicians that has hithertofore received little attention in the bioethics literature.

As a secular professional, the physician has an inescapable obligation to protect and promote the social-role, subjective, and deliberative interests of all patients. The implication of this obligation in the present context is that the physician has an inescapable obligation to refer such a patient to a colleague who would not have objections in private conscience to accepting the pregnant woman as a patient. To this extent the physician is obligated, as a secular professional, to accept whatever compromise of private conscience that may be involved in making such a referral, because patients come to physicians, not private individuals.[21]

The Virtues as the Basis for Obstetric Ethics in the Clinical Setting

The virtue of self-effacement erases the mere self-interests of the physician but not always legitimate self-interests, and the virtue of self-sacrifice blunts mere self-interests but not always legitimate self-interests.

Compassion and integrity sustain the physician's commitment to the patient. In doing so, these four basic virtues serve as the individually necessary conditions for the physician-patient relationship in obstetric practice. Together they provide the sufficient condition for that relationship because they have the effect in clinical practice of focusing the concern of the physician on, and moving the physician to protect and promote, the interests of the patient. Insofar as they are relevant, the social-role, subjective, and deliberative interests shape the interests of the pregnant patient, while only social-role interests shape the interests of the fetal patient. These shapings are done by the ethical principles of beneficence or respect for autonomy, in the case of the pregnant woman, and the principle of beneficence, in the case of the fetal patient. We thus turn to a consideration of these principles, along the lines in which they were considered in Chapter 1.

The Principle of Beneficence

The principle of beneficence shapes the physician's understanding of the interests of the patient in terms of the social-role interests of the patient: the prevention of premature or unnecessary death *and* the prevention, cure, or at least management of disease, injury, handicap, and unnecessary pain and suffering. The death of any fetal patient (*not* all fetuses) and the death of any pregnant woman count as premature deaths, because these deaths occur before normal life expectancy in our species. The death of any fetal patient without a nonlethal anomaly or complication and the death of any pregnant woman without an irreversible life-taking condition count as unnecessary death. As a rule, for fetal patients and pregnant women without such complications, the primary social-role interest of the patient will be the prevention of premature and unnecessary death, because death makes impossible any attempt to protect and promote the other social-role interests of these patients. Because all of the social-role interests of the patient must be considered in beneficence-based clinical judgment, that judgment can be variable, depending on trade-offs among those interests.

Beneficence-Based Obligations to Pregnant Patients

As a rule, beneficence-based obligations to the pregnant patient will give priority to preventing her death. This includes both premature and unnecessary death, because lethal maternal complications of pregnancy that are irreversible are very rare in those settings, such as that in the United

States and the rest of the developed world (at least), where aggressive obstetric management for maternal benefit is available. At the same time, it will also rarely be the case that obstetric management will either promote all of the pregnant patient's social-role interests or some of those interests without impairing others. More often, the patient's social-role interest in preventing premature or unnecessary death will be promoted at the price of impairing to some degree the social-role interest of preventing morbidity. That is, beneficence-based clinical judgment typically will aim to identify the range or continuum of obstetric interventions that are in the pregnant patient's social-role interests, a continuum that, as a whole, sets the boundaries on both what is reasonable in beneficence-based clinical judgment—all alternatives within the continuum—and what is unreasonable in beneficence-based clinical judgment—all alternatives outside the continuum. The latter are not in the pregnant patient's social-role interest, that is, insofar as beneficence-based clinical judgment is concerned.

Beneficence-Based Obligations to Fetal Patients

For fetal patients it is important to appreciate that beneficence-based obligations vary, depending on the presence and severity of fetal anomalies and complications. Some anomalies and complications are lethal in the sense that they are irreversibly life-taking. No known intervention will prevent death from occurring imminently in these cases. When it is impossible to seek what is usually the primary social-role interest of patients, the prevention of premature or unnecessary death, it is no longer obligatory to do so and the other social-role interests of the patient become primary. Preventing the death of such a patient is not in the interest of that patient; preventing morbidity is. This occurs when lethal fetal anomalies and complications can be diagnosed with certainty. In such cases, because there is no beneficence-based obligation to prevent the premature death of the dying fetus that is a fetal patient (i.e., a dying nonviable fetus deemed to be a patient by the pregnant woman), nonaggressive obstetric management is justified. For the dying fetus that is not a patient (i.e., a dying nonviable fetus denied the status of being a patient by the pregnant woman), both nonaggressive management and termination of the pregnancy are justified.

Some fetal anomalies and complications that can be diagnosed with very high probability involve either a very high probability of premature or unnecessary death before the end of the neonatal period or a very high probability of short-term survival with severe and irreversible deficit of central nervous system anatomy or physiology, of the sort that precludes or virtually precludes development of the neonate beyond primitive physical function, and precludes or virtually precludes cognitive development requisite to later achieving independent moral status. In such cases, aggressive obstetric and neonatal management—especially the latter—carry a high probability of iatrogenic impairment of the patient's social-role interest in preventing morbidity. Indeed, the burden of iatrogenic morbidity as the price for attempting to prevent premature death can be very substantial in these cases. More accurately, these cases should be described as attempts to postpone death at the price of overly burdensome iatrogenic morbidity. When this occurs, death may become no longer unnecessary, although it will still be premature.

When this sort of trade-off among the social-role interests of the fetal patient occurs, beneficence-based obligations to the fetal patient are minimal. This is because attempting to postpone premature death is in the fetal patient's interest, and preventing substantial morbidity as the price for postponing death—in qualitative beneficence-based clinical judgment at least and maybe even in quantitative beneficence-based clinical judgment—is just as much in the fetal patient's interest.

When beneficence-based obligations to the fetal patient are minimal, nonaggressive management of the pregnancy is justified. By aggressive management we mean delivery in a tertiary center as appropriate, as well as the use after viability occurs of tocolytic agents, fetal surveillance, cesarean delivery, and other interventions for fetal benefit. As the probability of achieving reasonable qualitative benefit for the fetal patient decreases, the strength of beneficence-based obligations to the fetal patient decrease. When those obligations decrease to a very great degree but do not disappear altogether, beneficence-based obligations to the fetal patient are minimal. Even so, the fetal patient retains an interest in preventing premature death, and so termination of pregnancy, when there are minimal beneficence-based obligations to the fetal patient, is not justified. This is an important implication of the strong, beneficence-based prohibition against killing the fetal patient. Minimal beneficence-based obligations to the fetal patient exist when there is a diagnosis with certainty of either a high probability of premature death before the end of the neonatal period, or a high probability of short-term survival with severe and irreversible central nervous system anatomical or physiological impairment such that later achievement of independent moral status is highly improbable.

All other trade-offs among the social-role interests of the fetal patient result, we believe, in more-than-minimal beneficence-based obligations to the fetal patient. Other than cases in which there are no or only minimal beneficence-based obligations to the fetal patient, uncertainty of diagnosis or less than high probability of outcomes not in the fetal patient's social-role interest make any qualitative or quantitative judgments about trade-offs among fetal interests subject to considerable variability. That is, more-than-minimal beneficence-based obligations exist when there is a range or continuum of management strategies that protect and promote the interests of the fetal patient to some degree and are thus variously in that patient's social-role interest. More-than-minimal beneficence-based obligations to the fetal patient exist, therefore, when there is uncertainty about diagnosis of a serious anomaly or when there is less than a high probability of either premature death before the end of the neonatal period or less than high probability of short-term survival with severe central nervous system impairment. Obviously, as the confidence in diagnosis of the absence of life-taking or central nervous system-impairing anomalies or complications grows, the more substantial become beneficence-based obligations, in particular, the overriding priority within beneficence-based clinical judgment to prevent the premature death of the fetal patient.

In general, then, when the fetus is a patient, the physician owes to it beneficence-based obligations. For the reasons explained above, the fetus is incapable of possessing subjective or deliberative interests and so there can be no autonomy-based obligations to the fetus. Thus, there are no fetal rights generated by subjective or deliberative interests. Recall from Chapter 1 that beneficence-based obligations are grounded in the competencies of medicine. These competencies can be understood entirely independently of the subjective and deliberative interests of patients. The intellectual and moral authority of beneficence-based obligations to the fetal patient for the physician are not, therefore, reduced or diminished in any way when they are the only type of ethical obligations that the physician has to a patient—which is the case when the fetus is a patient.

The Principle of Beneficence as a Set of Concrete Guides to Action in the Obstetric Management of the Pregnant Patient and the Fetal Patient

Considered by itself, the principle of beneficence on the account that we have provided constitutes more than a mere "checklist" of items to be considered in obstetric practice. It provides concrete action guides for the physician in obstetric practice—more than one of them, because of the heterogeneity of beneficence-based clinical judgment. Those guides are summarized in Table 3–1.

Table 3-1 Beneficence-Based Action Guides for Obstetric Practice

Beneficence-Based Action Guides Applied to Pregnant Woman

1. Management strategies based on clear-cut beneficence-based clinical judgments about what is in the pregnant patient's interest ought to be implemented *the social-role interests of the pregnant patient having been taken into account.*
2. Any one of the range or continuum of management strategies based on variable and uncertain beneficence-based clinical judgments about the interests of the pregnant patient may properly be implemented *the social-role interests of the pregnant patient having been taken into account.*
3. Management strategies that lie outside the range or continuum of those based on variable and uncertain but reliable beneficence-based clinical judgments about the interests of the pregnant patient ought not to be implemented *the social-role interests of the pregnant patient having been taken into account.*

Beneficence-Based Action Guides Applied to the Fetal Patient

4. When there are more-than-minimal beneficence-based obligations to the fetal patient, only aggressive obstetric management ought to be implemented.
5. When there are minimal beneficence-based obligations to the fetal patient, nonaggressive and aggressive obstetric management may be implemented, but termination of the pregnancy ought not to be implemented.
6. When there are no beneficence-based obligations to the dying fetus that is a fetal patient to prevent its death, nonaggressive obstetric management ought to be implemented.
7. When there are no beneficence-based obligations to the dying fetus that is not a fetal patient, both nonaggressive obstetric management and termination of the pregnancy may be implemented.
8. Any management strategy found in reliable beneficence-based judgment not to be in the fetal patient's social-role interests ought not to be implemented.

It is important to emphasize that these beneficence-based guides to the action of the physician in obstetric practice cannot be regarded as absolute, that is, always controlling of the clinician's behavior. The limited character of these guides is a direct function of several factors: (1) the limited scope of interests of pregnant patients taken into account by beneficence-based clinical judgment; (2) the presence of variable, non-clear-cut qualitative and quantitative judgments in the determination of minimal beneficence-based obligations to fetal patients; and (3) the inherently disputable nature of the account that we have given of minimal beneficence-based obligations to fetal patients.

The Principle of Respect for Autonomy

The principle of respect for autonomy shapes the physician's understanding of the interests of the patient in terms of the subjective and deliberative interests of the patient. As argued earlier, the fetus cannot meaningfully be thought to possess subjective or deliberative interests and so the principle of respect for autonomy plays no role in the identification of obligations to fetal patients.

Autonomy-Based Obligations to Pregnant Patients

In obstetric practice only the pregnant patient possesses such interests. Hence, the physician in obstetric practice owes autonomy-based obligations only to the pregnant patient.

Unlike the principle of beneficence, no content can be provided a priori, that is, without conferring with the pregnant patient, or reliable surrogates of formerly autonomous pregnant patients who now irreversibly lack the capacity for autonomous decision making, for the interests that give substance and meaning to autonomy-based clinical judgment. That content can only be provided by the pregnant patient or, when that patient is unable to do so, by those reliably thought to represent her subjective and deliberative interests. Autonomy-based clinical judgment about what is in the pregnant patient's interest concerns her judgment about which obstetric interventions protect and promote her subjective and deliberative interests.

It is important to note that there is nothing in the concepts of either subjective or deliberative interests, as we have developed them here, that excludes the possibility that they may include the pregnant woman's concerns, hopes, plans for, and sense of obligation to the fetus, the child it can become, and the morally independent individual that it could become. That is, subjective interests need not be exclusively self-regarding, although they can be.

Deliberative interests in obstetric ethics should probably be understood to be almost always both self-regarding and other-regarding. This is because in the process of forming her deliberative interests the pregnant woman must, as a conceptual matter and thus a matter of intellectual and moral seriousness and integrity, take account of the existence of beneficence-based obligations on her part to the fetal patient. This is particularly the case concerning viable fetuses, which are fetal patients partly as a function of the pregnant patient's acceptance of risks to her own interests—subjective, deliberative, and social-role interests alike. How the pregnant patient negotiates trade-offs in forming her deliberative interests depends vitally, therefore, on the physician's judgments about what is in the social-role interest of the fetal patient, especially beneficence-based action guide #8. These judgments are properly shared with the pregnant woman and are part of the information that she needs to take into account in forming her deliberative interests.

In addition, the deliberative interests of the pregnant patient will be formed in response to a consideration of her own social-role interests and the physician's beneficence-based judgment about what is in her social-role interest, especially beneficence-based action guide #3. Thus, the latter also play a vital role in the formation of the pregnant patient's deliberative interests.

As we shall see in Parts II and III of this book, the formation by the pregnant patient of her deliberative interests plays a crucial role in the strategies for both preventing and managing ethical conflict and crises in obstetric practice. Rather than get ahead of ourselves at this point, we return to the task of identifying autonomy-based obligations of the physician to the pregnant patient.

Chief among these will be to avoid paternalism. In terms of Chapter 1, paternalism involves the imposition of beneficence-based clinical judgment about what is in the pregnant patient's social-role interest on the autonomous pregnant patient without her consent. When the pregnant patient, by refusing intervention, in effect refuses any longer to be a patient, there is no intellectual or moral authority to any beneficence-based judgment regarding her social-role interests that she is obligated to remain a patient. Because of the limited scope of beneficence-based clinical judgment, it possesses no authority to mandate that someone become or remain a patient. This is a matter for courts to decide. (See Chapter 7.) To think otherwise is to misunderstand in a fundamental fashion the limited nature of the principle of beneficence in bioethics.

Whether the pregnant patient can be obligated to the fetal patient, particularly the viable fetal patient, to remain a patient is not a matter, strictly speaking, of paternalism. Rather, it concerns the harm principle applied to the pregnant patient in the following complex fashion: To what extent is the pregnant patient obligated to accept inconvenience or risk to herself to prevent risk, including greater risk in terms of the social-role interests of both, to the fetal patient? That is, what risks of impairment of her social-role, subjective, and deliberative interests is the pregnant patient reasonably obligated to accept as the price of protecting and promoting the social-role interests of the fetal patient?

These matters are shaped by the nature and limits of the moral-fiduciary, beneficence-based obligations of the pregnant patient to the fetal patient. How these limits ought to be negotiated involves the prevention and management of ethical conflict and crises in obstetric practice. This issue therefore constitutes a central theme of Parts II and III of this book.

Table 3-2 Autonomy-Based Action Guides for Obstetric Practice

1. The physician in obstetric practice is obligated in all cases to acknowledge and respect the integrity of the values and beliefs of the pregnant patient, even and especially when those values and beliefs lead to the expression of subjective or deliberative interests that are inconsistent with the pregnant patient's social-role interests or the physician's subjective and deliberative interests, including the physician's private conscience, that is, the physician's own religious beliefs or serious moral convictions.
2. The physician in obstetric practice is obligated to elicit from the pregnant patient her subjective-interests-based preferences about the management of her pregnancy.
3. Obstetric management strategies consistent with the subjective interests of the pregnant patient ought to be implemented.
4. The physician in obstetric practice is obligated to elicit from the pregnant patient her deliberative-interests-based preferences, with special attention to how they take account of her subjective interests and the social-role interests of the fetal patient.
5. Obstetric management strategies consistent with the deliberative interests of the pregnant patient ought to be implemented.
6. Obstetric management strategies inconsistent with the subjective interests of the pregnant woman, when these are the only interests expressed, ought not to be implemented, because they involve unjustified paternalistic interference with autonomy as legal self-determination.
7. Obstetric management strategies inconsistent with the deliberative interests of the pregnant patient ought not to be implemented, because they involve unjustified paternalistic interference with the pregnant woman's autonomy as moral autonomy.

The Principle of Respect for Autonomy as a Set of Concrete Guides to Action in the Obstetric Management of the Pregnant Patient

Considered by itself, the ethical principle of respect for autonomy on the account that we have provided constitutes more than a "checklist" of items to be considered. It provides action guides to the physician in obstetric practice—more than one of them because of the heterogeneity of autonomy-based clinical judgment. Those guides are summarized in Table 3–2.

The Relative Significance of the Principles of Beneficence and Respect for Autonomy in Obstetric Clinical Judgment

The relative significance of the ethical principles of beneficence and respect for autonomy in obstetric ethics concerns how the conflicts between action guides based on these two principles should be negotiated in clinical practice. This topic will be taken up in detail in Parts II and III of this book.

Our approach will be distinctive in that we shall emphasize the importance for the physician and pregnant patient alike of the expression of her deliberative, not just subjective, interests. This is one of the main implications of her beneficence-based obligations to the fetal patient. The pregnant woman's decisions about the management of her pregnancy are serious matters. Granted, they are not always entered into in a reflective fashion. However, to permit them to be entered into or, worse, continued in an unreflective fashion or to fail to take the opportunity to encourage reflective decisions—that is, to elicit expression of the woman's deliberative interests—sets up the physician-patient relationship for preventable, serious, even unmanageable (in some cases) ethical crises. This happens, in our judgment, too frequently. Hence, we emphasize preventive ethics in this book.

Moreover, to fail to prevent conflict or crisis is to show a profound disrespect for the pregnant woman, treating lightly in her life what she should not consider to be light matters, as one might if, in the language of Chapter 1, one equated respect for autonomy with respect for legal self-determination. Doing so is one of the most dehumanizing things the physician could do to a pregnant patient, because it paternalistically treats the pregnant woman as less than an adult.

Obligations to Third and Fourth Parties to the Physician-Patient Relationship

In general, the obligations of the physician in obstetric practice to third and fourth parties to the physician-patient relationship are the same as they are in clinical practice generally, although the family of the pregnant patient deserves particular consideration. This is especially true of the man who contributed a gamete to the pregnancy, what we term the "male gamete provider," and to the pregnant patient's spouse or partner, who may or may not be (and may not know whether or not he is) the male gamete provider.

The male gamete provider, unless he has explicitly waived such a stake (as in sperm donation), as well as the pregnant woman's spouse or partner, have a direct stake in the disposition and management of a pregnancy when the fetus is a patient. This is because the issue of such a pregnancy will be his issue, quite literally. His legitimate subjective and deliberative interests are therefore significantly at stake. As pointed out above, however, the primary moral relationship of the male gamete donor to the fetal patient is one of obligation, not freedom. Any subjective interests on his part must therefore take this obligation into account, as (obviously) deliberative interests must. Thus, those interests cannot be ignored by the physician, but must be taken into account.

The pregnant woman also needs to take account of such interests. In particular, she needs to judge what influence such interests should have in her determination of whether the risks to her of interventions for the benefit of the fetal patient are obligatory to assume. The most that can be said is that she ought to take the interests of the male gamete provider, spouse, or partner into account.[22] Because there is no accepted philosophical ethical theory about what the outcome of such reflection ought to be in any particular set of circumstances, nothing can be said authoritatively by her physician about what she should in fact conclude about how such obligations are to be taken into account. This conclusion has an important clinical implication: at most the physician can suggest that the pregnant woman may want to consider the interests of the male gamete donor, spouse, or partner but nothing more can be said or implied with moral authority.

The interests of the male gamete provider, spouse, or partner are variably at stake in the pregnant woman's decision about whether the previable fetus is a patient. Nonetheless, as we have argued, this decision is solely a function of her autonomy. This has an important clinical implication: the physician is obligated to the pregnant woman to explain to her and to the male gamete provider, spouse, or partner if necessary, that the decision is hers and hers alone to make.[23]

The Identification of Ethical Conflict and Crisis in Obstetric Practice

Based on the preceding discussion of the elements of a framework for obstetric ethics, we are now in a position to complete that framework by providing for the identification of ethical conflict in obstetric practice in terms of the following taxonomy, which we take to be exhaustive of the extent of such ethical conflict. That is, on the basis of the preceding discussion the identification of ethical conflict in obstetric practice can be summarized conveniently. (See Table 3–3.)

How This Framework Differs From Others

We have already touched on the differences between our framework for obstetric ethics and others in the bioethics literature. In closing this chap-

Table 3-3 The Identification of Ethical Conflict in Obstetric Practice

Areas of No Conflict

1. The physician in obstetric practice is obligated in all cases to acknowledge and respect the integrity of the values and beliefs of the pregnant patient, even and especially when those values and beliefs lead to the expression of subjective or deliberative interests that are inconsistent with the female patient's social-role interests or the physician's subjective or deliberative interests, including the physician's private conscience, that is, his or her own religious beliefs or serious moral convictions (autonomy-based action guide #1).
2. The physician in obstetric practice is obligated to elicit from the pregnant patient her subjective-interests-based preferences, as appropriate, about her health care (autonomy-based action guide #2).
3. The physician in obstetric practice is obligated to elicit from the pregnant patient her deliberative-interests-based preferences, with special attention to how they take account of her subjective interests and the social-role interests of the fetal patient (autonomy-based action guide #4).

Ethical Conflict

4. Beneficence-based management strategies in the pregnant woman's interest (beneficence-based action guides #1 or 2) vs. autonomy-based management strategies in the pregnant woman's interest (autonomy-based action guides #3 or 5).
5. Beneficence-based management strategies in the pregnant woman's interest (beneficence-based action guides #1 or 2) vs. beneficence-based management strategies in the fetal patient's interest (beneficence-based action guides #4 or 5).
6. Beneficence-based management strategies in the fetal patient's interest (beneficence-based action guides #4 or 5) vs. autonomy-based management strategies in the pregnant woman's interest (autonomy-based action guides #3 or 5).
7. Beneficence-based management strategies (beneficence-based action guides #1, 2, 4, 5, 6, or 7) vs. interests of third parties.
8. Autonomy-based management strategies (autonomy-based action guides #3 or 5) vs. interests of third parties.

Ethical Crisis

9. Implementation of management strategies outside the continuum of beneficence-based clinical judgment about the pregnant woman's interests (in violation of beneficence-based action guide #3) vs. implementation of management strategies inconsistent with the pregnant woman's subjective interests (in violation of autonomy-based action guide #6) or deliberative interests (in violation of autonomy-based action guide #7).
10. Implementation of management strategies outside the continuum of beneficence-based clinical judgment about the fetal patient's interests (in violation of beneficence-based action guide # 8) vs. implementation of management strategies inconsistent with the pregnant woman's subjective interests (in violation of autonomy-based action guide #6) or deliberative interests (in violation of autonomy-based action guide #7).
11. Implementation of management strategies outside the continuum of beneficence-based clinical judgment (in violation of beneficence-based action guides #3 or 8) or implementation of management strategies inconsistent with the pregnant woman's subjective interests (in violation of autonomy-based action guide #6) or deliberative interests (in violation of autonomy-based action guide #7) vs. interests of third parties.

ter we want to draw those differences more forcefully. There are three main alternatives:

The Fetus Never Has Moral Status

This view is straightforward and so can be summarized succinctly. The fetus has no moral status. Hence, the only obligations of the physician are owed to the pregnant woman. Indeed, autonomy-based obligations are paramount. As Annas puts it, ". . . the moral and legal primacy of the competent, informed pregnant woman in decision making is overwhelming," because of the inherent and ineliminable uncertainty of prognostic clinical judgment.[24]

Such a view thus relies heavily on the uncertainty of clinical judgment in obstetrics about fetal outcome. We pointed out in Chapter 1 how this view profoundly misunderstands the epistemology of clinical judgment. To this criticism we add the following.

Some proponents of this view make a great deal of the analogy to abortion, without arguing for the analogy.[25] The hidden assumption that they make is that the pregnant woman can deny moral status to any fetus at any time. In particular, she can deny the moral status of being a patient to the viable fetus. In *Roe* v. *Wade* and subsequent cases, the U.S. Supreme Court does not consider whether the viable fetus is a patient, only whether it is a person in the sense of the term as used in the U.S. Constitution.[26] But the two issues are not the same. Hence, the analogy to abortion as a way to dismiss the moral status of the fetus fails, unless the moral status of the fetus as patient is also excluded. But, one need not be a person to be a patient,[27] and so the analogy fails.

Because the analogy fails, it is therefore mistaken to think that the primary moral relationship of a pregnant woman to the fetal patient is one of freedom. This is not so, as we have argued above. The role of the pregnant woman as moral fiduciary of the fetal patient is, mistakenly, overlooked by such a view.

There is a further, important implication of this error: court-ordered obstetric intervention is seriously misunderstood. Annas, and those who follow a similar line of argument, fail to see the real issue here.[28] Only a court can decide to enforce legally the pregnant woman's ethical obligation to the fetal patient as its moral fiduciary. The issue is not a matter of interfering with the supposedly unfettered autonomy of the pregnant woman to benefit the fetus. Such an approach thus misconstrues fundamentally the issue that courts have yet to address.

The Fetus Has Graded Moral Status

We have also commented on our differences with the second alternative, that the fetus has graded independent moral status, especially our concern that the foundations of this view are ultimately theological. The fetus with graded moral status generates, it is thought, increasingly strong claims on the pregnant woman and her physician as the pregnancy progresses. Thus, there are justified limits on abortion and a justification for aggressive obstetric management.

Here we want to make a separate, philosophical criticism. The view that the fetus has graded moral status agrees with our framework that it is only sometime postpartum that a human being generates independent moral status. As we pointed out above, the noncontroversial time at which this occurs is during the second year of life. Evans, Fletcher, et al. seem to assume that the fetus achieves full independent moral status at term.[29] This is a mistake, because it assumes as uncontestable something that is hotly contested. Thus, any theory of graded moral status, if it is to be reliable, must set the time of achievement of independent moral status at a point beyond dispute, that is, sometime in the second year of life postpartum (for a statistically normal gestational length pregnancy).

Once this conceptual point is recognized, any theory of graded moral status of the fetus encounters a serious, disabling philosophical problem: there is no clear, unambiguous accrual of graded moral status during pregnancy. Just how much graded moral status is accrued at any moment?, is a question to which proponents of this view offer in response only undefined and unsupported intuitions. But more is required to establish reliably that the fetus at any particular time has *enough* of graded moral status to override the physician's beneficence-based and autonomy-based obligations to the pregnant woman. Thus, Evans and Fletcher's concept of graded moral status has no clinical applicability, especially since they do not take into account the presence and severity of fetal anomalies. By contrast, our framework provides an account of the qualitative differences and clinical implications of no, minimal, and more-than-minimal beneficence-based obligations to the fetal patient.

The Fetus Has Full Moral Status

We have commented in Chapter 1 and earlier in this chapter extensively on the serious shortcomings of the third alternative, that the fetus always possesses full moral status. These concerned the equivocation of "right to life," the inescapable theological origins of this view, and the profound misunderstanding of those theological origins. Obviously, on such a view there are substantive obligations to fetuses at all gestational ages on the part of the pregnant woman and her physician against abortion and in favor of aggressive obstetric management as a matter of routine.

Here we add two philosophical criticisms. First, this view takes no account of the presence and severity of fetal anomalies and their implications for variable beneficence-based obligations to the fetal patient. The conceptual error here is to assume that independent moral status entails maximal beneficence-based obligations regardless of anomalies. Second, this view assumes that, as the fiduciary of any fetus, in her uterus or elsewhere in her body, the pregnant woman is obligated to take any and every risk to protect and promote the unvarying, maximal interests of the fetus. Respect for the pregnant woman's autonomy is simply eliminated, as if her subjective and deliberative interests did not exist. This is simply philosophical nonsense.[30]

In summary, each of the other alternative frameworks for obstetric ethics is profoundly disabled. Each can be shown philosophically to suffer from disabling, internal, methodological flaws. Each is also inadequate when compared to our proposed framework.

Conclusion

Ethical conflicts and crises are surely intellectually provocative and engaging to discuss. Indeed, the obstetric ethics literature abounds with discussion of "four-alarm" cases and issues. However intellectually engaging it may be to consider such cases and issues, their ethically most significant feature for physicians and patients alike in clinical practice should be their prevention. It is thus to the strategies of preventive ethics in gynecologic and obstetric practice that we turn in Part II before addressing the management of ethical conflict and crisis in Part III.

NOTES

1. The reader will note that throughout this book we use the term "pregnant woman," not "mother." To be a mother, a woman must have a child, that is, an *ex utero* human being whom she bore, whom she adopted, or to whom contributed an ovum. A pregnant woman is not the mother of her fetus. Similarly, the male partner or spouse is not a father. In the same vein, we do not use the phrase, "unborn child." This phrase, if it is to be used at all, can only, we believe, be used in connection with the viable fetal patient. Its only use is to signal the interest of the viable fetal patient in becoming a child, and not either to signal independent moral status or to covertly assert dependent moral status.

2. See, for example, Maurice J. Mahoney, "Fetal-Maternal Relationship," in Warren T. Reich (ed.), *Encyclopedia of Bioethics* (New York: Macmillan, 1978), pp. 485–89; John C. Fletcher, "The Fetus as Patient: Ethical Issues," *Journal of the American Medical Association* 246 (1981):772–3; J.A. Pritchard, P.C. MacDonald, and N.F. Gant, *Williams Obstetrics,* 17th ed. (Norwalk, Conn.: Appleton-Century-Crofts, 1985), p. xi; Roger L. Shinn, "The Fetus as Patient: A Philosophical and Ethical Perspective," in Aubrey Milunsky and George J. Annas (eds.), *Genetics and the Law* (New York: Plenum Press, 1985), pp. 317–24; Thomas H. Murray, "Moral Obligations to the Not Yet Born: The Fetus as Patient," *Clinics in Perinatology* 14 (1987):313–28; Maurice J. Mahoney, "The Fetus as Patient," *Western Journal of Medicine* 150 (1989):517–40; E.R. Newton, "The Fetus as Patient," *Medical Clinics of North America* 73 (1989):517–40; and LeRoy Walters, "Ethical Issues in Intrauterine Diagnosis and Therapy," *Fetal Therapy* 1 (1986): 32–37.

3. See, for example, M.R. Harrison, M.S. Golbus, R.A. Filly, *The Unborn Patient* (New York: Grune and Stratton, 1984); A.W. Liley, "The Fetus as a Personality," *Australia New Zealand Journal of Psychiatry* 6 (1972):99–105; American Academy of Pediatrics Committee on Bioethics, "Fetal Therapy: Ethical Considerations," *Pediatrics* 81 (1988):898–99; American College of Obstetricians and Gynecologists Committee on Ethics, *Patient Choice: Maternal-Fetal Conflict* (Washington, D.C.: American College of Obstetricians and Gynecologists, 1987); and American College of Obstetricians and Gynecologists Technical Bulletin, *Ethical Decision-Making in Obstetrics and Gynecology* (Washington, D.C.: American College of Obstetricians and Gynecologists, 1989).

4. Charles E. Curran, "Abortion: Contemporary Debate in Philosophical and Religious Ethics," in Warren T. Reich (ed.), *Encyclopedia of Bioethics,* pp. 17–26; John T. Noonan (ed.), *The Morality of Abortion,* (Cambridge: Harvard University Press, 1970); and Andre E. Hellegers, "Fetal Development," *Theological Studies* 31 (1970):3–9.

5. See, for example: John T. Noonan, *A Private Choice: Abortion in America in the Seventies* (New York: The Free Press, 1979); James Bopp (ed.), *Restoring the Right to Life: The Human Life Amendment,* (Provo, Utah: Brigham Young University, 1984); and James Bopp (ed.), *Human Life and Health Care Ethics* (Frederick, Md.: University Publications of America, 1985).

6. Mark I. Evans, John C. Fletcher, I.E. Zador, et al., "Selective First-Trimester Termination in Octuplet and Quadruplet Pregnancies: Clinical and Ethical Issues," *Obstetrics and Gynecology* 71 (1988):289–96; and G.R. Dunstan, "The Moral Status of the Human Embryo: A Tradition Recalled," *Journal of Medical Ethics* 10 (1984):38–44.

7. George J. Annas, "Protecting the Liberty of Pregnant Patients," *New England Journal of Medicine* 316 (1988):1213–14; Sherman Elias and George J. Annas, *Reproductive Genetics and the Law* (Chicago: Year Book Medical Publishers, 1987), pp. 253–62; Sherman Elias and George J. Annas, "Perspectives on Fetal Surgery," *American Journal of Obstetrics and Gynecology* 145 (1987):807–12; George J. Annas, "Pregnant Women as Fetal Containers," *Hastings Center Report* 16 (1986):13–14; and George J. Annas, "Forced Cesareans: The Most Unkindest Cut of All," *Hastings Center Report* 12 (1982):16–17, 45.

8. See note no. 4 and B. Andrew Lustig, Baruch A. Brody, H. Tristram Engelhardt, Jr., and Laurence B. McCullough (eds.), *Theological Developments in Bioethics: 1988–1990* (Dordrecht, The Netherlands: Kluwer Academic Publishers, 1991).

9. See, for example, H. Tristram Engelhardt, Jr., *The Foundations of Bioethics* (New York: Oxford University Press, 1986); Carson Strong, "Ethical Conflicts between Mother and Fetus in Obstetrics," *Clinics in Perinatology* 14 (1987): 313–28; Garland Anderson and Carson Strong, "The Premature Breech: Cesarean Section or Trial of Labor?," *Journal of Medical Ethics* 14 (1988):18–24; Norman M. Ford, *When Did I Begin?: Conception of the Human Individual in History, Philosophy and Science* (Cambridge, England: Cambridge University Press, 1988); Carson Strong and Garland Anderson,

"The Moral Status of the Near-Term Fetus," *Journal of Medical Ethics* 15 (1989):25–27; and L. Fleming, "The Moral Status of the Fetus: A Reappraisal," *Bioethics* 1 (1987): 15–34.

10. Dame Edith Warnock, "Do Human Cells Have Rights?," *Bioethics* 1 (1987):1–4. See also Richard M. Hare, "An Ambiguity in Warnock," *Bioethics* 1 (1987):175–78. A human being need not have independent moral status in order to be a patient. See William Ruddick and W. Wilcox, "Operating on the Fetus," *Hastings Center Report* 12 (1982): 10–14.

11. See, for example, H. Tristram Engelhardt, Jr., *The Foundations of Bioethics*. The "virtually" is added to accommodate views such as those of Michael Tooley who would probably argue that some human beings, for example, those who are profoundly mentally retarded, never gain the moral status of a person, because they never attain the ability to have the self-consciousness and reflection that Tooley sees as requisite for personhood/independent moral status. See Michael Tooley, *Abortion and Infanticide* (Oxford: The Clarendon Press, 1983). A similar argument about rights and mental retardation has been made by McCullough. See Laurence B. McCullough, "The World Gained and the World Lost: Ethical Dimensions of Labelling the Mentally Retarded," in Loretta Kopelman and John C. Moskop (eds.), *Ethics and Mental Retardation* (Dordrecht, The Netherlands: D. Reidel Publishing Co., 1984), pp. 99–118.

12. The argument that we will make takes the following general form: If X can be reliably expected to reach future state Y, X has a stake in Y. If Y will benefit X, depriving X of Y sets back X's interests and, to this extent, harms X. If Y has a high probability on balance harming X, X has only a minimal stake in Y. Metaphysically speaking, X does not exist as wholly present but also as future. [For an account of how this can be the case, see Irwin C. Lieb, *Past, Present, and Future: A Philosophical Essay about Time* (Springfield, Ill.: University of Southern Illinois, 1992)]. The metaphysical questions regarding the dependent moral status of the fetus are two: (1) When is there good reason to treat the fetus as if it were wholly present?, and (2) When is there good reason to treat the fetus as both present and future? In the first case the fetus is not a patient. In the second case, the fetus is a patient. On the account we have given of fetal interests, the views of Mathieu that the fetus has no present interests is, simply, conceptually mistaken. Metaphysically, she treats the fetus as wholly future, a curious view. See Deborah Mathieu, *Preventing Prenatal Harm* (Dordrecht, The Netherlands: Kluwer Academic Publishers, 1991): pp. 19–21.

13. Mary Mahowald, "Beyond Abortion: Refusal of Cesarean Section," *Bioethics* 3 (1989):106–121.

14. M. Hack and A.A. Fanaroff, "Outcomes of Extremely-Low-Birth-Weight Infants between 1982 and 1988," *New England Journal of Medicine* 321 (1989):1642–47. We therefore disagree with Justice O'Connor of the U.S. Supreme Court that the trimester scheme of *Roe* v. *Wade,* at least with respect to viability, is no longer applicable. See *Webster* v. *Reproductive Health Services,* 109 SCt 3040 (1989).

15. In particular, obstetric ultrasound imaging does not make the fetus a patient.

16. See note no. 14.

17. See Chapter 5 for a discussion of selective termination of multifetal pregnancies.

18. Pascal's wager concerns whether God exists, more precisely, whether on balance one ought to believe that, and act as if, God exists. If one does so and one turns out to be wrong, one has lost little. If one does not do so and turns out to be wrong, one stands to lose a great deal indeed. See Richard H. Popkin, "Pascal, Blaise," in Paul Edwards (ed.), *Encyclopedia of Philosophy* (New York: Macmillan, 1967), vol. 6, pp. 51–55.

19. Biological variability applies here. Thus, we do not define lethality as the 100 percent probability of death either in utero, during the intrapartum period, or early in

the postpartum period. Anencephaly and triploidy are paradigms of lethal fetal anomalies.

20. John Gregory, *Lectures on the Duties and Qualifications of a Physician* (London: W. Strahan, 1772), p. 18.

21. In effect, because patients come to physicians for their medical care, not to individuals with a particular private conscience, one's obligations as a physician, as a rule, take precedence. The obligation to see to the protection and promotion of the patient's interests in the form of an effective referral thus takes precedence. To this extent, the private individual who is primarily a physician to patients may have to associate with evil. One way to avoid this problem and stay in practice is for the physician to declare one's private conscience and its complete implications *before* accepting anyone as a patient and securing explicit consent of a patient to these terms, including consent to the moral and medical risks to the patient of these terms. Whether this can be done without contradicting philosophical, secular medical ethics is not, in our minds, a settled matter, however. Thus, routinely adopting this strategy is not, we believe, ethically justified until further inquiry is undertaken.

22. The language we use eschews the use of "father," just as we eschew the use of "mother." See note no. 1.

23. This is an important consideration in teenage pregnancy and the decision of the pregnant teenager about the disposition of her pregnancy, especially situations in which the teenager may have been manipulated into having sexual intercourse without contraception.

24. George J. Annas, "Protecting the Liberty of Pregnant Patients," 1213.

25. Sherman Elias and George J. Annas, *Reproductive Genetics and the Law,* pp. 253–62.

26. A "person" in the philosophical sense of this term does not have the same meaning as "person" in the U.S. Constitution. The latter seems to mean a member of the human species who is alive and ex utero and within the jurisdiction of the U.S. Constitution. The philosophical concept requires more, for example, rationality or self-consciousness, and requires less, for example, it does not require being under any legal jurisdiction.

27. See note no. 10.

28. See Chapter 7 for further discussion of this line of argument.

29. See note no. 6.

30. It strikes us that this total neglect of obligations to the pregnant woman will be found to be theological nonsense, as well.

II | *The Prevention of Ethical Conflict and Crisis in Gynecologic and Obstetric Practice*

4 General Strategies for Preventing Ethical Conflict and Crisis in Clinical Practice

In the previous three chapters, we provided a series of frameworks for the identification of ethical conflict in gynecologic and obstetric practice. In general terms, our findings can be summarized as follows: there can be conflicts between or among beneficence-based obligations to the female or fetal patient, between beneficence-based and autonomy-based obligations to the female patient or pregnant patient, between beneficence-based and autonomy-based obligations to the pregnant woman and beneficence-based obligations to the fetal patient, and conflicts between obligations to the patient and obligations to third-parties and fourth-parties to the physician-patient relationship. This is certainly a formidable array, and it only states the conflicts in abstract terms.

Sometimes ethical conflict counts as ethical crisis. This occurs when there is a conflict between the beneficence-based action guide not to implement clinical management strategies that are not in the patient's social-role interest and autonomy-based action guides not to implement clinical management strategies that are not in the female or pregnant patient's subjective or deliberative interests.

There can also be crisis between ethical obligations owed to the patient and ethical obligations owed to third parties to the physician-patient relationship. We will consider these separately from the prevention of ethical conflict and crisis within the physician-patient relationship.

Virtually all recent ethical and legal analyses of conflict resolution in gynecologic and obstetric ethics have employed an acute-care model of ethics, in which the *solution* of ethical conflict is sought. There has been precious little attention paid to the clinically more relevant task of preventing ethical conflicts and crises in gynecologic and obstetric practice.[1] We believe that virtually all ethical conflicts and most ethical crises can be prevented and that—far more frequently than now occurs—attempts therefore should be made to prevent them in clinical practice. The principal contribution of this book to ethics in obstetrics and gynecology and to bioethics generally is to emphasize the centrality of preventive ethics to clinical practice.

Practicing preventive ethics is surely in the social-role interest of the patient. As we shall see, making preventive ethics a priority in clinical practice is also a powerful autonomy-enhancing strategy. Finally, by making the strategies of preventive ethics routine in gynecologic and obstetric practice, the only remaining ethical conflicts should be ethical crises and these will be more developed and mature and thus more amenable to management. This is because conflicts that remain after the application of preventive ethics strategies will involve conflicts only between beneficence-based obligations, on the one hand, and, on the other, autonomy-based obligations that are informed by deliberative interests or between such obligations and third-party interests. Preventive ethics strategies thus produce a moral common ground as the basis for managing remaining ethical crises. Absent this common ground, the resolution of ethical crises is little more, we believe, than a corrosive power struggle.

Preventive ethics is the topic for Part II of this book. In this chapter we will provide an account of general strategies for the prevention of ethical conflict and crisis in clinical practice. Chapters 5 and 6 provide more detailed, specific approaches for preventing ethical conflict and crisis in gynecologic and obstetric practice, respectively.

The three main strategies of preventive ethics in the physician-patient relationship are informed consent as an ongoing dialogue with the patient, negotiation, and respectful persuasion. An additional, fail-safe strategy is the proper use of ethics committees. Informed consent is the main clinical strategy for preventing ethical conflict in our account, a hitherto unappreciated clinical and ethical dimension of informed consent. This is because the informed consent process produces a moral common ground between the physician and the patient and frequently results in a mutually agreed-upon care plan for the patient.

If the informed consent process fails to produce a mutually agreed upon plan for the care of the patient, the response should be to prevent the evolution of the remaining ethical conflict into an ethical crisis through the preventive ethics strategies of negotiation, respectful persuasion, and the proper use of ethics committees. Negotiation is designed to address and resolve differences that emerge from the informed consent process, to prevent them from evolving further into ethical crises. Respectful persuasion and the use of ethics committees are designed to prevent existing conflicts from persisting and becoming worse. These strategies of preventive ethics take their meaning and justification from how we understand the interaction of beneficence and respect for autonomy in clinical judgment. We therefore begin with this consideration and then turn to a discussion of each of the four strategies of preventive ethics. We will then consider preventive ethics strategies for conflicts and crises between obligations to patients and obligations to third parties.

Preventive Ethics Strategies for Conflicts and Crises Within the Physician-Patient Relationship

The Interaction of Beneficence and Respect for Autonomy in Clinical Judgment

It is obvious from the discussion of beneficence and respect for autonomy in the previous chapters why ethical conflict occurs in clinical practice (See Table 1–4, page 72, Table 2–3, page 93, Table 3–3, page 123): the clinical perspective and the patient's perspective on the patient's interests and on what is in the patient's interest can and do differ. Most of the time, however, beneficence-based and autonomy-based clinical judgments are in synergy. For example, a woman may present with an adnexal mass of 10cm. The gynecologist would explain this diagnostic finding and the potential for malignancy and torsion of the mass as well as the unlikelihood of spontaneous resolution. In beneficence-based clinical judgment, surgical management provides a clear-cut greater balance of goods over harms for the patient, while nonsurgical management provides a clear-cut greater balance of harms over goods, in terms of the social-role interests of the patient. Beneficence-based clinical judgment requires a careful explanation of these matters[2] to the patient and supports a definitive recommendation for surgical management. Respect for the patient's autonomy also requires explanation of these matters, but goes further and obligates the physician to elicit the patient's value-based preferences for managing this condition, which almost always coincide with beneficence-based clinical judgment. In other words, the patient incorporates the clear-cut beneficence-based clinical judgment of the physician into her own perspective on her subjective and deliberative interests and how they best can be protected and promoted. This is the way that beneficence-based and autonomy-based clinical judgments are in synergy with each other.

The same occurs when a pregnant woman at term, informed that her pregnancy is complicated by well-documented, complete placenta previa,[3] accepts a recommendation for cesarean delivery. This intrapartum strategy is life-saving for the at-term fetal patient in a clear-cut fashion in beneficence-based clinical judgment.[4] The same is the case for beneficence-based clinical judgment applied to the pregnant woman: her mortality risks are essentially eliminated, whereas vaginal delivery poses a near 50 percent mortality risk.[5] The pregnant woman who accepts the recommendation for cesarean delivery to manage well-documented, complete placenta previa at term incorporates the physician's beneficence-based clinical judgment about her interests and the interests of her fetus into her own perspective on her subjective and deliberative interests concerning the management of what has suddenly become a high-risk pregnancy.

The synergy between beneficence-based and autonomy-based clinical judgments in both the physician's and the woman's thinking may be a fortuitous accident. In routine matters (in the sense of this phrase explained in Chapter 2), such as those in which the patient's social-role interests are not vitally at stake, this accidental synergy suffices. When matters are not routine, conflict is more likely, because the patient's social-role interests or fiduciary ethical obligations to the fetal patient are more likely to collide with her subjective or deliberative interests.

At this point one might argue that respect for autonomy in such circumstances is always the appropriate conflict management strategy. We think not. In obstetric practice, the pregnant woman has fiduciary ethical obligations to the fetal patient that she is not, as an *ethical* matter (but *not,* therefore, in all cases as a legal matter; see Chapter 7), free to ignore. She must as a matter of intellectual and moral integrity on her part take such obligations into account in the formation of her own interests. To deny this and simply insist that any expression of her subjective or deliberative interests on her part is as good as any other,[6] is to say that respect for autonomy in its moral sense does not require the physician to take the pregnant woman seriously as a person in the sense of moral agent.[7] Respect for autonomy as legal self-determination makes no such requirement, exposing yet another dimension of its ethically abstract character. The preceding considerations are sufficient, we also believe, to say that the pregnant woman has an ethical obligation to the physician to be serious when her social-role interests or her fiduciary ethical obligations to the fetal patient's social-role interests are vitally at stake, that is, when these interests are at risk for being set back in a serious, far-reaching, and irreversible fashion. This obligation is realized in the informed consent process.

The same holds true for gynecologic practice. When the female patient's social-role interests are vitally at stake, she is surely free under autonomy as legal self-determination to make a decision simply on the basis of her subjective interests. But this is, again, to say that respect for autonomy does not require the physician to take the female patient seriously as a person, in the sense of a moral agent. Here, too, the patient has an ethical obligation to her physician to be serious when matters are serious. This obligation is realized in the informed consent process.

In short, the patient in both gynecologic and obstetric practice has an ethical obligation to her physician to be serious when her social-role interests are at risk for being set back in a serious, far-reaching, and irreversible fashion. To be serious means that the patient moves from the expression of her subjective interests to the formation and expression of her deliberative interests. When matters are serious, she is also prudent to understand her role in the physician-patient relationship in this fashion. At the same time, the physician always has an autonomy-based obligation to the patient to acknowledge and respect the integrity in the patient's moral life of her values and beliefs, as is plain from the previous three chapters. As shown consistently in Chapters 1 through 3, there is no ethical conflict about this aspect of respect for the patient's autonomy. (See Chapter 1, Table 1–4, p. 72, Chapter 2, Table 2–3, p. 93 and Chapter 3, Table 3–3, p. 123) This obligation cannot be realized if respect for the patient's autonomy never goes beyond respect for her subjective interests. This is because subjective interests may or may not be a function of the patient's values and beliefs, whereas deliberative interests must be a function of the patient's values and beliefs, by definition.

The patient's deliberative interests, recall, are formed on the basis of subjective interests that are adequately informed about her medical condition and that of the fetal patient and their prospects under different clinical management strategies. Such information necessarily includes the physician's beneficence-based clinical judgment about such matters. That is, the formation of her deliberative interests by any female patient necessarily involves consideration of her social-role interests, particularly when her social-role interests and, therefore, her deliberative interests are vitally at stake.

The formation of deliberative interests by any pregnant patient necessarily involves consideration of her and the fetal patient's social-role interests, particularly when those social-role interests, and, therefore, her deliberative interests are vitally at stake. The formation of deliberative interests by the female patient or pregnant woman is the process through which the possibility of synergy between beneficence-based and autonomy-based clinical judgment evolves from a largely accidental to a largely deliberate occurrence. Deliberate synergy between beneficence-based and autonomy-based clinical judgment constitutes the aim of the strategies of preventive ethics. Each, in turn, builds on the area in which, as we saw in the previous three chapters, there is never ethical conflict: respect for autonomy in the form of acknowledging the integrity of the values and beliefs of the female or pregnant patient and eliciting her subjective-interests-based and deliberative-interests-based preferences.

The Informed Consent Process: A Preventive Ethics Strategy for Ethical Conflict

Informed consent is the process that puts these two autonomy-based action guides into clinical practice. Because it is a process, informed consent is not a form or piece of paper and it is not the signature of the female patient or pregnant woman on a form or piece of paper. These are only assurances or evidence—of varying reliability—that the informed consent process took place. Moreover, focusing on forms or pieces of paper—epitomized in the frequently heard request or even order "go get the consent"—reduces what should be a thoughtful and ongoing dialogue with the patient to a bureaucratic ritual[8] that, at best, misses the point and, at worst, dehumanizes the patient and physician alike. What is this process, then?

The Law as a Useful Reference Point

The law provides a useful reference point and has already been considered in Chapter 1. The law of informed consent is part of the law of malpractice. This is an important consideration because malpractice law concerns the enforcement of the *physician's* behavior. It therefore does not concern itself with the regulation of the patient's behavior, much less with possible ethical obligations that the patient may have to the physician in the informed consent process. In the law, the informed consent process is typically understood to involve three steps: (1) disclosure by the physician to the patient of an adequate amount of information; (2) understanding of that information by the patient; and (3) a voluntary choice by the patient regarding the management of her condition.

What does the law require of the physician? Basically two things: in relation to (1), the provision of an adequate amount of information to the patient; and, in relation to (3), noninterference with the patient's exercise of her autonomy as legal self-determination in choosing for or against diagnostic or therapeutic management plans. An adequate amount of disclosure meets one of two standards.[9] The first, the professional community standard, requires that the physician disclose what the relevantly trained and experienced physician would disclose to the patient about her condition and alternatives for managing it. The second, the reasonable person standard, requires the physician to disclose what the hypothetical reasonable person—an individual capable of thinking things through in a rational manner—would want to know in the patient's situation. The state courts that have adopted this second standard (about a third of the states) have criticized the professional community standard for placing the patient at risk for systematic underdisclosure of information that the patient can reasonably be expected to find relevant to her situation.[10] The reasonable person standard requires that the physician disclose to the patient an accurate and as complete as possible an account of the patient's condition, the alternatives—including doing nothing—available to manage the patient, and the benefits and risks—*not* risks alone with no information about benefits as a context in which to assess risks—of each alternative, including doing nothing. The physician is then obligated not to interfere with the exercise of the patient's autonomy.

The law does not require that the patient understand well or completely what is disclosed, only that the information is disclosed in a manner and at a level that the patient can reliably be expected to grasp. This obligation is satisfied in the law even if the patient only "roughly" comprehends the information that has been disclosed.[11] The law makes a further, implicit assumption: patients will be uniformly able to understand and evaluate this information without the physician's assistance. This assumption, we believe, can be dangerous, because it invites the physician routinely to leave the patient alone in situations where the patient might very much appreciate assistance in understanding and evaluating the information that has been disclosed, in particular, those situations in which the patient's social-role interests, and therefore deliberative interests, are vitally at stake.

The law also makes a further, implicit assumption: informed consent begins with something that the physician does, namely, giving information to the patient, as if there were no preparation required for doing so. That is, the law assumes that the patient has a ready context in her existing fund of knowledge into which the new information can be integrated, even if only in a "rough" way. The law also assumes that either the physician already is aware of this context or, worse, is free to pay no attention to it. This is a mistake, because the patient can sometimes bring to her care incomplete or incorrect understanding of her condition, its causes, its consequences, or what medical care has to offer to her. This phenomenon cuts across differences of education, income, or race among patients.

The law is nonetheless a useful reference point, because it underscores the nature of informed consent as a process and because it highlights some of the physician's obligations to the patient in this process. However, the law does not fully account for the physician's ethical obligations, because it does not concern itself with what the patient needs to do in this process and with possible obligations that the patient may have to her physician in this process. The law, in other words, ignores what is involved in the *patient's* understanding the information provided to her by her physician. This is no surprise, as we noted above; the law regulates only the physician's, not the patient's behavior. As a consequence, legal models of informed consent are inadequate to capture its ethical dimensions.

The Ethical Dimensions of Informed Consent

Informed consent as a process obviously involves *both* the physician and the patient. To gain a fuller picture of what this process involves, we need to turn to the ethical dimensions of informed consent. There are several.

The first concerns the principle of respect for the autonomy of the patient. There is widespread agreement in the literature on the ethics of informed consent that respect for the patient's autonomy is a bedrock ethical dimension of informed consent. There is less said about how to put this principle into clinical practice, so that it can actually be applied in clinical practice. To do so, we identify four sequential autonomy-based behaviors on the part of the patient: (1) absorbing and retaining information about her condition and alternative diagnostic and therapeutic responses to it; (2) understanding that information cognitively, namely, that each such response has likely consequences;[12] (3) understanding that information evaluatively, namely, rank ordering those responses on the basis of an evaluation of their consequences, now understood in terms of benefits and risks;[13] and (4) expressing subjective-interests-based or deliberative-interests-based preferences as the outcome of the previous three steps.

The fourth of these behaviors presupposes the first three. For the expression of subjective-interests-based preferences, the first three behaviors can indeed be "rough." Most of the time in gynecologic practice the expression of a subjective-interests-based preference will do, because the female patient's social-role interests are not vitally at stake. When those interests are vitally at stake, for example, in the diagnosis and management of gynecologic cancers, the female patient has at least an interest in the formation and expression of her deliberative interests. Too, if she is to be a genuine partner in the process, she is ethically obligated in such circumstances to her physician to make her expression of such interests part of the informed consent process. In obstetric practice, the expression of subjective-interests-based preferences will do, until the fetus is a patient. When this is the case, the pregnant patient, as a matter of intellectual and moral integrity, needs to take account of her obligations to the fetal patient. This necessarily involves the formation of deliberative interests. That is, a pregnancy going to viability is a morally serious matter. Hence, the pregnant patient surely has an interest in the formation of her deliberative interests in such circumstances. Too, if she is to be a genuine partner in the process, she is ethically obligated to her physician to make her expression of such interests part of the informed consent process.

There are behaviors on the part of the physician that correspond to each of the four above behaviors on the part of the patient. First, the physician is obligated to recognize the capacity of each patient to deal with health care information—and *not* to underestimate that capacity. The patient frequently depends on the physician to a considerable extent for accurate and complete information. At the same time, the physician must recognize that patients can and do seek out information on their own, including sometimes quite technical information. Too, the physician must attend to the possibility that the patient is beginning the informed consent process with incomplete or even inaccurate information about her condition and how it might effectively be managed.

The second ethical dimension of the informed consent process is that the physician is not to interfere—though the physician can, when necessary, assist the patient—with her cognitive and evaluative understanding of information that has been provided to her. The law assumes that patients can readily undertake these tasks. An important ethical dimension of informed consent is that patients sometimes need or will ask for assistance in doing so. Patients may need assistance when social-role interests are vitally at stake. Patients may at any time ask for assistance. Indeed, an important autonomy-enhancing strategy is to encourage patients to do so, as they see fit. We underscore the point that in this process the physician is in the counseling and recommending roles, not the deciding role, with the goal being the exercise by the patient of her autonomy. Thus, the physician is more than simply a technician who imparts information to the patient, which is all that the law would seem to require him or her to be. The effective counselor helps the patient, when necessary, to interpret and evaluate information, according to the patient's need or request to do so.

The third ethical dimension of informed consent is that the physician is to elicit the patient's subjective-interests-based preferences or deliberative-interests-based preferences, as appropriate. The patient's preferences are correctly understood to be value-based when the patient at some level has engaged in evaluative understanding of the information provided by the physician. In routine matters, those in which the patient's social-role interests are not vitally at stake, evaluative understanding probably only requires reference by the patient to her subjective interests, for example, in consenting to an annual Pap smear after the age of 40. When matters are not routine, that is, when the patient's social-role and, therefore, deliberative interests are vitally at stake, evaluative understanding requires reference by the patient to her deliberative interests. She needs to give her situation and its management serious consideration, for example, in response to a diagnosis of uterine cancer or of a multiple gestation pregnancy of a high order.

In short, the ethical dimensions of the informed consent process take account of the behaviors of *both* the physician and the patient. The law takes account of only the first, underscoring the significant difference between ethics and law in this clinical context.

Nine Steps of the Informed Consent Process

We are now in a position to spell out the informed consent process in a step-wise fashion. Although at first these nine steps may seem burdensome, each is clinically ethically significant and worth distinguishing. These steps begin with the recognition that the patient needs an accurate and as complete as possible fund of knowledge as the starting point of the process and proceed on the assumption, elaborated above, that the patient may need or request assistance in her participation in the informed consent process. There are nine steps in making the informed consent process an ethical, not merely legal, undertaking.[14]

1. The physician initiates the process by eliciting from the patient what she believes about her condition, its diagnosis, alternatives available to manage it, and her prognosis under each alternative.
2. The physician corrects factual errors and incompleteness in the patient's fund of knowledge. This does not require that the patient receive a complete medical education.
3. The physician provides and explains his or her clinical judgment about the patient's condition and all available management strategies (including doing nothing, i.e., watchful waiting).
4. The physician works with the patient, as needed or requested, to help her to develop as complete as possible a picture of her condition and alternatives available (including doing nothing, i.e., watchful waiting) to manage it.
5. The physician works with the patient, as needed or requested, to help her identify her relevant values and beliefs.
6. The physician, as needed or requested, helps the patient, *in a nondirective fashion,* to evaluate her alternatives in terms of those values and beliefs.
7. The patient undertakes to cognitively and evaluatively understand her condition, the available management strategies (including doing nothing, i.e., watchful waiting), and their prognoses and expresses her subjective-interests-based or deliberative-interests-based preferences.
8. The physician makes a recommendation, based on the clinical judgment already explained in step 3.
9. A mutual decision is reached and it is implemented.

Implementing the Nine Steps of the Informed Consent Process

There are two ethically and clinically attractive features of this approach to informed consent. First, this approach takes both the female patient and pregnant patient seriously, by treating her as a unique individual with her own personal informational needs and desires regarding her level of participation in the clinical decision making process. This prevents the dehumanization of the patient. Second, this approach signals to patients the need to be serious when matters are indeed serious. When matters are serious, the physician-patient relationship works much better when it is symmetrical, that is, when the patient takes an active part in making and implementing clinical decisions. This prevents the dehumanization of the physician. We want to amplify a bit on some of the key steps in this process.

DISCLOSING AN ADEQUATE AMOUNT OF INFORMATION. Step 2 involves disclosing an adequate amount of information to the patient. There are some especially important considerations along these lines in the care of both obstetric and gynecologic patients. Each will be considered in turn.

Adequate information in gynecologic practice. An area of particular concern for adequate disclosure of information in gynecologic practice concerns chronic illness. Patients with chronic gynecologic problems or disease, for example, all gynecologic cancers and HIV infection, need to understand several important features of their health status. First, chronic conditions and diseases cannot usually be cured. Instead, management is the goal, where management aims at secondary prevention[15] and tertiary prevention.[16] Second, there may be locally or regionally available research protocols that are enrolling subjects. Third, acute events can frequently result in accelerated deterioration of the chronic condition. Fourth, advance planning for end-of-life interventions should be introduced and the patient encouraged to consider the value of advance directives. (See Chapter 5.)

Adequate information in obstetric practice. In obstetric practice the pregnant woman who is taking her pregnancy to viability and thus to term needs to be made aware of a number of clinical issues. The basis upon which we identify the following items is that each involves a built-in potential for significant ethical conflict, because the woman's deliberative interests may be vitally at stake. From the perspective of preventive ethics, the potential for ethical conflict overrides objections that the physician need not inform all pregnant women about them. Moreover, informing women about them enhances their autonomy and their ongoing role in preventive ethics. Any adverse psychological reactions can be addressed over time, with far greater confidence about their successful alleviation than occurs in the midst of unanticipated obstetric emergencies. To disclose the possibility of such events occurring is directly analogous to the routine announcements of airline personnel of procedures to be followed in case of an emergency. There is no evidence that would cause one to think that such routine warnings produce unmanageable psychological stress.

First, the pregnant woman should be given information about the variable but substantial rate of cesarean section in the United States, in the hospital in which she will deliver and the physician's rate of performing cesarean section.[17] The physician should also explain personal, experienced-based beliefs about certain obstetric practices, such as repeat cesarean section and breech delivery.

Second, the physician should explain that fetal anomalies occur in 2–3 percent of all pregnancies and that certain diagnostic tests,[18] including ultrasound, maternal serum alpha-fetoprotein screening, chorion villus sampling, and amniocentesis, all exist. The benefits and harms of these procedures to the pregnant woman and to the fetus should be explained.[19] The physician should explain that, while some fetal anomalies might be detected by these methods, some might not.

Third, the physician should explain that intelligence is a multifactorial trait and that even optimal obstetric care cannot guarantee normal intelligence or even freedom from central nervous system defects such as cerebral palsy.[20]

Fourth, the pregnant woman needs to be made aware that a routine pregnancy can become a high risk pregnancy quickly and without warning as, for example, in the case of premature rupture of membranes or premature labor. Should this occur the woman may rapidly confront a series of complex and difficult decisions.

Fifth, for women who are considering a delivery at home there should be an objective presentation of the benefits and harms of this mode of delivery and need for backup should untoward events occur.

Sixth, the woman should be made aware of the legal right to an abortion. Federal or state requirements to the contrary[21] are unethical, because they are contradictory to informed consent requirements. The precise gestational age at which abortion is in fact unavailable will as a result of clinical practice patterns vary from state to state; information about practices in the local area should be provided.

Providing the patient with an adequate information base is not limited to only routine pregnancies, but also applies to clinical settings in which complications might arise. For example, if preterm labor occurs that is arrested with tocolysis, there should be a plan for mode of delivery in case the tocolysis subsequently fails. Although this disclosure of information primarily serves autonomy-based obligations to the pregnant woman, beneficence-based obligations are not absent. Information about adverse outcomes should be presented in a sensitive and supportive manner so as to minimize trauma to the pregnant woman.

This information should be disclosed at a level and at a pace appropriate to the intellectual capacity of the pregnant woman to understand it. The authors caution against underestimating this capacity in pregnant women, including teenagers. For non-English speaking patients a competent translator should be provided at this and the next two stages of the informed consent process.

Strengthening the disclosure process. The process of disclosing information in both obstetrics and gynecology could be usefully strengthened in a number of ways. Physicians could provide written or audiovisual materials to the patient and the patient could also be encouraged to seek out information from reliable, publicly available sources, including medical libraries. For chronic gynecologic conditions, for example, physicians could provide the patient with a list of questions that the physician, on the basis of careful reflection on experience with other patients with the same disease, believes the patient may find important. Chronic conditions allow considerable time for decision making and this chronicity should be taken advantage of in the informed consent process. Providing the patient with a list of such questions enhances the patient's autonomy by providing a structure for the patient's process of cognitive and evaluative understanding and focusing her attention and reflection on key technical aspects of care. In addition, reviewing the questions regularly with the patient can assist the physician to monitor the patient's progress in cognitively and evaluatively understanding her condition. Finally, except in emergent situations, this nine-step informed consent process need not be completed in a single visit, but can be stretched out over several. The physician should, however, beware the pitfalls of procrastination, for example, the loss of competence before the informed consent process can be completed for a patient with gynecologic cancer associated with metastases to the brain.

Two notable failures to provide adequate disclosure. There is a striking and important example in modern gynecology of the breakdown of the disclosure requirements of the informed consent process. This occurred in New Zealand, where an authority on cervical dysplasia believed mistakenly that carcinoma in situ would not progress to true cervical malignancy and, therefore, definitive surgical management was not warranted.[22] It was therefore not offered as an alternative, even though there was significant beneficence-based justification for doing so: the risk of death would be reduced by surgical management. There was also an obvious autonomy-based justification for doing so: informing a women about surgical management enhances her autonomy by providing her with the opportunity to cognitively and evaluatively understand the full range of management strategies, not an artificially truncated range. Thus, step 3 above was egregiously violated. Twenty-nine (22 percent) of the 131 patients who were followed with carcinoma in situ and continuing abnormal cytology did develop invasive carcinoma.[23] This disastrous outcome should eliminate any skepticism about the importance and direct clinical applicability of the informed consent process in clinical practice.

A second, more subtle, example of failure to obtain informed consent involved a study of a mandatory perinatal ethics committee on abortion.[24] This committee was established to "consider and decide requests by physicians for their patients who seek abortions,"[25] to be sure that abortions were performed consistent with the institution's religiously-based policy. Apparently, the physician-generated requests were reviewed by the committee without the knowledge or consent of the pregnant women who sought abortions. The committee blocked access to abortions on a number of occasions. While these women were free to go elsewhere, their autonomy was plainly violated by the institution's practice and some may have faced additional, unnecessary complications as a consequence. The investigators who studied the committee's work seemed unaware of its ethically unjustified policy of reviewing abortion requests by an institutional committee without the pregnant woman's consent to such review.

UNDERSTANDING THE INFORMATION DISCLOSED. Steps 5, 6, and 7 of the informed consent process involve the patient with the assistance of the physician as necessary or as requested, in assessing the information in terms of her values and beliefs. The goal in these steps should be to encourage and, as necessary, assist the patient to articulate, over time, a value-based framework that makes sense to her for the management of her gynecologic condition or her pregnancy. In obstetrics, the focus at this stage should not be just on particular decisions but also on the woman's expectations, hopes, and plans for her pregnancy. The authors believe that there is far greater likelihood of common commitment at this value-based level between the pregnant woman and the physician than there might be if potentially conflicting decisions were the initial focus. Common commitments lay the foundation for a physician-patient relationship that is meaningful and rewarding for both parties. This positive benefit of the informed consent process has been overlooked by the approach to obstetric ethics emphasizing the pregnant woman's autonomy.

A central value-related concern that must be addressed by the pregnant woman, one that appropriately shapes her understanding about pregnancy, is that, if the pregnancy continues to viability, the fetus is also a patient, in the sense discussed in Chapter 3. Pregnant women need to understand the ethical implications of the fetus as patient.

Two such implications are inescapable. First, the woman incurs beneficence-based ethical obligations to the fetus as a patient, as explained in Chapter 3. These ethical obligations are variable and do not translate readily into legal obligations, a fact of which the woman should be made aware. (See Chapter 7.) These ethical obligations on her part are directly parallel to the beneficence-based obligations of the physician to the fetus as a patient. Acknowledging this common moral ground is an indispensable element of the informed consent process.

The second implication is that these beneficence-based obligations to the fetal patient may appropriately place ethical limits on the exercise of her autonomy and on the relative weight that her physician appropriately places on beneficence-based and autonomy-based obligations to the pregnant woman. These two implications together are what make obstetric practice and obstetric decision making by pregnant women and their physicians ethically unique in medicine.

The goals of this stage of the informed consent process are to assist the pregnant woman to articulate in as clear and as coherent a fashion as possible her values and beliefs, to identify areas of shared values and commitments between the patient and the physician, to acknowledge differences, and to negotiate a general framework within which those differences can be managed in a mutually respectful fashion.

MAKING RECOMMENDATIONS. The above account of the informed consent process is distinctive in yet another way, namely, its explicit provision for and emphasis upon the physician's making a recommendation in step 8, after the patient's expression of value-based preferences. Step 8, of course, relies on step 3, which involves the formation of the physician's clinical judgment about the management of the patient. Clinical judgment ultimately concerns the protection and promotion of the interests of the patient, including social-role, subjective, and deliberative interests. Clinical judgment therefore ultimately involves an interaction between the principles of beneficence and respect for autonomy, because these principles interpret social role, subjective, and deliberative interests.

We argued in Chapter 1 that neither of these two principles can be routinely assigned greater priority than the other and that any such priority must be worked out in the particular clinical context. This is obviously relevant to step 3, which concerns the formation and explanation of the physician's clinical judgment about the patient's management. We therefore consider here when in practice one of the principles may be assigned greater priority than the other.

When beneficence is justifiably accented in clinical judgment and recommendations. Sometimes beneficence is justifiably accented in clinical judgment. A beneficence-based recommendation can therefore be made with confidence in step 8 of the informed consent process. We believe that there are three circumstances in which this is the case.

The first occurs when there is only one management strategy that protects and promotes the patient's social-role interests. Consider again the example, from the beginning of this chapter, in which a woman presents with an adnexal mass of 10 cm. The physician would, as part of step 3, explain this finding and the potential for malignancy and torsion of the mass as well as the very small likelihood of spontaneous resolution. In beneficence-based clinical judgment, surgical management provides a clear-cut greater balance of goods over harms for the patient, while nonsurgical management provides a clear-cut greater balance of harms over goods for the patient. Step 3 requires a careful explanation of these matters to the patient. Step 8 therefore would justifiably involve a definitive recommendation for surgical management.

Second, when the information being discussed with the patient is primarily technical in nature, clinical judgment is also justifiably beneficence-based. The identification of the range of antibiotics effective for a particular bacterium or the selection of an intraoperative technique is primarily technical in nature. These matters are justifiably managed in beneficence-based clinical judgment because they concern the determination of the social-role interests for aggregates of patients with a particular diagnosis and treatment plan. Obviously, the individual values and beliefs of a particular patient, whether her subjective or deliberative interests, cannot be taken account of in this process. The recommendation of a selection from a range of antibiotics in step 8 is therefore beneficence-based. The selection of intraoperative technique is beneficence-based and this should be explained to the patient in step 3.

Third, when the probability that the patient's social-role interests will be protected and promoted is high, for example, chemotherapy for gestational trophoblastic disease, or surgical correction of a prolapsed uterus, beneficence-based clinical judgment is also justified. This is because in such circumstances the net benefit to the patient's social-role interests is clear-cut.

When beneficence is not justifiably accented in clinical judgment and recommendations. In other circumstances, recommendations made in step 8 should be based on both beneficence and respect for autonomy. Two such circumstances are worth identifying.

When the patient's subjective or deliberative interests are likely to be at stake in ways important to her, as they frequently are, for example, in the management of infertility or in the consideration of an elective abortion, the patient's subjective or deliberative interests should be of greater importance to the physician than her social-role interests. This is because a judgment must be made about the priority of those social-role interests vis-à-vis the patient's subjective and deliberative interests. Because of the limited scope of beneficence-based clinical judgments, the physician possesses no moral authority to make any judgment about what priority ought to be assigned in such matters. The decision must therefore be left up to the patient, inasmuch as it is solely a function of her autonomy. Therefore, when the patient's subjective or deliberative interests are likely to be at stake in ways important to her, the physician should be careful to emphasize the limits of beneficence-based clinical judgment in step 3 and to be nondirective with respect to step 8, by not making a definitive recommendation.

The second circumstance occurs when the probability that the patient's social-role interests will be protected and promoted is low, for example, experimental chemotherapy for advanced ovarian malignancy or prophylactic oophorectomy at 40–45 years of age.[26] In such circumstances, there are alternative reasonable management strategies, that is, a variety of strategies—including doing nothing—that to some extent protect and promote the social-role interests of the patient. There is no clear-cut benefit to any one of the alternatives, and perhaps significant risks associated with each. This should be carefully explained to the patient in step 3. Step 8 should involve the presentation of the full range of reasonable alternatives, with the patient free to select any one of them. This would be the case, for example, in the case of surgery versus radiotherapy for management of stage 1A cervical cancer[27] or in the case of the method of contraception. In the absence of clear-cut benefit, no one alternative can exclude the others as unreasonable in beneficence-based judgment. To think otherwise is to fall prey to a form of paternalism that is ethically unjustified on beneficence-based grounds, as pointed out in Chapters 1 through 3.

MAKING A VOLUNTARY DECISION BY THE PATIENT. The seventh step of the informed consent process involves the patient in making voluntary decisions about gynecologic or obstetric care when the need for specific decisions arise. "Voluntary" means uncoerced and free of controlling influences.[28] A process of arriving at carefully considered, explicit, value-based preferences increases the likelihood of a voluntary decision occurring in a crisis. It is certainly part of this process, if there is time after the woman has expressed her value-based preference, for the physician to recommend other approaches and to explain the values that support them. This opens the opportunity for negotiation about differences in terms of underlying values and beliefs that justify them.

CREATING MORAL COMMON GROUND. It is crucial to recognize that the informed consent process aims to create common moral ground between the physician and the patient concerning the patient's interests and how they can effectively be protected and promoted. This is because in the informed consent process, as it is described above, the patient must to some extent take account of the physician's clinical judgment and recommendations in the formation of her deliberative interests. The deliberative interests that the patient thus identifies will take into account *both* her subjective interests—her own values and beliefs about what is in her interest—and her social-role interests—the physician's beneficence-based judgment(s) about what is in her interest. The formation by the patient of her deliberative interests thus creates the basis for creating a common moral ground between the patient and her physician. In other words, the informed consent process, correctly understood in terms of its ethical dimensions, is a powerful antidote to the malignant concept, discussed in Chapter 1, of patients and physicians as strangers to each other. This common moral ground is essential for preventing conflicts that emerge from the informed consent process from evolving into crises, which occur precisely when it is not possible to establish common moral ground.

Negotiation: A Preventive Ethics Strategy for Ethical Conflict and Crisis

The informed consent process need not and therefore may not in some cases (a rare event, we believe) result in a mutually agreed upon plan for the care of the gynecologic or obstetric patient. A preventive ethics strategy is required to address such differences and attempts to resolve them before they evolve further into an ethical crisis. Negotiation is such a strategy, because it builds logically on the common moral ground that should emerge from the informed consent process. That is, the informed consent process has the virtue of obliging the patient to move toward the formation of her deliberative interests, especially when matters are serious, rather than remaining simply at the level of subjective interests, as the basis for her preference(s) regarding her clinical management. The formation of her deliberative interests by the patient obliges the physician, in turn, to identify, acknowledge, and take into account the values and beliefs of the patient as expressed in her deliberative interests.

The key feature of the patient's deliberative interests is that they must, at some level, take into account the patient's social-role interests, which are the basis for steps 3 and 8 of the informed consent process. Thus, the patient's deliberative interests, as she develops them during the informed consent process, provide the basis for negotiation as a preventive ethics strategy.

It is important to appreciate that negotiation is *not* a zero-sum game, a process in which every gain or advantage for one party comes at the price of a loss or disadvantage for the other party. This cannot be the case, because the patient's deliberative interests already include elements of both beneficence-based and autonomy-based clinical judgment. Both the patient and her physician therefore have a stake in the content of the patient's deliberative interests. If the conflict evolves into a crisis, its resolution does become a zero-sum game. (See Chapter 7.)

The negotiation process thus should begin with the physician requesting the female patient or pregnant patient to express her deliberative interests clearly. That is, in gynecologic practice the physician should ask the patient what is most important to her in the management of her condition and the maintenance of her health. In obstetric practice the physician should ask the patient what is most important to her about the management of her pregnancy, the maintenance of her health, and the maintenance of the health of the fetal patient. The patient should be encouraged to express herself in some detail and as clearly as possible.

The physician should be listening for two things. First, does the patient have a coherent formulation of her deliberative interests? If the physician does not gain a coherent picture of the patient's values, the physician should point out where matters are unclear and ask the patient to explain. If the patient has expressed what appear to be inconsistent values, this should be respectfully and sensitively pointed out to the patient and she should be provided an opportunity to reflect on whether she meant to be inconsistent. The presumption of rational discourse is that she did not mean to be inconsistent. It seems reasonable as part of the negotiation to ask the patient to choose between frankly inconsistent values. If she does not do so, respectful persuasion should be employed, as described in the next section.

Second, the physician should review with the patient all beneficence-based clinical judgments that are consistent with her deliberative interests. Here the variability of beneficence-based clinical judgment and the need to keep that variability always in mind, as discussed in Chapters 1 through 3, should come to the fore. If the patient has formed her deliberative interests clearly and with reflection on the sort of information provided in steps 1, 2, and 3 of the informed consent process, then it is highly unlikely that those deliberative interests will be inconsistent with the *full-range* of beneficence-based clinical judgment about the management alternatives for the patient. Should the patient elect an alternative that is unreasonable in beneficence-based clinical judgment, triggering a crisis, the response should be respectful persuasion, as described in the next section.

This analysis of negotiation indicates that the common moral ground between the physician and the patient that should emerge from the informed consent process can be exploited and strengthened as the basis for negotiation, should the informed consent process fail to produce a mutually agreed upon care plan. This common moral ground should be the starting point of negotiation, rather than the expressed clinical preferences of the physician or of the patient.

Taking this common moral ground as the starting point also helps, we believe, to foster an atmosphere of good will and mutual respect, thereby encouraging negotiation as a preventive ethics strategy. An example would be when the physician recommends cesarean delivery for failure to progress during labor. Should the pregnant woman disagree, negotiation would point to the common ground of mutual concern for the well being of both the pregnant woman and her fetal patient. This would naturally lead to consideration of extended labor for a specified period. That is, the pregnant woman would be asked to accept continuing labor on a trial basis, with an agreement to reconsider her preference not to have a cesarean delivery should the fetal patient's condition or her own deteriorate in a way that could set back or even doom the fetal patient's or her social-role interests. Thus, the negotiating process stays focused throughout on the patient's considered values and beliefs, which have been informed and made more deliberative in part by the patient attending to and taking account of her physician's clinical judgment and recommendation. On this basis, disagreement that results from the informed consent process can be prevented from evolving further into a crisis.

Respectful Persuasion: A Preventive Ethics Strategy for Ethical Conflict and Crisis

Negotiation as a preventive ethics strategy for ethical conflict and crisis may fail. Consider again the example just above. This clinical situation becomes ethically more difficult for the physician if the woman wants to continue trial of labor after the specified period has elapsed and the fetal patient's condition, or her own, deteriorates further. At this point or at some point thereafter, obstetricians will typically become uncomfortable about permitting trial of labor to continue. Trial of labor will come to be seen in beneficence-based clinical judgment as increasingly difficult to justify and perhaps even impossible to justify, especially in terms of the fetal patient's social-role interest in avoiding unnecessary morbidity, as well as a death that would be both unnecessary and premature. In this situation, the probability for more divisive ethical conflict, indeed, an ethical crisis, between the pregnant woman and her physician increases. In the authors' view, these conflicts will, in obstetric practice, be mainly of two kinds.

First, there can be differing interpretations about how to balance beneficence-based obligations to the fetal patient against autonomy-based and beneficence-based obligations to the pregnant woman. Second, there can be differing interpretations of how best to fulfill beneficence-based obligations to the fetal patient or to the pregnant woman. The patient's religiously-based beliefs may play a role in both types of conflict. Sooner or later, however, the physician's threshold of discomfort will be crossed—when the physician believes that the pregnant woman's choice is inconsistent with the beneficence-based obligations the physician has to the fetal patient or to the pregnant woman—triggering a crisis. When the threshold of unreasonable beneficence-based clinical judgment for the physician is crossed, it is important to recognize that there is a clinical strategy that does not involve simply acquiescing to the pregnant woman's decision or simply seeking to coerce her compliance, namely, respectful persuasion, or an attempt to talk the pregnant woman into accepting the physician's recommendation.

In the authors' view, respectful persuasion involves the physician in the following steps:

1. Review with the woman information about diagnosis, management alternatives, prognoses, and her values about these matters that were disclosed during the informed consent process.
2. Explain one's reasoning for taking the position one has taken.
3. Explain how other physicians may disagree.
4. Explain how one meets these objectives.
5. Show how the patient's values and beliefs, including values and beliefs she could reasonably adopt if she has expressed inconsistent values, support the recommendation.
6. Urge the patient to reconsider.

Identifying these elements of persuasion enables us to draw the ethically significant distinction between respectful persuasion and disrespectful persuasion. If any step is not satisfied, the physician is engaging in disrespectful persuasion, because the physician is seeking to impose values on the patient and persuade her to accept their implications. Respectful persuasion starts with and builds on the patient's own values and beliefs, on her deliberative interests.

Uncertainty occurs when conditions 2–4 can be satisfied completely or nearly so. In this circumstance it is possible for the physician to give a well-founded account of beneficence-based obligations to the fetal patient or pregnant woman. It is also possible for the pregnant woman to come to a competing account on these matters, based on her values and beliefs. In these cases, autonomy-based obligations may not always be ethically overriding because in some cases there can be beneficence-based obligations to the fetal patient of potentially equal, or even greater, weight than autonomy-based obligations to the pregnant woman.

We have in mind here the case of well-documented complete placenta previa[29] at term and a woman's reluctance to accept cesarean section. The risks to the pregnant woman of cesarean section are, for the most part, not life-threatening and are reversible. Indeed, cesarean delivery reduces the risks of maternal mortality dramatically. The harms to the fetal patient of an attempted vaginal delivery are life-threatening and irreversible and are virtually eliminated by cesarean delivery. Moreover, as pointed out earlier, the preventive ethics strategies of informed consent and negotiation would have included a discussion with the pregnant woman of her beneficence-based ethical obligations to the fetal patient and that those obligations bind her now and should shape her deliberative values. When there is such a clear-cut balance in favor of beneficence-based obligations to the fetal patient, persistent efforts at persuasion count as respectful persuasion.

The Proper Use of Ethics Committees: A Fail-Safe Preventive Ethics Strategy for Ethical Conflict and Crisis

While ethics committees are useful forums for discussion of ethical conflict in gynecologic and obstetric care,[30] they can appear to patients as inherently coercive mechanisms unless they are utilized carefully. In their crisis prevention role ethics committees should be asked to review the processes of informed consent, negotiation, and respectful persuasion, to determine if they were thorough and, if not, whether it might be useful to attempt them again. If the committee makes such a recommendation, it should make specific criticisms and suggestions. That is, the ethics committee should first be asked to engage in quality assurance of informed consent, negotiation, and respectful persuasion. In addition, the committee's educational activities and policies should emphasize preventive ethics, so that only genuine, that is, unpreventable, ethical crises occur, those in which the choice is between disrespect for the autonomy of the patient or violation of beneficence-based judgment. This implies that ethics committees should be considered only in response to medical uncertainty.

To prevent the patient from perceiving a committee as potentially coercive, resort to the committee should occur only with her consent and she should be invited to participate in all of the deliberations by the committee about her case. The virtue of this strategy is that it permits the frank discussion of disagreement without simply acquiescing to her autonomy while, at the same time, it reinforces at an institutional level respect for each pregnant woman's autonomy.

Preventive Ethics Strategies for Conflicts Between Obligations to the Patient and Obligations to Third Parties

Conflicts with Family Members or Partners of the Patient

In Chapters 2 and 3 we pointed out that the interests of family members or partners of the patient as third parties are something for the patient to assess. Conflicts with family members can be prevented by reminding them, as necessary, that they are not the patient and by supporting the female or pregnant patient in her judgment of the place of those interests in the formation of her subjective and deliberative interests. Two further strategies can also be used.

First, simply to assert, "My patient always comes first," won't do, because this assertion assumes that obligations to family members and partners need never be taken into account. In particular, it assumes that the obligation of the physician to avoid unnecessary harm to the social-role, subjective, and deliberative interests of such third parties could never take precedence over beneficence-based and autonomy-based obligations to the patient. This assumption is difficult to sustain, particularly in situations where the avoidable harm to the third party in question is serious, far-reaching, and irreversible. This is certainly the case when a physician discovers that a patient is HIV+ and has not notified sexual partners of this fact. These individuals, obviously, are at unwitting and unconsented to risk of lethal infection—which surely counts as serious, far-reaching, and irreversible. The harm to the patient of disclosing such information to the endangered third party (in cases where the patient autonomously declines to do so) is somewhat serious and perhaps somewhat far-reaching, but not necessarily irreversible. Rigorous clinical judgment should conclude that the harm to the third party, therefore, is far graver. Thus, the general obligation to prevent gratuitous harm that is serious, far-reaching, and irreversible from befalling innocent others (the "harm principle") properly takes precedence over beneficence-based obligations to the patient. That obligation also takes precedence over autonomy-based obligations to the patient, because they are usually understood to be limited by the harm principle.[31]

Second, family members, as third parties to the physician-patient relationship, should not be involved in the decision-making process about the patient's care without the patient's permission. For example, results of gynecologic surgery should not be shared with family members before the patient recovers and can consent to doing so, unless the patient has consented in advance to such disclosure. Preventive ethics underscores that respect for autonomy, at a minimum, requires this, because the patient may not want these third parties to be involved. Since these third parties have no standing *within* the physician-patient relationship, they have no independent claim to be involved in that decision-making process. At the same time, the patient may value family involvement in decision making, especially in the formation of deliberative interests. This will have important implications for assisted reproduction technologies and abortion, which will be discussed in Part III.

Conflicts with Institutional Third and Fourth Parties

As pointed out in Chapter 1, institutional third and fourth parties loom ever larger in the clinical landscape. Ethical conflicts of this type, as pointed out in Chapter 1, involve justice and the allocation of health care resources. Conflicts with third parties should be prevented. Indeed, increased efforts must be expended toward this important goal, lest those ethical conflicts unnecessarily evolve into ethical crises. (See Chapter 7.)

Disputes about the management and distribution of private and public health care resources are structured and managed by the ethical principle of justice, which requires generally that we give each individual that individual's due, where "due" is understood in terms of fairness. This is a necessarily abstract principle and there is no settled philosophical theory about *the* principle of justice that all reasonable people must accept. Rather, there are competing theories, the details of which will not concern us here. Enough can be said about justice and health care, we think, and its links to bioethics in the clinical setting without having to resolve the centuries-old philosophical debates about the nature of justice and its moral demands on us and our social institutions. Clinical judgment need not be impaired by this lack of closure.

We begin with two useful and important distinctions. The first concerns substantive versus procedural principles of justice. Substantive principles of justice concern the *outcome* of the process of allocating health care resources, that is, who will get what. The questions of whether antenatal care should be available to all pregnant women or whether there should be universal access to assisted reproductive techniques are, for example, questions of substantive justice. Procedural principles of justice concern the *process* of decision making about the distribution of resources. The question of whether Medicaid recipients should be more extensively involved in the process of deciding what Medicaid will cover in a particular state is, for example, a question of procedural justice.[32] Some theories of justice accent one of these at the expense of the other, while others attempt to address both. The impact of third and fourth parties on the physician-patient relationship, as we shall see shortly, raises issues of both substantive justice—how much medical care a particular patient will receive—and procedural justice—the physician's role in the process of deciding how much medical care that particular patient will receive. Because of the ongoing disputes about substantive justice, our approach to the issues will accent procedural justice.

The second distinction concerns two different ways in which the allocation of health care resources can be addressed, two different levels, really. The first way is at the macro-level of public policy. It concerns, for example, whether universal access to some basic, decent minimum of health care services should be assured as a matter of justice.[33] We term this the issue of the *horizontal* distribution of health care resources. It is at this level of justice and health care that the United States is presently engaged in health care policy debates about such matters as a universal right to health care and the appropriate response of private and public owners of health care resources to such a right. Different concepts of substantive justice, obviously, can lead to quite different understandings of what a right to health care should involve, because they disagree about what "just health care" should mean in substantive terms.[34]

The second level at which the distribution or allocation of health care resources arises is "at the bedside," in the day-to-day care of patients in clinical practice, in-patients and out-patients alike. The issues here concern the different levels of intensity of resources that could be employed.

We term this the *vertical* distribution of resources. It is at this level that there are debates in the clinical setting about how much to provide for a particular patient, knowing that the provision of high intensity care for that particular patient may distort both vertical and horizontal distribution of resources, in turn resulting in possibly adverse impact on other patients or those who want or need to be patients.

In our experience, issues of justice and medical care seem remote to the clinical practice of most physicians, matters about which they commonly believe that they can do very little. After all, justice and health care concerns mainly the third and fourth areas of bioethics identified at the beginning of Chapter 1: What ought morality to be for the social institutions that organize, deliver, or pay for health care?; and, What ought morality to be for health care policy? These are macro-level bioethical issues and will ultimately be settled, if at all, in the democratic process. There have been few successful attempts in the literature to identify links between such macro-level considerations and the micro-level of bioethics: What ought morality to be for health care professionals and for patients?

In our view, the most successful such attempt to date has been undertaken by Morreim.[35] Her proposals address how physicians ought to prevent ethical conflict at the bedside about the vertical distribution of resources. Morreim's proposal is based on the need to make a distinction between two distinct standards of care, rather than a single standard of care. Her argument is directed to the common law of torts and malpractice, but can be readily adapted to bioethics in the clinical setting, we believe.

Instead of a single standard of care, which is defective because it conflates professional competence with an assumed ability always to gain access to resources the clinician and patient do not always own, Morreim proposes two standards. The first she terms the "Standard of Medical Expertise."[36] This standard, Morreim correctly believes, holds independently of the resources that might in fact be available for the care of a particular patient. That is, independently of limited resources, society can and should hold the physician to standards of expertise concerning the identification of the interests of a particular patient and which interventions are in that patient's interest. Limited resources are thus never an excusing condition for clinical judgment that does not take into account the social-role, subjective, and deliberative interests of a patient. Clinical judgment is a function of the clinician's fund of knowledge and experience, clinical acumen, and time spent with the patient—all of which are under the control of the clinician.

Morreim's second standard she terms the "Standard of Resource Use."[37] This standard recognizes that neither the clinician nor the patient owns most of the resources consumed in patient care. Moreover, we would add, issues about the vertical distribution of resources are raised in the context in the United States, at least, where there is no consensus account of what the horizontal and vertical distribution of resources should be. The physician, therefore, cannot simply claim that "My patient comes first," as if this would settle the matter, because this is precisely what is now in dispute. Such an approach is perceived now to be possibly injurious to the legitimate interests of institutional third parties. By the same token, such third parties cannot simply claim—either directly or indirectly through fourth parties—that their interests come first, because this is also in dispute, because the rigorous pursuit of those interests is perceived to place patients at risk for impairment, not protection and promotion, of their legitimate interests.

Morreim's proposal in response to this ethical conflict is right on target: the clinician can and ought to be held to a standard of reasonable advocacy on behalf of the patient. We adopt this as the main preventive ethics strategy for ethical conflict with third and fourth parties to the physician-patient relationship.

Notice that this standard is not one of substantive justice, namely, that the physician should always succeed in procuring the resources that a particular patient is reliably thought to need. Rather, this standard is one of procedural justice: The physician should actively engage third and fourth parties—from insurance companies to hospitals and case managers—in advocacy on behalf of the patient. The physician, as advocate for the patient, has an inescapable justice-based procedural obligation to be engaged in, and seek to influence the outcome of, the process of deciding about the vertical distribution of resources. Such advocacy, obviously, will require that the physician has reached defensible, well worked-out clinical judgments about what is in a particular patient's interest. Such clinical judgments, we believe, will be based on a rigorous account of what is in the patient's interest, the patient's social-role and deliberative interests being taken into account. We do not believe that the patient's subjective interests have a strong claim in matters of horizontal and vertical distribution of resources, because these matters involve the obligation of third and fourth parties to satisfy the positive rights of patients to health care. The subjective interests of patients do not provide the stability for such a right that deliberative and social-role interests provide. These are large and complex matters, however, and, because they are beyond the scope of bioethics in the clinical setting, we defer a more systematic account of them to another time.

Reasonable advocacy for the interests of the patient may fail. That is, institutions of health care may not respond to such advocacy. In the clinic or hospital setting, we believe that the response of the clinician should be to persist, appealing to the traditional, fiduciary mission of clinics and hospitals, namely, to protect and promote the interests of patients under the care of the clinic or hospital.

When payers, private and public fail to respond, matters are different. Private payers have contracted obligations to pay for services as specified in their approved benefits "package." Beyond this, it is not at all clear that, in justice, private payers bear any justice-based obligation. Indeed, such payers can justifiably respond that the patient should, in her own interests, have prudently saved for noncovered costs. There is no such (relatively clear-cut) contract, however, between patients and public payers, except as specified in authorizing legislation. In both cases, however, patients and their physicians may confront a situation in which the assertion of third party interests puts the interests of the patient at risk of serious, far-reaching, and irreversible harm. This would seem to trigger an ethical crisis, which will be addressed in Chapter 7.

Advantages of Preventive Ethics

There are a number of important advantages to the preventive ethics approach to conflict resolution in gynecologic and obstetric care. First, the primary focus of preventive ethics is on underlying values and beliefs of both parties rather than specific decisions, as has been pointed out in other ethically conflictual contexts in health care.[38] There is a greater likelihood of discovering areas of commonality and negotiating disagreements if values and beliefs are the starting point of the informed consent process rather than specific decisions.

Second, this approach reduces the emotional stress and ethical risks of decision making in emergent situations in obstetric practice wherein the pregnant woman is at risk for experiencing all at once the unexpected burdens of beneficence-based obligations to the fetal patient. The role of the pregnant woman as the moral fiduciary of her fetal patient is ethically complex in itself as are also its ethical implications for the physician-patient relationship. Complex matters require time and reflection if they are to be managed successfully and are therefore at high risk for being badly managed in a rush.

Third, preventive ethics focuses the physician-patient relationship on underlying matters of deep significance to both parties. It thus furthers the aim of humanizing gynecologic and obstetric care by avoiding the steering of women's choices under a false banner of respect for autonomy. This can occur, for example, when the physician offers cesarean section as a valid alternative when it is not justified on maternal or fetal-patient beneficence-based grounds. Respect for autonomy does not create a positive obligation on the physician's part to perform risky medical and surgical procedures when they are not indicated. Flying such a false banner of autonomy becomes even more ethically troublesome when the physician's real motivations are those of mere self-interest, for example, convenience and higher fees.

Fourth, like all preventive strategies it is hoped that preventive ethics in this context will reduce the incidence of disvalued events, in the present context ethical conflicts and unresolved ethical conflicts that evolve into ethical crises. This should significantly reduce the need to resort to court orders to manage ethical crises.

Finally, a preventive ethics approach will enhance the opportunity for the early detection of irreconcilable value-based differences between a particular pregnant woman's subjective and deliberative interests and a particular physician's subjective and deliberative interests, or private conscience. In these cases, the physician will have ample time and opportunity to help the pregnant woman find a physician whose values are more compatible with her own and arrange for the transfer of her care with a minimum of bad feelings and a maximum of mutual respect, if she decides to choose another physician.

Conclusion

The preventive ethics strategies discussed in this chapter enjoy strong ethical justification. First, they acknowledge and incorporate the distinct and complementary perspectives on the interests of the patient that are captured by the principles of beneficence and respect for autonomy. Second, they create and build on a common moral ground between the physician and patient. They are thus powerful antidotes to the notion that physicians and patients are, and must remain, moral strangers to each other. Third, these strategies are systematically antipaternalistic, on both beneficence-based and autonomy-based grounds. Finally, they enhance the roles of physician and patient alike as true partners. The physician neither "makes decisions" nor is reduced to a technocratic automation. To the contrary, these preventive ethics strategies preserve and encourage the physician's virtue of integrity. Indeed, integrity provides a significant moral underpinning of these strategies. Respect for the patient's autonomy, at risk for being little more than a slogan, is made substantive and clinically meaningful. This is all the more the case for the topics in preventive ethics in gynecologic practice, discussed next, and topics in preventive ethics in obstetric practice, discussed in Chapter 6.

Conflicts with third-parties in both gynecologic and obstetric practice pose no distinct challenges beyond those discussed in this chapter, except that in obstetric practice the physician may need to make reasonable advocacy for the fetal patient or for two patients, the pregnant woman and the fetal patient. Thus preventive ethics strategies for third-party conflicts are not separately discussed in the next two chapters.

NOTES

1. See Frank A. Chervenak and Laurence B. McCullough, "Clinical Guides to Preventing Ethical Conflict between Pregnant Women and their Physicians," *American Journal of Obstetrics and Gynecology* 162 (1990):303–7, and "Preventive Ethics Strategies for Drug Abuse during Pregnancies," *Journal of Clinical Ethics* 1 (1990):157–58.

2. It is sometimes assumed that beneficence-based clinical judgment opposes such disclosure of information. Not so. There is a strong tradition of beneficence-based obligation to make such disclosure. See Ruth Faden and Tom L. Beauchamp, *A History and Theory of Informed Consent* (New York: Oxford University Press, 1986), especially pp. 53–113.

3. By "well-documented, complete placenta previa" we mean the following: (1) Transabdominal or transvaginal ultrasound examination is performed by individuals competent in the technique and interpretation of its results; (2) The placenta is clearly visualized on ultrasound examination to cover the cervical os completely; (3) To maximize reliability, ultrasound examination should be performed shortly before delivery. The reliability of the examination varies inversely with the time remaining before expected date of delivery, because of increased variability of data regarding outcome the earlier the examination is performed. Satisfaction of these three criteria makes a false positive diagnosis of complete placenta previa highly unlikely. See William J. Ott, "Placenta Previa," in Frank A. Chervenak, Stuart Campbell, and Glenn Isaacson (eds.), *Textbook of Ultrasound in Obstetrics and Gynecology* (Boston: Little Brown, 1993), pp. 1493–1502; and D. Farine, H.E. Fox, and I.E. Timor-Tritsch, "Placenta Previa: Transvaginal Approach," in *Textbook of Ultrasound in Medicine,* pp. 1503–8.

4. C. Crenshaw, D.E.D. Jones, and R.T. Parker, "Placenta Previa: A Survey of Twenty Years Experience with Improved Survival by Expectant Therapy and Cesarean Delivery," *Obstetrical & Gynecological Survey* 28 (1973):461–70.

5. J.A. Pritchard, P.C. MacDonald, and N.F. Gant (eds.), *Williams Obstetrics,* 17th. ed. (Norwalk, Conn.: Appleton-Century-Crofts, 1985), p. 409; D.B. Cotton, J.A. Read, R.H. Paul, et al., "The Conservative Aggressive Management of Placenta Previa," *American Journal of Obstetrics and Gynecology* 137 (1980):687–95.

6. This view of matters is held implicitly by Annas (and Elias). See George J. Annas, "Protecting the Liberty of Pregnant Patients," *New England Journal of Medicine* 316 (1988):1213–14; Sherman Elias and George J. Annas, *Reproductive Genetics and the Law* (Chicago: Year Book Medical Publishers, 1987), pp. 253–62; Sherman Elias and George

J. Annas, "Perspectives on Fetal Surgery," *American Journal of Obstetrics and Gynecology* 145 (1987):807–12; George J. Annas, "Pregnant Women as Fetal Containers," *Hastings Center Report* 16 (1986):13–14; and George J. Annas, "Forced Cesareans: The Most Unkindest Cut of All," *Hastings Center Report* 12 (1982):16–17, 45.

7. There may be some parallels here to Baruch Brody's view of respect for persons in his *Death and Dying Decision Making* (New York: Oxford University Press, 1988), *passim*.

8. For a critical account of informed consent as a bureaucratic ritual, see Stephen Wear, *Informed Consent: Patient Autonomy and Physician Beneficence Within Clinical Medicine* (Dordrecht, The Netherlands: Kluwer Academic Publishing, 1992), Ruth Faden and Tom L. Beauchamp, *A History and Theory of Informed Consent,* and Jay Katz, *The Silent World of Doctor and Patient* (New York: The Free Press, 1984).

9. See Ruth Faden and Tom L. Beauchamp, *A History and Theory of Informed Consent.*

10. ibid.

11. *Canterbury* v. *Spence,* 446 f. 2d 1772, 785 ID.C. Cir. (1972). We rely on the edited version of the case in Judith Areen, Patricia A. King, Steven Goldberg, and Alexander Morgan Capron (eds.), *Law, Science and Medicine,* (Mineola, N.Y.: The Foundation Press, 1989), pp. 372–85.

12. Becky C. White, *Competence to Consent* (Dordrecht, The Netherlands: Kluwer Academic Publishers, 1994).

13. ibid.

14. These steps are based on Laurence B. McCullough, "An Ethical Model for Improving the Physician-Patient Relationship," *Inquiry* 25 (1988):454–65.

15. "Secondary prevention" means the prevention of first appearance of symptoms of pathology.

16. "Tertiary prevention" means the prevention of recurrence of symptoms, especially more serious symptoms, of pathology.

17. G.L. Goyert, S.F. Bottoms, M.C. Treadwell, and P.C. Nehra, "The Physician Factor in Cesarean Birth Rates," *New England Journal of Medicine* 320 (1989):706–9.

18. J.L. Simpson, "Genetic Counseling and Prenatal Diagnosis," in S.G. Gabbe, et al. (eds.), *Obstetrics: Normal and Problem Pregnancies* (New York: Churchill Livingstone, 1986), pp. 211–14.

19. Frank A. Chervenak and Laurence B. McCullough, "Prenatal Informed Consent for Sonogram: An Indication for Obstetric Ultrasound," *American Journal of Obstetrics and Gynecology* 161 (1989):857–60.

20. K.B. Nelson and J.H. Ellenberg, "Antecedents of Cerebral Palsy," *New England Journal of Medicine* 315 (1986):81–86.

21. *Rust* v. *Sullivan,* 59 U.S. L.W. 4451, 23 May 1991. President Clinton rescinded these restrictions upon taking office in January, 1993.

22. *The Report of the Committee of Inquiry Into Allegations Concerning the Treatment of Cervical Cancer at National Women's Hospital and Into Other Related Matters* (Auckland, New Zealand: Government Printing Office, 1988).

23. ibid.

24. John La Puma, Cheryl A. Darling, Carol B. Stocking, and Katy Schiller, "A Perinatal Ethics Committee on Abortion: Process and Outcome in 31 Cases," *The Journal of Clinical Ethics,* 3 (1992):196–203.

25. ibid.

26. C. Thomas Griffiths, "The Ovary," in Robert W. Kistner (ed.), *Gynecology: Principles and Practice,* 3rd. ed. (Chicago: Year Book Medical Publishers, 1979), pp. 325–426.

27. C. Thomas Griffiths, "The Cervix," in Robert W. Kistner (ed.), *Gynecology: Principles and Practice,* 3rd. ed., pp. 105–173.

28. See Tom L. Beauchamp and Laurence B. McCullough, *Medical Ethics: The Moral Responsibilities of Physicians* (Englewood Cliffs, N.J.: Prentice-Hall, Inc., 1984), and Ruth R. Faden and Tom L. Beauchamp, *A History and Theory of Informed Consent.*

29. See note no. 3.

30. For a guide to the literature on ethics committees, see Pat M. McCarrick and Judith Adams, "Ethics Committees in Hospitals" (Washington, D.C.: National Reference Center for Bioethics Literature, Kennedy Institute of Ethics, 1987).

31. How best to inform at-risk third parties is a matter of some controversy. See Suzanne E. Landis, Victor J. Schoenbach, David J. Weber, et al., "Results of a Randomized Trial of Partner Notification in Cases of HIV Infection in North Carolina," *New England Journal of Medicine* 326 (1992):101–110.

32. The state of Oregon has proposed a priority system for health care benefits for Medicaid recipients. This system is known as the "Oregon Health Plan." A concise description is provided by Paige R. Sipes-Metzler, "Oregon Update," *Hastings Center Report* 21 (1991):13.

33. This is the recommendation on the President's Commission for the Study of Ethical Problems in Medicine and Biomedical and Behavioral Research, *Securing Access to Health Care, Volume One: Report* (Washington, D.C.: U.S. Government Printing Office, 1983).

34. For a useful discussion of the right to health care, see Thomas J. Bole and William B. Bondeson (eds.), *Rights to Health Care* (Dordrecht, The Netherlands: Kluwer Academic Publishers, 1991).

35. E. Haavi Morreim, *Balancing Act: The New Medical Ethics of Medicine's New Economics* (Dordrecht, The Netherlands: Kluwer Academic Publishers, 1991); "Stratified Scarcity: Redefining the Standard of Care," *Law, Medicine and Health Care* 17 (1989):356–67; and "Rationing and the Law," in Robert Baker (ed.), *Rationing America's Health Care* (Washington, D.C.: The Brookings Institution, 1994).

36. E. Haavi Morreim, *Balancing Act.*

37. ibid.

38. Emily A. Agree, Steven Lipson, Beth J. Soldo, and Laurence B. McCullough, "Long-Term Care Decision-Making," in William Reichel (ed.), *Clinical Aspects of Aging,* 3rd ed. (Baltimore: Williams and Wilkins, 1989), pp. 617–26.

5 | Preventive Ethics Topics in Gynecologic Practice

More can be said about preventing ethical conflict in gynecologic practice than was said in the previous chapter about general strategies for preventing ethical conflicts in clinical practice. In this chapter we therefore provide a more detailed account of the prevention of ethical conflict in gynecologic practice. Our focus will be primarily on Steps 3 and 8 of the informed consent practice, particularly whether recommendations are justified and, when they are, what they should be. Our approach will be to analyze topics pertinent to gynecologic practice in terms of the framework for gynecologic ethics set out in Chapter 2. On this basis we shall present arguments about whether and what recommendations may be made by the physician as part of the informed consent process.

Gynecologic practice concerns only one patient, the female patient. We therefore consider the following topics: contraception and family planning; ectopic pregnancy; abortion before viability; gynecologic diseases; critical care management of the female patient; and care of the terminally ill female patient.

Contraception and Family Planning

Contraception and family planning concern decisions about when, how many, and at what interval to have children. These are matters that do not fall within the competencies of medicine. Medicine is competent only to address the health-related dimensions of such decisions. Obviously, such information should be disclosed to any woman contemplating contraception as part of Step 3 of the informed consent process.

Some of this information may be of considerable moral significance to women who, for religious or other reasons of moral conviction, believe that the conceptus possesses moral status, even independent moral status. Medicine has no reliable grounds for believing that such status exists for all conceptuses and so must stay neutral on the issue of the independent moral status of the conceptus, an inescapable implication of the argument in Chapter 3. The female patient, however, is under no such restriction, and may believe that the conceptus possesses significant independent moral status.

This is a relevant consideration in contraceptive decision making, because some forms of contraception are abortifacients (or might be), while others prevent ovulation. This fact should be explained to the female patient as part of Step 3 of the informed consent process. For women who believe that the conceptus possesses significant independent moral status, this information is crucial to their evaluative understanding of alternatives available to them. Steps 5, 6, and 7 are therefore the responsibility of the female patient to undertake, inasmuch as physicians are not competent to advise patients regarding theological or other matters of private conviction. Obviously, physicians are competent to inform women about the health benefits and risks of various forms of contraception and so may be involved in Steps 5 and 6 in this respect. Barrier techniques of contraception may also raise similar concerns for some female patients, for example, those who subscribe to theological views on the unity of sexual intercourse and procreation.[1]

For patients with moral objections to abortifacient contraceptives, Step 8 should be a recommendation for a selection among a range of contraceptive approaches that are not abortifacients, or, as the case may be, that do not involve barrier techniques.

The preceding presumes that the female patient is capable of participating in the informed consent process. Some patients may pose questions in this regard, in particular, mentally retarded patients and chronically mentally ill patients.

Mentally Retarded Patients

Mental retardation is understood to mean: "significantly subaverage mental functioning."[2] Mentally retarded patients do not constitute a homogeneous group. Like all human traits, mental retardation exhibits variability. Mental retardation is divided into four levels: mild, moderate, profound, and severe.

There is nothing about mild mental retardation per se that deprives a mildly retarded female patient of the ability to participate in the informed consent process.[3] This is probably also the case for moderately retarded female patients.

This is not the case, however, for profoundly and severely retarded female patients.[4] Someone else must decide for them because it is difficult if not impossible to speak meaningfully of profoundly or severely mentally retarded individuals as autonomous, in the sense of possessing the capacity to form subjective or deliberative interests about reproduction. Moreover, these individuals may be at risk for sexual exploitation or abuse, the results of which may be compounded by a pregnancy. Thus, it is not surprising that parents of profoundly or severely mentally retarded daughters seek means to prevent pregnancy.

In this situation, parents are making a beneficence-based judgment for the never-autonomous patient. In doing so, they need to carefully distinguish the patient's social-role interests from their own, including what they may reasonably identify as a legitimate interest in avoiding financial or childbearing responsibility for a grandchild. The physician should point out the importance of this distinction for the parents' task of making a reliable judgment about the care of their child.

This judgment will concern the social-role interests of the patient. The following matters are relevant: the likely occurrence of unprotected sexual intercourse, the reliability of various nonsurgical contraceptive techniques, the reversibility of techniques, and the morbidity and mortality risks of various techniques. There is strong support in the literature for the use of "least restrictive" techniques.[5] Implantable contraceptive drugs such as Norplant[6] should therefore be given careful consideration.

The role of the physician should be nondirective in Step 8 of the informed consent process. This is because any one of the full range of contraceptive techniques, from abstinence to surgical sterilization, fall within the bounds of protecting and promoting the social-role interests of the patient. Surgical sterilization, for example, ensures that the severely or profoundly mentally retarded female patient will not become pregnant. This may be in her social-role interest, given the difficulty that such women can experience with pregnancy itself. In addition, the legitimate interests of the patient's parents in avoiding undue burdens on themselves may be protected by sterilization. On the other hand, sterilization is usually irreversible and, in comparison to implantable devices such as Norplant, is not the least restrictive alternative. Moreover, it is difficult to predict which severely or profoundly mentally retarded women are at risk for experiencing serious difficulty with pregnancy. Then too, there are many, often subtle, qualitative trade-offs among the alternatives, so that it would be unjustified to think that one stands out clearly as "the best." The physician should afford parents time and assist them to make appropriate inquiries, for example, with other parents or religious advisers.

Chronically Mentally Ill Patients

Family planning interventions to prevent pregnancy with female chronic mental patients pose unique ethical challenges to the gynecologist.[7] Respect for the patient's autonomy is difficult to implement for patients with chronic mental illness. The definition of chronic mental illness is still evolving, but established criteria include the diagnosis of a major mental disorder such as schizophrenia, major affective disorder, or personality disorder; disabilities in social, physical, or employment related areas; and a prolonged duration (usually two years or more) of treatment and illness.[8] Patients with chronic mental illness differ in an ethically significant fashion from the mentally retarded. Hence, existing guidelines and previous work on the ethics of family planning for mentally retarded patients are not conceptually adequate for patients with chronic mental illness. For example, the guidelines of the American College of Obstetricians and Gynecologists (ACOG) for mentally handicapped patients treat informed consent issues in terms of a dichotomy between those capable of consent and those not capable of consent.[9] This applies to mentally retarded patients, as is plain in the preceding section. By contrast, patients with chronic mental illness fall between the extremes of this dichotomy. They therefore are justifiably treated as an ethically and clinically distinct group.

To deal effectively with the ethically unique nature of chronic mental illness, we will utilize the concept of chronically and variably impaired autonomy[10] as the basis for whether and what recommendations regarding contraception and family planning for such patients should be made.

It is important to note that up to 2.4 million people are seen in community mental health clinics. Schizophrenia itself exhibits a lifetime prevalence of about 1 percent. Female patients with chronic mental illness may present to family planning clinics or be brought to the physician by concerned family members, as is the case with mentally retarded patients. Hospitalized patients may also be seen on a consultation basis, including pregnant patients. Chronic mental illness involves cognitive impairment, poor judgment, affective instability and impulsivity. These can result in behaviors that include unsafe sexual practices and intravenous drug use.[11] Thus, chronically ill female patients are at risk for sexually transmitted diseases, including HIV-related diseases, and for unwanted pregnancies.[12] Such patients are also unlikely to comply with a recommendation of abstinence as a family planning strategy.

The informed consent process described in Chapter 4 presupposes that the female patient: attends to information disclosed to her in Steps 2 and 3; absorbs, retains, and recalls this information; appreciates that this information has significance in her life and the lives of others, which is pertinent to Steps 4–7; evaluates information in some orderly way, Step 7; and communicates preferences at some meaningful level, Step 7. Patients with chronic mental illness can have these capacities variously affected by such factors as attentional deficits, denial, paranoid or grandiose ideas, delusions, affective disturbances, and disrupted communication skills.

Chronically and Variably Impaired Autonomy

The obstetric, pediatric, and psychiatric outcomes associated with chronic mental illness include the possibility of significant obstetric and mental health complications,[13] possible adverse consequences in child development,[14] and potential adverse consequences for chronic mental patients and their partners.[15] The decision making process for chronic mental patients includes, as noted just above, many factors that can impair or disrupt that process. There is, unsurprisingly, a tendency for physicians to approach the family planning interventions for chronically mentally ill, fertile, sexually active female patients in a paternalistic fashion, that is, to strongly influence or even take over the patient's autonomous decision making process to avoid significant adverse consequences.

We noted just above that for chronic mental patients, one or more of the capacities required to participate in the informed consent process is likely to be impaired and that this is a permanent feature of their mental illness. In addition, this impairment may vary for each of the relevant steps of the informed consent process to differing degrees, including differing degrees over time in the same patient. This clinical ethical phenomenon has been termed chronically and variably impaired autonomy.[16]

This phenomenon characterizes the chronic mental patient. A chronic mental patient may at any one time be above a threshold for one capacity, for example, to attend to what is being said or cognitive understanding, while being below a threshold for another capacity, for example, evaluative understanding or communicating a decision based on cognitive and evaluative understanding. That patient's decisions are indeed substantially autonomous,[17] but only in some respects and not in others, with variation over time.

We have emphasized in earlier chapters the presumption in clinical practice that the patient possesses adequate decision making capacity. Indeed, the informed consent process that we set out in the previous chapter would be meaningless in the absence of such a presumption. This capacity may seem, at first, to be called into question by the patient's chronically and variably impaired autonomy. Interestingly, the variability of chronically and variably impaired autonomy calls into question two common assumptions about such patients: (1) that the capacity to make decisions is always absent; and (2) that attempts at informed consent can be justifiably omitted. This helps to illuminate further the unique character of chronically and variably impaired autonomy, and one of its important implications: these patients should not be judged uniformly to be without decision making capacity.

Ethically Justified Recommendations

Chronically and variably impaired autonomy, then, means that there is always some one or more aspects of impaired autonomy present in chronic mental patients. The variable aspects of impaired autonomy may be responsive to ameliorative interventions. This clinical reality serves as the basis for a series of ethically justified guidelines for family planning interventions to prevent pregnancy in female chronic mental patients.

The first-line response should therefore be to treat chronically and invariably impaired autonomy, with the aim of restoring all aspects of impaired autonomous decision making to a degree at or above a nominal threshold. Each of the first seven steps of the informed consent process has its own threshold. These thresholds are patient- and decision-specific. Substantially autonomous decision making occurs when the patient can exercise all of the capacities at or above their threshold with respect to the decision at hand, for example, to use contraceptive barriers.

In some cases chronic mental patients will meet or exceed all of these thresholds. Since clinical judgment about such matters concerns the patient's mental illness and its effects on decision making capacity, the involvement of a psychiatrist in working with chronically mentally ill patients to bring them to substantial autonomy may be very helpful. Securing such involvement in most hospital settings should not be difficult, inasmuch as consultation-liaison psychiatric services are generally available. In other settings, especially family planning centers, appropriate liaison should be established to psychiatric centers, including community mental health programs.[18]

When the patient's decision making capacities are at or above their thresholds, the patient is capable of participating in the informed consent process. The physician's recommendation in Step 8 should therefore be a choice from among the full range of contraceptive techniques, including surgical sterilization and Norplant.[19]

Sometimes efforts to ameliorate chronically and variably impaired autonomy will not succeed, but the patient is nonetheless near thresholds for substantially autonomous decision making as a result of efforts to bring the patient to substantial autonomy. Such patients may meet some thresholds but not others. Simply making a recommendation, that is, in effect deciding for such patients what is to be done, may impose on the patient values different than those held by the patient, a subtle form of paternalism. Chronically and variably impaired autonomy does not in all cases necessarily imply that such values are unknown or unknowable to the physician. They may have been expressed or utilized by the patient, for example, in steps of the informed consent process. The patient's values are therefore, in principle, available as the basis for a response to chronically and variably impaired autonomy irreversibly near but not at thresholds for substantially autonomous decision making. A patient irreversibly near the thresholds for decision making can at least assent to medical care and can do so meaningfully if the care plan implemented respects her values. The strategy of this response is to present alternatives to the patient that are reliably judged to be consistent with her values and ask her to select from among them.

Special Considerations

Sometimes efforts to bring a patient to or near thresholds for substantially autonomous decision making may fail. Such patients are irreversibly substantially below one or more thresholds. They may therefore be irreversibly below all thresholds. In the literature, the scope of ethical concern is typically expanded beyond the patient's interests to include the interests of possible future children and social costs.[20] How should each of these three factors shape clinical ethical judgment?

THE PATIENT'S INTERESTS. The interests of the patient concern whether pregnancy can be reliably judged to pose significant mental health and physical benefits and risks to the patient. While the mental health and physical risks may be serious, for example, disruption of psychiatric treatment or self-destructive behavior, this is not always the case. Fewer still of these risks are irreversible. Mental health risks brought on by pregnancy can be addressed through rigorous biopsychosocial interventions, as can risks to physical health. It is rarely the case that those risks are predictable with reliability, even in patients with documented history of the occurrence of such risks in a prior pregnancy. Making recommendations on paternalistic grounds seems therefore not to be justified.

RISKS TO POSSIBLE FUTURE CHILDREN. The risks to possible future children involve the ethical issues of harm to others than the patient. Those risks involve both genetic and social risks. There are some circumstances in which a possible future child is at significant risk for the incidence of genetic mental illness, for example, schizophrenia.[21] Schizophrenia is certainly a serious disease and there is some intuitive appeal to saying that children born with schizophrenia to two parents with the disease might well be better off having never existed. This intuition, in our view, rests on a contended concept, namely, wrongful life. This is the concept that life under certain circumstances is worse than being dead.[22] The problem here is that being dead is not a benefit to someone, because there is no "someone" to be benefited. Thus, this intuition fails to be conceptually well-grounded in beneficence-based clinical judgment.

There are social risks to the children of one or two parents with chronic mental illness. These range along a continuum from disrupted or even impaired development to court-ordered removal from the home. These risks may be reversible over time and unpredictable in many cases. Thus, serious irreversible social risks to such children are difficult to predict with certainty or even high probability. If the preceding analysis is correct, making reproductive decisions for these patients cannot be justified on the basis of avoiding harm to possible future children.

SOCIAL COSTS. Social costs, however, of pregnancy, birth, and childbearing by women with chronic mental illness do exist. The ethical issue here is whether society can reasonably invoke a justice-based claim to avoid such costs. Society has declined to do so thus far. There is a good reason for this social policy. These women are not the only people at risk for incurring social costs to society from their reproductive decisions. Teenage women, and men, for example, constitute a group whose reproductive decisions cause considerable social costs. Yet no attempt is made to restrict their reproductive decisions. Picking out only women with chronic mental illness for restriction of their reproductive decisions because of social costs would therefore constitute arbitrary discrimination and would be patently unjust. Picking out all women, but not men, whose reproductive decisions involve social costs, would constitute wholesale violation of their constitutional and civil rights, the right to privacy in particular, which is also patently unjust. Thus, appeals to avoiding harm to society cannot be justified.

The social costs to parents, spouses, and sexual partners of chronic mental patients may be legitimate considerations. For example, the strong preference of parents who bring the patient for treatment not to be responsible for rearing a grandchild are understandable. This can certainly count as a legitimate interest. However, harm to these legitimate interests is not inevitable, inasmuch as other alternatives are available, for example, should she became pregnant, the woman elects abortion or raises her child by herself or places her child for adoption. The strong preference of a husband or sexual partner to avoid a pregnancy for the patient can be readily satisfied by his undertaking appropriate measures to ensure his own sterility. Thus, harm to his legitimate interests is not inevitable either.

When appeals to paternalism and harm to others cannot succeed, there is no ethical justification for overriding contraceptive choices. Thus, for this third group of patients, the approach to Step 8 should be the same as for the second group of patients.

Reproductive Decision Making by Adolescents and HIV-Infected Patients

Reproductive decision making by adolescents and HIV-infected patients is becoming ethically conflictual, because of the political debate about abstinence-based and safer-sex-based counseling. We believe that in gynecologic ethics this should be viewed as a false dichotomy. Indeed, failing to provide information about *both* will increase, not prevent, ethical conflict.

The central ethical requirement of step 3 of the informed consent process is clear: the female patient must be informed about all available responses to the control of reproduction. Obviously, abstinence is an effective form of reproductive control when it is followed without fail. This should be explained to the female patient, along with the fact that human nature is such that abstinence is not always followed without fail. When it is not, there are other means to prevent pregnancy. Informing the female patient about these other means in a nondirective fashion is not equivalent to encouraging those means—the claims in the political debate to the contrary notwithstanding. Ultimately the patient must decide for herself based on her values and beliefs, including religious values. These values must be respected.

HIV infection is a documented risk of unprotected sexual intercourse. Step 3 of the informed consent process requires that this fact be explained to all sexually active female patients and to female patients who are contemplating becoming sexually active. The gravity of the consequences of HIV infection serve only to underscore and lend urgency to this obligation. Obviously, the alternative of sexual abstinence should be discussed. Given its effectiveness in preventing HIV infection when rigorously followed, abstinence should be recommended as the most effective measure to prevent HIV infection, as part of step 8 of the informed consent process. When the female patient is or wants to be sexually active, step 3 of the informed consent process also requires that techniques of safer sex ("safe" sex is a misnomer and dangerously misleading, especially to adolescents) also be explained, again in a nondirective fashion. Given the gravity of the consequences of unprotected sexual intercourse, safer sex techniques should be recommended as part of step 8 of the informed consent process. A recommendation here means what any recommendation means, namely, that the female patient who is or wants to be sexually active needs to take account of the physician's beneficence-based judgment in her evaluation of her alternatives and her decision about which to adopt for herself. In this context a recommendation is not equivalent to approval of sexual activity, particularly in the case of adolescents.

The response of physicians to the political debate on these matters should be to make clear what gynecologic ethics, especially preventive ethics in gynecologic practice, requires of physicians. Any public policy that restricts the information provided as part of step 3 of the informed consent process should be vigorously resisted as unethical. Moreover, failing to fulfill one's obligations under step 3 for reasons of private conscience is also ethically unjustified. The female patient comes to a physician for well-considered medical, that is, beneficence-based, not private-conscience-based or biased clinical judgment.

Ectopic Pregnancy

An ectopic pregnancy, with the exclusion of some rare forms of abdominal pregnancy, cannot be successfully taken to viability, much less to term. There is, therefore, no way for the female patient meaningfully to assert a link between the ectopic conceptus/fetus and a future possible human being with independent moral status and thus confer the status of being a patient on such a conceptus/fetus. This is the fundamental moral significance of ectopic pregnancy.

There is, therefore, only one patient in cases of ectopic pregnancy. This condition poses only health risks to the female patient. Her social-role interests are only going to be set back if the ectopic pregnancy continues. The longer it continues, the more likely will her social-role interests be at risk for being set back in a serious, far-reaching, and irreversible fashion. In short, her social-role interests are, or soon will be, vitally at stake. There is thus a valid beneficence-based ground for recommendation to terminate ectopic pregnancy in Step 8 of the informed consent process.

Abortion Before Viability

Abortion ranks as one of the most divisive issues affecting contemporary American society. This divisiveness has the potential to extend to the medical profession because physicians counsel pregnant women and perform abortions. The voluminous literature on the ethics of abortion can be accurately described as a controversy for which closure on a common moral ground is impossible.[23] As noted in Chapter 3, this is because of the markedly varied arguments about when, why, and by whom there might be ethical obligations owed to the fetus.

Clinical Management

The first response of many persons to the abortion controversy is to try to establish theological or philosophical grounds for the independent moral status or lack of independent moral status of the fetus.[24] As explained in Chapter 3, independent moral status would mean that the fetus in and of itself generated its own moral status, including moral rights, which would have to be acknowledged and respected by everyone. The disabling problem with these responses is that they are so varied that no common moral ground has emerged and clinical application therefore has been impossible. Theological traditions are marked by deep disagreement, both intramurally and transmurally. In these matters, moreover, theological traditions have been unable to agree on a single perspective from which their disputes can be universally and authoritatively settled. Philosophical traditions have fared no better. Indeed, the voluminous philosophical literature on the ethics of abortion is markedly heterogeneous in its methodologies and results. Thus, no single philosophical perspective can claim with legitimacy a primacy over any other. In 1973, the Supreme Court in *Roe* v. *Wade* correctly observed that philosophers and theologians have been unable to settle the question of when human life begins, that is, when the fetus has moral status. There has been no progress in the intervening years.[25] Indeed, there seems to be no common moral ground available.

The implication for physicians of this lack of progress is that they should be deeply suspicious of any responses to the abortion controversy that assert an indisputable account about the independent moral status or lack of independent moral status of the fetus. Suspicion is justified, because no such account can claim final intellectual or moral authority, given the necessarily disputable nature of all accounts of the independent moral status of the fetus.

Physicians in gynecologic practice need not be morally paralyzed, however, because medicine does not need an account of the *independent* moral status of the fetus, as we argued in Chapter 3. This is because gynecologic ethics asks the question, "When is the fetus a patient?" This question is not about the independent moral status of the fetus. Instead, it is a question about the *dependent* moral status of the fetus. That is, the moral status of the fetus is a function of whether the fetus always has the moral status of being a patient, as explained in Chapter 3.

We shall argue the following: when the previable fetus is not a patient, the response of physicians to the abortion controversy is clear. Pregnant women in consultation with their physicians should be permitted to make their own decisions for or against the moral status of the previable fetus and therefore about abortion. However, when the previable fetus is a patient, the response of physicians to the abortion controversy is that this freedom sometimes can be justifiably limited, as discussed in Chapter 6.

Recall from Chapter 3 that no link can be established via biomedical technological capacity between the previable fetus and the endpoint of the moral continuum of human development, independent moral status. This is simply what "previable" means. The only possible remaining link is the pregnant woman's choice about the disposition of her pregnancy. However, because that link is solely a function of her autonomous choice, the pregnant woman is under no ethical obligation to regard the previable fetus as a patient. The physician is therefore under no such obligation for the same reason. Thus, before viability, a pregnant woman is free to withhold, confer, or, having once conferred, withdraw the status of being a patient from the fetus. In other words, for secular gynecologic ethics, the abortion controversy regarding previable fetuses is resolved for physicians by the autonomous decision of the woman regarding her pregnancy and the dependent moral status of the fetus as a patient.

There is in the literature an approach that holds that all of obstetric ethics is essentially a function of the pregnant woman's autonomy.[26] On this approach, the distinction among viable, nonviable, and previable fetuses that we made in Chapter 3 would not be made. From this it would follow that the pregnant woman is free to withhold, confer, or once having conferred, withdraw the status of being a patient on the fetus throughout pregnancy. With respect to previable and nonviable fetuses, therefore, this approach to gynecologic ethics and that of the authors are in agreement on the response of gynecologic ethics to the abortion controversy.

Some might object at this point that physicians have an obligation not to be an agent of harm to the previable fetus, independently of what a pregnant woman may choose. That is, the principle of "*Primum non nocere*," or nonmaleficence, may be violated. The authors have two responses to this objection. First, "*Primum non nocere*" is neither an absolute nor, indeed, a first principle of medical ethics in general or of obstetric ethics in particular. Instead, nonmaleficence is secondary to beneficence, as we argued in Chapter 1. Second, even if "*Primum non nocere*" were admitted as a primary consideration, it would only show that a physician should not harm a patient. It cannot be invoked to show that a particular human being *is* a patient. The principle of beneficence cannot be used for this purpose either. As argued in Chapter 3, both beneficence and respect for autonomy figure in answers to the question of when the fetus is a patient.

In summary, the response of gynecologic ethics to the abortion controversy regarding previable fetuses is the following. The abortion of previable fetuses, the central focus of the abortion controversy because virtually all abortions are performed before viability, involves no violation of the principles of secular gynecologic ethics. Neither does the abortion of nonviable third trimester fetuses, those with lethal anomalies. In both cases abortion does not involve violation of beneficence-based obligations. "*Primum non nocere*" is not violated either. Hence, no recommendation about the disposition of a previable pregnancy should be made as part of Step 8 of the informed consent process. Physicians should engage in Steps 5 and 6 only to the extent that beneficence-based clinical judgment is competent to do so, viz, regarding health risks of pregnancy vis-à-vis abortion.

The Abortion Controversy and the Distinction Between Professional and Private Conscience

Gynecologic ethics, as understood in this book, generates the ethical obligations that a physician in gynecologic practice has to the female patient. Gynecologic ethics transcends differences of private morality because it binds the conduct of *all* gynecologists, as physicians. Gynecologists, however, also have private consciences, which are shaped by the private morality of each individual. Private morality is a function of such individual factors as personal experience, family upbringing, and religious tradition. In contrast to professional conscience, private conscience is variable because of the striking heterogeneity of these and other sources of private conscience. Professional conscience governs the response to the abortion controversy of the gynecologist as a physician bound by the obligations of a professional role. Patients come to *physicians,* not private individuals, for their medical care, as we argued in Chapter 3. Private conscience cannot bear on the professional role but governs only the gynecologist's responses in nonmedical roles of lay person and private citizen.

Professional conscience governs the gynecologist's obligations to the patient. Private conscience governs whether continuing to serve as a gynecologist to a particular patient obligates the physician to act in such a way as to produce intolerable burdens on the physician's private moral convictions, values, and beliefs, including those of theological origin. We pointed out in Chapter 3 that self-effacement and self-sacrifice do not require the routine abandonment of such moral convictions, values, and beliefs. Respect for the integrity of the private conscience of each individual gynecologist on the part of patients means that some women justifiably cannot become, or justifiably cannot continue for particular purposes to be, patients of a particular gynecologist. Thus, asserting respect for autonomy in the form of respect for the moral convictions, including religious convictions, of private conscience can sometimes be a legitimate ethical claim on the part of the gynecologist. That is, gynecologic ethics underscores the legitimate role of religious belief and other forms of moral conviction that count as deliberative interests in the formation of the private conscience of the gynecologist.

There are important limits on such a claim. Matters of private conscience do not govern the physician's response to the abortion controversy in gynecologic ethics, only the morality of abortion in one's private moral life, that is, in terms of one's response to one's roles other than that of being a gynecologist. Thus, on the basis of private conscience, one has no intellectual license to judge the morality of pregnant women who contemplate termination or continuation of their pregnancies, or to judge adversely behavior of colleagues that is consistent with gynecologic ethics. Private conscience justifies only withdrawing from particular cases. When withdrawal is undertaken, professional conscience requires that the physician see to it that the pregnant woman's care is transferred in an orderly and safe manner to a colleague whose private conscience is not violated by the pregnant woman's decisions. No judgments about the morality of those decisions should be expressed to the pregnant woman, for whom, as pointed out above, the gynecologist acts exclusively in the role of physician, not a private person. Hence, private-conscience-based ethical judgments have *no* place in the informed consent process. To think or act otherwise undermines the virtue of integrity.

While private-conscience-based moral objections to a pregnant woman's decision should never be used to judge her, it does not follow that physicians as citizens have no freedom to add their private-conscience-based views on the morality of abortion to the ongoing public debates about abortion and public policy in our country. In doing so, however, when they invoke the professional mantle, their contribution must be governed in its moral content by gynecologic ethics. Otherwise, gynecologists can join the political fray as interested lay persons or citizens, with no special or authoritative perspective *as physicians* on the abortion controversy. When gynecologists contribute as physicians to public debate on topics such as abortion, they are constrained by the secular, philosophical character of bioethics and its response to the question, "When is the fetus a patient?"

Implications for Obstetric Residency Programs

The preceding has important implications for obstetric residency programs. The authors, like many others, have heard anecdotal reports that applicants to some residency programs sometimes learn, in one way or another, that all residents in those programs are required to perform abortions. The authors have asked ACOG and CREOG for data on this subject and the authors were told that no data have been collected.

Such an educational policy raises troubling ethical issues because it denies the integrity of private conscience and misinterprets gynecologic ethics and its implications for professional conscience. As to the latter, all that gynecologic ethics can show is that, when the fetus is not a patient, a pregnant woman possesses unrestricted freedom regarding the disposition of the pregnancy. Gynecologic ethics does not show, therefore, that every gynecologist should carry out a pregnant woman's request for an abortion, because doing so may violate the physician's private conscience in some cases. Any educational program that requires all residents to perform abortions rests on a misunderstanding of the limits of professional conscience and the obligation to respect private conscience. Indeed, such a policy unjustifiably violates private conscience, although a policy of offering training in abortion procedures as an option would not.

This is different from a policy that, on the basis of the religious traditions of the sponsoring institution, prohibits residents from performing abortions at that institution. This is because there is a well-established tradition in our society that religious institutions have the right to protect the integrity of their traditions so long as no harm befalls innocent, nonconsenting human beings. Because such a policy does not tell residents what to believe as a matter of private conscience, because such a policy is consistent with the limits of gynecologic ethics, and when such a policy does not eliminate access to abortion in a community, it is ethically justified.

The authors are fully cognizant of the possibility of abuse of a policy that permits exceptions on the grounds of private conscience. The best remedy to prevent such abuse is to require residents (1) to document the basis of their objections to performing abortions in a way analogous to the requirement imposed upon citizens who seek conscientious objector status regarding military service, and (2) to define clearly the additional duties expected of residents in lieu of not performing abortions. We fully support additional duties for residents who do not perform abortions, in order to be fair to all residents in a program.

Selective Termination of Multifetal Pregnancies

Selective termination of multifetal pregnancies has recently emerged as an effective and, increasingly in tertiary centers, a management option for multiple gestations.[27] Evans, et al., in a landmark article, first addressed the ethical implications of this clinical intervention.[28] There is widespread agreement to support their general view that selective termination of multiple pregnancies of high order (four or more) (fetal reduction) to twins or of an anomalous fetus should be an option for the pregnant woman.[29] The current ethical debate centers on the justification of selective termination to a singleton either from a multiple gestation of high order or from a triplet or even twin pregnancy.

Recently reported data suggest that selective termination is regarded as ethically acceptable for high order pregnancies but not for twin and triplet pregnancies.[30] By themselves, such data are not decisive ethically, because they *describe* moral views about selective termination to a singleton; they do not *justify* such views. That is, descriptive ethics cannot perform the task of normative ethics. That task involves arguments. There are arguments in the literature that oppose reduction of a multifetal pregnancy to a singleton.[31] These arguments, however, fail, as we show just below. Therefore, selective termination to a singleton is ethically justifiable and therefore should be presented as an option in Step 8 of the informed consent process to pregnant women with multiple gestations, whether they are of high order or triplets or twins.

Evans, et al., have made the most important argument against selective termination to a singleton.[32] They base their argument on the principle of proportionality. As they put it, "Proportionality is the source of the duty, when taking actions involving risks of harm, to balance risks and benefits so that actions have the greatest chance to cause the least harm and the most benefit to persons directly involved."[33] They clearly intend to include the human fetus, or, at least the fetus without anomalies, in the category of persons, because they take the view that the fetus possesses what they call "graded" moral status.[34]

As should be plain from our analysis of graded moral status in Chapters 1 and 3, this argument is based on questionable assumptions. One is that Evans, Fletcher, et al., assume but do not argue that the fetus has independent moral status, even if only to some degree. This assumption is hotly contested in the literature on abortion and therefore should be defended. Evans, et al., nowhere argue against views, such as Engelhardt's,[35] that it is incoherent to treat the fetus as possessing independent moral status.

Claims about the independent moral status of the fetus necessarily involve the further claim that some characteristic of the fetus that it possesses in and of itself, independently of the pregnant woman or any other factor, grounds obligations to the fetus on the part of the pregnant woman and her physician. Among these obligations, on the principle of proportionality, would be the prevention of unnecessary death. In particular, independent moral status means that terminating a multiple pregnancy to a singleton is not justified unless there is some overwhelming reason. Since mortality risks for a twin pregnancy do not greatly exceed those for a singleton pregnancy, Evans, Fletcher, et al. conclude that no such reason exists. Hence, selective termination to a singleton, they conclude, is ethically unjustifiable.

The problem with this argument is that any claim that the fetus possesses independent moral status, whether graded or not, is made against a background of the striking inability to reach closure on a single authoritative account of the independent moral status of the fetus in the history of either philosophical or theological ethics.[36] This outcome is not surprising, because there is no single methodology that would be authoritative for all of the profoundly diverse, indeed, inconsistent, schools of thought involved in this endless debate. For closure ever to be possible a single, universally accepted methodological authority for philosophical and/or theological traditions would have to be irrefutably established, an inconceivable event. Evans, Fletcher, et al. offer an argument that in effect presumes that this inconceivable event has occurred, and so their argument does not succeed.

Zaner, et al. basically support the position of Evans, et al. Zaner, et al. add the additional argument that a woman who undergoes ovulation induction "is desirous of becoming pregnant and would incur an increased risk of aborting both fetuses of a twin gestation by selective termination."[37] Any objection to taking such a risk assumes some degree of independent moral status of the fetus, an assumption that, as we have just shown, cannot be sustained. Alternatively, the argument of Zaner, et al. implicitly assumes that beneficence-based ethical judgment is the sole basis for analyzing the ethical issues involved. That is, they assume that availing herself of assisted reproduction techniques means that the pregnant woman has irrevocably conferred the status of being a patient on at least two of the fetuses in a multiple gestation. In effect, Evans, Fletcher, et al. share this assumption.

The fundamental problem with this assumption is that its adherents misunderstand the concept of the fetus as patient and the relationship between that concept and the autonomy of the pregnant woman. We pointed out in Chapter 3 that any attempt to understand the moral status of the fetus in terms of independent moral status of the fetus is bound to fail. We therefore take the only alternative approach, one that is based on the recognition that being a patient does not require that one possess independent moral status.[38] Instead, the fetus should be understood in terms of dependent moral status.

Selective termination involves previable fetuses, and the only link between the previable fetus and its later achieving independent moral status is the pregnant woman's autonomy. The link between a previable fetus and later achieving independent moral status therefore can be established *only* by the decision of the pregnant woman to confer the status of being a patient on her previable fetus. Because independent moral status of the fetus cannot be reliably established, the previable fetus has no independent claim to the status of being a patient and therefore the concern of beneficence-based clinical judgment independently of the pregnant woman's autonomy. That is, a pregnant woman is free to withhold, confer, or, having once conferred, withdraw the status of being a patient on or from the previable fetus according to her own values and beliefs. Overall has recently provided a useful account of the sort of considerations that women might find relevant in making such a decision.[39] The previable fetus is presented to the physician as a potential beneficiary of obstetric management solely as a function of the pregnant woman's autonomy. Beneficence-based clinical judgments about what is in the fetus's interest therefore come into play only *after* the woman confers the status of being a patient on the fetus(es) that she intends to take to term.

In contrast, Evans, Fletcher, et al. assume that the fetus can have moral status independently of the pregnant woman's autonomy. Zaner, et al. assume that once the moral status of being a patient is conferred by the pregnant woman on a previable fetus she is not free to withdraw such status. Both assumptions, we have now shown, are unfounded.

The pregnant woman does confer the status of being a patient on the fetus that survives selective termination to the singleton that she intends to take to term. As a consequence, there are beneficence-based obligations on her part and her physician's part to the singleton fetal patient to avoid significant harm that might result from the selective termination procedure. The medical facts at this time do not support the clinical judgment that harm will occur with high probability. In fact, it recently has been suggested that there might be biologic *advantages* in terms of survival and lower risk of premature birth for a multiple gestation of a high order reduced to a singleton versus reduction to twins.[40] In the case of selective termination of twins to a singleton, a randomized clinical trial would be necessary to clearly assess whether the survivor would fare slightly better or slightly worse than twins without intervention. Given that the alternative to reduction of twin gestation is often complete termination, any minor risk of harm of the procedure becomes moot under beneficence-based judgment when balanced against 100 percent mortality. Hence, there are no beneficence-based obligations to the surviving singleton fetus not to terminate the pregnancy to a singleton.

Evans, Fletcher, et al. also consider the benefits and burdens of selective termination to parents, including the benefits of having one child versus having two. Medicine possesses no competence to reach a beneficence-based judgment about whether it is better for prospective parents to have two children rather than just one child resulting from a pregnancy. There are therefore no grounds for including such a benefit in a beneficence-based clinical judgment and in Steps 3 and 8 of the informed consent process. Such matters are solely a function of the autonomy of the prospective parents and therefore in this respect autonomy-based obligations of the physician to them are decisive.

Nothing in what we have argued obliges the physician in all cases to carry out the request of a pregnant woman for selective termination of her pregnancy to a singleton. As argued above, no patient has a positive right to oblige a physician to act in a way that violates the physician's private conscience, that is, those moral convictions and beliefs that the physician possesses independently of being a physician. At the same time, it is not justified to impose one's private conscience on the pregnant woman or to base claims of professional ethics on private conscience.

The implications of our argument for clinical practice are the following. The informed consent process ethically requires physicians to inform pregnant patients about available alternatives for managing their condition. Since selective termination of a multifetal pregnancy of any order to a singleton is ethically justifiable, this alternative should be described in Step 3 and presented as an option along with the other options, for example, selective termination to twins or continuing the pregnancy without intervention, in Step 8 of the informed consent process. A pregnant woman's request for selective termination to a singleton should be respected and implemented. Obviously, physicians who object to selective termination to a singleton in private conscience are bound by the above disclosure obligations. At the same time, they should not feel compelled to perform the procedure but are obligated to make an appropriate referral.

The abortion controversy in our country will not disappear. It seems to intensify with each new Supreme Court ruling and actions of state legislatures and governors on the subject. Gynecologic ethics, precisely because of its philosophical, secular character, equips physicians to respond to this ongoing controversy in the disciplined, reasoned fashion expected of members of a learned profession. By submitting to the intellectual discipline of secular gynecologic ethics, physicians can act to prevent the divisiveness of the abortion controversy from extending to the medical profession.

Gynecologic Diseases

Gynecologic diseases, gynecologic cancers in particular, deserve special mention as a preventive ethics topic in gynecologic practice. This is because gynecologic cancers can place the social-role interests of the female patient vitally at stake. For example, surgical management of bilateral ovarian or uterine cancers entails loss of reproductive capacity, which may affect subjective and deliberative interests. Gynecologists should be especially sensitive to this often unappreciated ethical dimension of gynecologic cancers. Step 3 of the informed consent process, for example, can result in the patient having to confront the implications of serious gynecologic disease for her subjective and deliberative interests. Some patients may therefore struggle at first with Steps 4–7 and the physician may be asked for assistance with them.

Sometimes there will be a clear-cut net benefit of a clinical management strategy, with all others only on balance not protecting or promoting the social-role interests of the female patient. This should be recommended in Step 8. An example is surgical management for carcinoma *in situ* of the cervix. At other times there will be a range or continuum of reasonable alternatives and Step 8 should be a recommendation of a choice among these alternatives. An example is surgery versus radiation therapy for Stage I carcinoma of the cervix.

This last point is important in situations where the physician has a strong preference among such a range or continuum of alternatives, for example, for surgical management rather than radiotherapy for cervical cancer Stage I. Failing to recommend the full range of reasonable alternatives by recommending only the one favored sets up the unwitting physician for unnecessary and totally avoidable ethical conflict. One needs to beware of illegitimate monetary self-interest as an influence on what is recommended in such cases.

It is also important to appreciate that with progressive, ultimately terminally gynecologic diseases, especially cancers, the logic of beneficence-based clinical judgment can change over time. This has important implications for recommendations that are ethically justified in step 8 of the informed consent process. Aggressive management in its early stages, for example, the first debulking surgery for ovarian cancer, usually confers more than minimal benefit on the female patient by preventing premature and unnecessary death, because the iatrogenic burden of aggressive management is usually not great or severe. Thus, it is ethically justified to recommend aggressive management as an initial response to gynecologic cancers. Over time, however, the iatrogenic burden of aggressive management, for example, experimental trial of chemotherapy for advanced ovarian malignancy, may increase, such that the benefit to be expected is only minimal. When this is the case, the recommendation should be for a choice between aggressive and nonaggressive management. As the disease progresses still further, the physician must be open to the possibility that continued aggressive management confers no benefit on the patient. The patient's imminent death cannot be prevented and iatrogenic burden of aggressive management increases. In such circumstances, the physician should point out that further aggressive management is now reliably thought to be futile in curing the patient's disease, for example, failure of surgical and chemotherapeutic management for advanced ovarian cancer. Finally, when aggressive management is not beneficial and when the burden of iatrogenic disease, injury, handicap, pain, and suffering mount, aggressive management may be rightly viewed in beneficence-based clinical judgment as only harmful. In these circumstances, for example, severe and uncontrollable pain due to advanced ovarian malignancy after failure of surgery and chemotherapy, the physician should recommend against aggressive management of the underlying disease process.

This continuum of beneficence-based clinical judgment and recommendations applies directly to "last ditch" trials of therapy, especially various experimental therapies for gynecologic cancers. The physician must keep clearly in mind that experimental therapies, especially Phase 1 chemotherapies, cannot be represented as beneficial to the patient or the patient's surrogate, when the patient can no longer participate in the informed consent process. This is precisely what is not known. The main benefit, if any is established, will be to future patients. Thus, no recommendation for the use of such experimental therapy can be made. At most, such therapy can be offered to the patient or her surrogate.

Obviously, as recommendations are based on minimal or no benefit to the patient, or net harm to the patient, the role for the female patient's autonomy increases. These are serious matters, in response to which the female patient needs to form her deliberative interests with care. Patients may welcome assistance in this process and so it should be offered to them, in particular, the opportunity to talk to other patients and their families.

It is crucial in all cases of terminal disease that will be allowed to take its course without aggressive response for the physician to identify and act upon ethical obligations to the dying patient. Of these, the beneficence-based obligation to prevent unnecessary pain and suffering is paramount. Patients should be thoroughly informed about aggressive pain management, including self-administered narcotic analgesia. That such medication might be addicting is ethically irrelevant in the case of dying patients, because whatever handicap that might result is worth the relief of pain and suffering. Furthermore, working with each female patient to help her achieve effective pain relief is a powerful preventive ethics strategy for avoiding the ethical conflict of physician-assisted suicide.

Physician-assisted suicide involves the physician in either providing the means that the competent patient uses to kill herself or, when she is unable to do so, administering those means oneself. In the first case the beneficence-based prohibition against killing is threatened, while in the second case it is violated. Is either ethically justified?

In our view, physician-assisted suicide will arise mainly in rare cases in which effective pain relief cannot be achieved or can be achieved only with effects on mental status that the female patient disvalues. In such circumstances, it seems that patients may well have a negative right to be left alone to kill themselves, to avoid a dying process that they reasonably judge to be unacceptable. It is less clear that patients have a positive right to obligate their physicians to act in ways that threaten or violate the beneficence-based prohibition against killing. The latter consideration raises the issue of whether, as a matter of public policy, the intellectual and moral integrity of beneficence-based clinical judgment should be protected or sacrificed in these agonizingly difficult—though, fortunately, rare—cases. We believe that a prudent society should protect the integrity of beneficence-based clinical judgment, as a way to protect the general life-preserving orientation of medicine. It follows from this that, while there may be a right of such patients to commit suicide, there seems to be no compelling ethical obligation of physicians to assist them to do so and a beneficence-based obligation not to assist them to do so. Our beneficence-based prescription is no less weak than one based in nonmaleficence.

We close this section with a consideration of innovations in gynecologic surgery for the management of gynecologic diseases. As is usually the case in surgery and in contrast to pharmacologic therapy, innovations in surgery develop without formal peer-review mechanisms, for example, institutional protocols or FDA review and approval. Obviously, there are powerful economic incentives for gynecologic surgeons to master new techniques as they are introduced. This has been especially the case with the recent introduction of minimal site or laparoscopic surgery. Step 3 bears directly on the prevention of ethical conflict in this situation. The newness of the procedure should be explained to the patient, as well as benefits and risks that have been documented in the scientific literature. If no such documentation exists, this should be explained to the female patient. The physician's own experience with the procedure, including training on animal models and experience with other patients, should be disclosed. The benefits and risks that the physician's own patients have experienced should also be explained. The patient should also be informed about centers or physicians whose experience is much greater. In the absence of such disclosure, the exercise of the patient of her autonomy in steps 4–7 of the informed consent process becomes meaningless and is therefore ethically unacceptable. The virtue of self-sacrifice plays an important role in preventive ethics in this context, because it serves to blunt the effect of the physician's understandable—but potentially dangerous—interest in remuneration. Self-sacrifice also serves as an important antidote to self-aggrandizement in the form of charging surgical fees that are egregious. We condemn this practice. Patenting surgical procedures should be regarded as ethically unjustified for the same reason and because patenting procedures could place the social-role interests of patients in jeopardy.

Critical Care of the Gynecological Patient

The management of some gynecologic diseases is thought to benefit from critical care interventions, in particular, when those diseases become life-threatening. This assumption requires close examination.

Sometimes critical care intervention prevents the patient's death without setting back the social-role interests of the patient in a serious, far-reaching, and irreversible fashion. More frequently, however, such setbacks are the unavoidable, iatrogenic consequences of critical care intervention. When that is the case, the benefit of critical care intervention is not clear-cut. Indeed, it is highly uncertain. As critical care intervention continues, the balance of risk may come to *exceed* the benefit of preventing death, eliminating any beneficence-based obligation to continue critical care intervention. In most cases, therefore, critical care intervention should be seen as a *trial* of intervention, an attempt to use critical care interventions to then determine reliably if they can be expected, on balance, to protect and promote the interests of the patient. This fundamental feature of critical care should be explained to the patient in Step 3. In doing so, the physician should make clear to the patient the continuum of beneficence-based clinical judgment about aggressive management that we described in the previous section: from more-than-minimal benefit, through minimal and no benefit, to only harmful. Critical care management of seriously and terminally ill patients can often follow this pattern.

In Steps 4–7 the physician should work with the patient to help her identify, if she wishes, limits on critical care intervention. In Step 8 the recommendation should be for trial of critical care intervention with agreed-upon stopping rules, either autonomy-based that the patient articulates, for example, regarding her expected quality of life, or beneficence-based, for example, regarding unnecessary pain and suffering or futility. These are, to be sure, clinically complicated matters. However, given their inescapable impact on the patient's subjective and deliberative interests, these matters cannot adequately be accommodated within beneficence-based judgment alone. The physician who thinks and acts to the contrary sets up oneself for totally unnecessary ethical conflict.

Advance Directives

A particularly important dimension of informed consent in gynecologic practice involves what have come to be known as "advance directives." Spurred by the famous case of Karen Quinlan in New Jersey in 1976,[41] almost all 40 legislatures have enacted "living will" legislation and, in as many states, there is legislative or common law authority for durable power of attorney for health care.

The basic idea of an advance directive is that a patient, when autonomous, can make decisions regarding her medical management in advance of a time during which she becomes incapable of making health care decisions. The ethical dimensions of autonomy that are relevant here are the following:

1. a patient may exercise her autonomy now in the form of a refusal of life-prolonging interventions;
2. autonomy-based refusal, expressed in the past and left unchanged, remains in effect for any future time during which the patient becomes nonautonomous;
3. that past autonomy-based refusal should therefore translate into physician obligations at the time the patient becomes unable to participate in the informed consent process; and
4. in particular, refusal of life-prolonging medical intervention should translate into the withholding or withdrawal of such interventions.

The living will is an instrument that permits the patient to make a direct decision to refuse life-prolonging medical intervention in the future. The living will becomes effective when the patient is a "qualified patient," usually terminally or irreversibly ill, and is also not able to participate in the informed consent process. Obviously, terminally or irreversibly ill patients who are able to participate in the informed consent process retain their autonomy to make their own decisions. Some states prescribe the wording of the living will, while others do not. The physician should become familiar with the legal requirements in the physician's particular jurisdiction. Living wills, to be useful and effective, should be as explicit as possible. Thus, some have proposed addenda to them, such as the "Values History"[42] or the "Medical Directive."[43] The legal basis for the living will is the legal right of self-determination, the right of any competent adult to determine what shall be done to her body. A number of state courts have made it clear that this right extends to the refusal of both hydration and nutrition. The recent U.S. Supreme Court ruling in the famous *Cruzan* case is ambiguous about whether there is such a right based in the U.S. Constitution.[44] As a consequence, hospitals and other health care institutions have begun to reconsider the refusal of hydration and nutrition based on a living will. The reader should become familiar with those institutional policies that affect one's patients.

The concept of a durable power of attorney is that any autonomous adult, in the event that that person later becomes unable to participate in the informed consent process, can assign decision making authority to another person. The advantage of the durable power of attorney for health care is that it applies only when the patient becomes nonautonomous. It does *not,* as does the living will, also require that the patient also be terminally or irreversibly ill. However, unlike the living will, the durable power of attorney does not necessarily provide explicit direction, only the explicit assignment of decision making authority to an identified individual or "agent." Obviously, any patient who assigns durable power of attorney for health care to someone else has an interest in communicating her values, beliefs, and preferences to that person. The physician can play a facilitating role in this process. Indeed, in order to protect the patient's autonomy, the physician should play an active role in encouraging this communication process, so that there will be minimal doubt about whether the person holding durable power of attorney is faithfully representing the wishes of the patient.

The main clinical advantages of these two forms of advance directives are that they encourage patients to think carefully in advance about the refusal of medical intervention and that these directives, therefore, help to prevent ethical conflicts and crises in the management of nonautonomous patients and nonautonomous and terminally or irreversibly ill patients. Unfortunately, the use of advance directives is not as widespread as it should be. This may change as a result of the Patient Self-Determination Act of 1990. This federal legislation applies to all hospitals receiving medicine funds and to health maintenance organizations and took effect December 1, 1991.[45] They are legally obligated to notify patients on admission or enrollment of their legal rights about informed consent and advance directives.

The reader is encouraged to think of advance directives as powerful, practical strategies for preventive ethics and to encourage patients to consider them carefully, especially patients with gynecological diseases—particularly gynecological cancers—that could become or are life threatening. That is, for all patients with gynecologic diseases that could become life-threatening or that would take away the patient's ability to participate in the informed consent process, Step 8 should involve a recommendation that the patient acquaint herself with the living will and durable power of attorney and consider executing them according to the legal requirements in the relevant jurisdiction. The risks of not doing so should be explained: a decision may have to be made for the patient that might be different than what she would decide for herself or be made by individuals other than the one she might prefer to name. Not having advance directives is not benign for patients.

Conclusion

Because of possible differences among the social-role, subjective, and deliberative interests of the female patient, there is an inherent potential for ethical conflict in gynecologic practice. This is surely true of the topical areas addressed in this chapter. This potential is realized in clinical practice too frequently, in our view. The informed consent process, especially information disclosed in Step 3 and recommendations made in Step 8, is an underutilized clinical strategy to prevent ethical conflict and crisis in gynecologic practice. In this chapter we have attempted to provide concrete and comprehensive preventive ethics proposals for gynecologic practice. We turn to the same task for obstetric practice in the next chapter.

NOTES

1. Congregation on the Doctrine of the Faith, "Instruction on Respect for Human Life in its Origin and on the Dignity of Procreation," *Origins* 16 (1987):697–711. Usually known by its abbreviated Latin title, *Donum Vitae*. See Joseph Boyle, "The Roman Catholic Tradition and Bioethics," in B. Andrew Lustig, Baruch A. Brody, H. Tristram Engelhardt, Jr., and Laurence B. McCullough (eds.), *Theological Developments in Bioethics: 1988–1990* (Dordrecht, The Netherlands: Kluwer Academic Publishers, 1991), pp. 5–21.
2. H.J. Grossman (ed.), *Manual on Terminology and Classification in Mental Retardation* (Washington, D.C.: American Association on Mental Retardation, 1977).
3. Committee on Ethics, American College of Obstetricians and Gynecologists, "Sterilization of Women who are Mentally Handicapped," Technical Bulletin No. 63 (Washington, D.C.: American College of Obstetricians and Gynecologists, 1988).
4. Laurence B. McCullough, "The World Gained and the World Lost: Ethical Dimensions of Labelling the Mentally Retarded," in Loretta Kopelman and John Moskop (eds.), *Ethics and Mental Retardation* (Dordrecht, The Netherlands: D. Reidel Publishing Co., 1984), pp. 99–118.

5. See Ruth Mackin and Willard Gaylin (eds.), *Mental Retardation and Sterilization: A Problem of Competency and Paternalism* (New York: Plenum Press, 1981); and Loretta Kopelman and John Moskop (eds.), *Ethics and Mental Retardation*.

6. D.R. Mishell, Jr., "Contraception," *New England Journal of Medicine* 320 (1989):777–85.

7. Laurence B. McCullough, John Coverdale, Timothy Bayer, and Frank A. Chervenak, "Ethically Justified Guidelines for Family Planning Interventions with Female Chronic Mental Patients," *American Journal of Obstetrics and Gynecology* 167 (1992):19–25.

8. A.P. Schinnar, A.B. Rothbard, R. Kanter, and Y.S. Jung, "An Empirical Literature Review of Definitions of Severe and Persistent Mental Illness," *American Journal of Psychiatry* 147 (1990):1602–8.

9. See note no. 3.

10. See note no. 7.

11. E. Carmen and S.M. Brady, "AIDS Risk and Prevention for the Chronic Mentally Ill," *Hospital and Community Psychiatry* 41 (1990):652–57.

12. H.V. Grunebaum, V.D. Abernethy, E.S. Rofman, and J.L. Weiss, "The Family Planning Attitudes, Practices, and Motivations of Mental Patients," *American Journal of Psychiatry* 128 (1971):740–43; V. Abernethy, "Sexual Knowledge, Attitudes, and Practices of Young Female Psychiatric Patients," *Archives of General Psychiatry* 30 (1974):180–82; and John H. Coverdale and J. Aruffo, "Family Planning Needs of Female Chronic Psychiatric Outpatients," *American Journal of Psychiatry* 146 (1989):1489–91.

13. M.E. Casiano and D.R. Hawkins, "Major Mental Illness and Childbearing: A Role for the Consultation-Liaison Psychiatrist in Obstetrics," *Psychiatric Clinics of North America* 10 (1987):33–35; B. Rudolph, C.L. Larson, S. Sweeny, E.E. Hough, and K. Adrian, "Hospitalized Pregnant Psychotic Women: Characteristics and Treatment Issues," *Hospital and Community Psychiatry* 41 (1990):159–63; and G. Wrede, S.A. Mednick, M.O. Hutteren, and C.G. Nilsson, "Pregnancy and Delivery Complications in the Births of an Unselected Series of Finnish Children with Schizophrenic Mothers," *Acta Psychiatrica Scandanavica* 62 (1980):369–81.

14. M.M. Weissman, E.S. Gershon, K.K. Kidd, et al., "Psychiatric Disorders in the Relatives of Probands with Affective Disorders: The Yale University-National Institute of Mental Health Collaborative Study," *Archives of General Psychiatry* 41 (1984):13–21; N.F. Watt, E.S. Anthony, L.C. Winn, J.E. Rolf (eds.), *Children at Risk for Schizophrenia: A Longitudinal Perspective* (Cambridge: Cambridge University Press, 1984); M.M. Silverman, "Children of Psychiatrically Ill Parents: A Prevention Perspective," *Hospital and Community Psychiatry* 40 (1989):1257–64.

15. L.J. Miller, "Psychotic Denial of Pregnancy: Phenomenology and Clinical Management," *Hospital and Community Psychiatry* 41 (1990):1233–37; T.F. McNeil, L. Kaij, and A. Malmquist-Larsson, "Women with Nonorganic Psychosis: Mental Disturbances During Pregnancy," *Acta Psychiatrica Scandanavica* 70 (1984):127–39; T.F. McNeil, L. Kaij, and A. Malmquist-Larsson, "Women with Nonorganic Psychosis: Pregnancy's Effect on Mental Health During Pregnancy," *Acta Psychiatrica Scandanavica* 70 (1984):140–48.

16. See note no. 7.

17. Ruth R. Faden and Tom L. Beauchamp, *A History and Theory of Informed Consent* (New York: Oxford University Press, 1986), pp. 237–41.

18. John H. Coverdale, J. Aruffo, and H. Grunebaum, "Developing Family Planning Services for Female Chronic Mentally Ill Outpatients," *Hospital and Community Psychiatry* 43 (1992):475–78.

19. See note no. 6.

20. Karen Lebacqz, "Sterilization: Ethical Aspects," in Warren T. Reich (ed.), *En-*

cyclopedia of Bioethics (New York: Macmillan, 1978), pp. 1609–13; and J.M. Friedman, "Sterilization: Legal Aspects," in Warren T. Reich (ed.), *Encyclopedia of Bioethics,* pp. 1613–18.

21. See note no. 14.

22. Warren T. Reich, "Life: Quality of Life," in Warren T. Reich (ed.), *Encyclopedia of Bioethics,* pp. 829–40.

23. Charles E. Curran, "Abortion: Contemporary Debate in Philosophical and Religious Ethics" in Warren T. Reich (ed.), *Encyclopedia of Bioethics,* pp. 17–26.

24. David M. Feldman, "Abortion: Jewish Perspectives," in Warren T. Reich (ed.), *Encyclopedia of Bioethics,* pp. 5–9; John R. Connery, "Abortion: Roman Catholic Perspectives," in Warren T. Reich (ed.), *Encyclopedia of Bioethics,* pp. 9–13; J.B. Nelson, "Abortion: Protestant Perspectives," in Warren T. Reich (ed.), *Encyclopedia of Bioethics,* pp. 13–17. See also B. Andrew Lustig, Baruch A. Brody, H. Tristram Engelhardt, Jr., and Laurence B. McCullough (eds.), *Developments in Theological Bioethics* (Dordrecht, The Netherlands: Kluwer Academic Publishers, 1991), *passim.*

25. Sydney Callahan and Daniel Callahan, *Abortion: Understanding Differences* (New York: Plenum Press, 1984); Daniel Callahan, "The Abortion Debate: Can this Chronic Public Illness be Cured?," *Clinical Obstetrics and Gynecology* 35 (1992): 783–91.

26. See Sherman Elias and George J. Annas, *Reproductive Genetics and the Law* (Chicago: Year Book Medical Publishers, 1987); and George J. Annas, "Protecting the Liberty of Pregnant Patients," *New England Journal of Medicine* 316 (1987):1213–14.

27. Mark I. Evans, John C. Fletcher, I.E. Zador, et al., "Selective First-Trimester Termination in Octuplet and Quadruplet Pregnancies: Clinical and Ethical Issues," *Obstetrics and Gynecology* 71 (1988):289–96; Y. Dumez and J.F. Oury, "Method for First Trimester Selective Abortion in Multiple Pregnancy," *Contributions to Gynecology and Obstetrics* 15 (1986):50–53; American College of Obstetrics and Gynecology, *Multifetal Pregnancy Reduction and Selective Fetal Termination: ACOG Committee Opinion 94* (Washington, D.C.: American College of Obstetricians and Gynecologists (April 1991); Ronald J. Wapner, G.H. Davis, A. Johnson, et al., "Selective Termination of Multifetal Pregnancies," *Lancet* 335 (1991):90–93; Richard L. Berkowitz, L. Lynch, U. Chitkara, et al., "Selective Reduction of Multifetal Pregnancies in the First Trimester," *New England Journal of Medicine* 318 (1988):1043–47; Mitchell S. Golbus, N. Cunningham, J.D. Goldberg, et al., "Selective Termination of Multiple Gestations," *American Journal of Medical Genetics* 31 (1988):339–48; John C. Hobbins, "Selective Reduction—A Perinatal Necessity?," *New England Journal of Medicine* 318 (1988):1062–63; Mark I. Evans, A. Drugan, S.F. Bottoms, et al., "Attitudes on the Ethics of Abortion, Sex Selection, and Selective Pregnancy Termination among Health Care Professionals, Ethicists, and Clergy likely to Encounter such Situation," *American Journal of Obstetrics and Gynecology* 164 (1991):1092–99; Richard M. Zaner, F.H. Boehm, G.A. Hill, "Selective Termination in Multiple Pregnancies: Ethical Considerations," *Fertility and Sterility* 54 (1990):203–5; Mark I. Evans, Y. Dumez, Ronald J. Wapner, et al., "Efficacy of Multifetal Pregnancy Reduction (MFPR): Collaborative Experience of the World's Largest Centers, *Society of Perinatal Obstetricians Abstracts* 164 (1990):225; and Christine Overall, "Selective Termination of Pregnancy and Women's Reproductive Autonomy," *Hastings Center Report* 20 (1990):6–11.

28. Mark I. Evans, John C. Fletcher, I.E. Zador, et al., "Selective First-Trimester Termination in Octuplet and Quadruplet Pregnancies: Clinical and Ethical Issues." More recently Fletcher and Evans state that "we are re-evaluating a position opposed to termination of all but one fetus." See John C. Fletcher and Mark I. Evans, "Ethics in Reproductive Genetics," *Clinical Obstetrics and Gynecology* 35 (1992):763–82.

29. See note no. 27.

30. Mark I. Evans, A. Drugan, S.F. Bottoms, et al., "Attitudes on the ethics of Abor-

tion, Sex Selection, and Selective Pregnancy Termination among Health Care Professionals, Ethicists, and Clergy likely to Encounter such Situation."

31. See notes nos. 28 and 30 and Richard M. Zaner, F.H. Boehm, and G.A. Hill, "Selective Termination in Multifetal Pregnancies: Ethical Considerations."

32. See note no. 28.

33. ibid., 295.

34. ibid., 294.

35. H. Tristram Engelhardt, Jr., *The Foundations of Bioethics* (New York: Oxford University Press, 1986).

36. See notes nos. 23, 24, and 25.

37. See note no. 31, 204.

38. William Ruddick and W. Wilson, "Operating on the Fetus," *Hastings Center Report* 12 (1982):10–14.

39. Christine Overall, "Selective Termination of Pregnancy and Women's Reproductive Autonomy," *Hastings Center Report* 20 (1990):6–11.

40. Mark I. Evans, Y. Dumez, Ronald J. Wapner, et al., "Efficacy of Multifetal Pregnancy Reduction (MFPR): Collaborative Experience of the World's Largest Centers."

41. *In re Quinlan,* 70 N.J. 10, 355 A.2d 647 (1976).

42. David J. Doukas, Steven Lipson, and Laurence B. McCullough, "Value History," in William Reichel (ed.), *Clinical Aspects of Aging,* 3rd. ed. (Baltimore: Williams and Wilkins, 1989), pp. 615–16; and David J.Doukas and Laurence B. McCullough, "The Values History: The Evaluation of the Patient's Values and Advance Directives," *The Journal of Family Practice* 32 (1991):145–51.

43. Linda Emanuel and Ezekiel J. Emanuel, "The Medical Directive: A New Comprehensive Advance Care Document," *Journal of the American Medical Association* 261 (1989):3288–93; and Ezekiel J. Emanuel and Linda Emanuel, "Living Wills: Past, Present, and Future," *Journal of Clinical Ethics* 1 (1990):9–19.

44. *Cruzan* v. *Director, Missouri Department of Health* 110 S.Ct. 2841, 2852 (1990).

45. The Patient Self-Determination Act of 1990 took effect December 1, 1991. It was part of the Omnibus Budget Reconciliation Act of 1990, Public Law 101–508, sec. 4207 and 4751.

6 | Preventive Ethics Topics in Obstetric Practice

More can be said about preventing ethical conflict in obstetric practice than was said in Chapter 4 about general strategies for preventing ethical conflict in clinical practice. In this chapter we therefore provide a more detailed account of the prevention of ethical conflict in obstetric practice. Our focus will primarily be on Steps 3 and 8 of the informed consent process, particularly whether recommendations are justified and, when they are, what they should be. Our approach will be to analyze topics pertinent to obstetric practice in terms of the framework for obstetric ethics set out in Chapter 3. On this basis we shall present arguments about whether and what recommendations may be made by the physician as part of the informed consent process.

Obstetric ethics concern two patients: the pregnant woman and the fetal patient. We will be concerned with the justification of recommendations regarding management that will protect and promote the interests of *both* patients. We will therefore consider the following topics: assisted reproduction; directive versus nondirective counseling for fetal benefit; routine offering of antenatal diagnosis; management of fetal anomalies; management of prematurity; HIV infection during pregnancy; and critical care obstetrics.

Assisted Reproduction

Assisted reproduction involves a variety of techniques, some of which do not necessarily involve physicians, for example, artificial insemination by donor. They will not be addressed in this book, inasmuch as they are primarily matters of public policy. Here we will consider two forms of assisted reproduction that are particularly ethically significant: in vitro fertilization and "surrogate" pregnancies. These topics have been addressed extensively in the bioethics literature.[1] Our framework for obstetric ethics permits us to address them concisely.

In Vitro Fertilization

We addressed the moral status of the in vitro embryo and its ethical implications for clinical practice in Chapter 3. There we argued that the in vitro embryo is a patient only if the woman into whose uterus it will be transferred confers upon it that status. This has important implications for Steps 3 and 8 of the informed consent process.

First, the woman must be informed, as part of Step 3, that the likelihood of a successful transfer is a function, to some extent, of the number of embryos that are transferred and that, the greater the number transferred, the greater the likelihood of a multifetal pregnancy. The latter piece of information is especially important, because, for women for whom the in vivo embryo is thought to possess significant independent moral status, there can be a moral risk of a multifetal pregnancy in the form of confronting a decision about whether to selectively terminate some fetuses to increase the likelihood of a successful pregnancy.

Second, any recommendation made in Step 8 about the particular number of in vitro embryos to be transferred should include discussion with the woman about several matters. The first is the morality of selective termination of a subsequent multifetal pregnancy, which the woman may find to be morally problematic. Additionally, because the in vitro embryo cannot reliably be thought in beneficence-based clinical judgment to possess independent moral status, no in vitro embryo has a claim on the physician to be transferred. Then too, medicine possesses no competence in beneficence-based clinical judgment to decide what number of children ought to issue from a pregnancy, as we argued in the previous chapter in the context of selective termination of multifetal pregnancies.

Third, no recommendation should be made in Step 8 about what to do with unused in vitro embryos, because their moral status as future possible patients is for the pregnant woman to decide. The recommendation should therefore be for the woman to decide whether unused embryos are to be preserved or discarded.

"Surrogate" Pregnancies

This topic has also been considered previously in Chapter 3. We argued there that the woman bearing the pregnancy is not a "surrogate"—this term is ethically misleading. If in vitro fertilization is also to be used, the number of embryos to be transferred is up to the woman who is attempting to become pregnant, not the female or male gamete donor. The informed consent process should thus make it clear to the woman that the decisions to be made are just like those of any other pregnancy. Obviously, Step 8 should be nondirective about whether the woman should undertake the pregnancy for others.

Directive Versus Nondirective Counseling for Fetal Benefit

In clinical practice directive counseling for fetal benefit involves one or more of the following: recommending against termination of pregnancy; recommending against nonaggressive management; or recommending aggressive management. Aggressive obstetric management includes interventions such as fetal surveillance, tocolysis, cesarean delivery, or delivery in a tertiary-care center when indicated. Nonaggressive obstetric management excludes such interventions. Directive counseling for fetal benefit, however, must take account of the presence and severity of fetal anomalies, extreme prematurity, and obligations to the pregnant woman.

The strength of directive counseling for fetal benefit of the viable fetus varies according to the presence and severity of anomalies. As a rule, the more severe the fetal anomaly, the less directive counseling should be for fetal benefit.[2] In particular, when there is "a very high probability of death as an outcome of the anomaly diagnosed or a very high probability of severe irreversible deficit of cognitive developmental capacity as a result of the anomaly diagnosed"[3] counseling should be nondirective in recommending between aggressive and nonaggressive management, but directive in recommending against termination. This is because, as we argued in Chapter 3, minimal beneficence-based obligations to such fetuses exist to provide aggressive obstetric management.

By contrast, when lethal anomalies can be diagnosed with certainty there are no beneficence-based obligations to provide aggressive management.[4] When such fetuses are dying patients the counseling should be nondirective in recommending between nonaggressive management and termination of pregnancy, but directive in recommending against aggressive management, for the sake of maternal benefit.

The strength of directive counseling for fetal benefit in cases of extreme prematurity of viable fetuses does not vary. In particular, this is the case for what we term just-viable fetuses, those with a gestational age of 24–26 weeks, for which there are significant rates of survival but also significant rates of mortality and morbidity.[5] These rates of morbidity and mortality can be increased by nonaggressive obstetric management while aggressive obstetric management may favorably influence outcome. Thus it would appear that there are substantial beneficence-based obligations to just-viable fetuses. This is all the more the case in pregnancies beyond 26 weeks gestational age.[6] Therefore, directive counseling for fetal benefit is justified in all cases of extreme prematurity of viable fetuses, considered by itself. Of course, such directive counseling is only appropriate when it is based on documented efficacy of aggressive obstetric management for each fetal indication. For example, such efficacy has not been demonstrated for routine cesarean delivery.[7]

The only possible link between the previable fetus and the child it can become is the pregnant woman's autonomy. Counseling the pregnant woman regarding the management of her pregnancy when the fetus is previable should be nondirective in terms of continuing the pregnancy or having an abortion, if she is unsettled about conferring the status of being a patient on her fetus. This is the ethical basis of the ethos of nondirective genetic counseling (before viability). If she does confer such status in a settled way, at that point beneficence-based obligations to her fetus come into existence and directive counseling for fetal benefit becomes appropriate for these previable fetal patients. Directive counseling against smoking, poor nutrition, and alcohol and other substance abuse is therefore justified. Just as for viable fetal patients, such counseling must take account of the presence and severity of fetal anomalies, extreme prematurity, and obligations owed to the pregnant woman.

For pregnancies in which the woman is uncertain about whether to confer such status, we argued in Chapter 3 that the fetus be *provisionally* regarded as a patient. This justifies directive counseling against behavior that can harm a fetus in significant and irreversible ways, for example, substance abuse, until the woman settles on whether to confer the status of being a patient on the fetus.

In particular, nondirective counseling is appropriate in cases of what we term near-viable fetuses, that is, those that are 22–24 weeks gestational age for which there are anecdotal reports of survival.[8] In the authors' view, aggressive obstetric and neonatal management should be regarded as clinical investigations, that is, a form of medical experimentation—not standard of care. There is no obligation on the part of a pregnant woman to confer the status of being a patient on a near-viable fetus, because the efficacy of aggressive obstetric and neonatal management has yet to be proven.

For viable fetal patients, then, recommendations in Step 8 are justifiably directive. Thus, the physician is justified in recommending against substance abuse and other forms of fetal neglect and abuse. Since family members, the spouse or partner in particular, may assist or even encourage fetal neglect or abuse, for example, by providing drugs to the pregnant woman, the physician's recommendations are justifiably directed to spouses and partners. This is because their relationship to the fetal patient, as we argued in Chapter 3, is primarily one of obligation, not freedom, to the pregnant woman and viable fetal patient. The management of fetal anomalies and prematurity will be considered in greater detail later in this chapter.

For previable fetuses Step 8 involves a recommendation that the pregnant woman decide the issue of whether the fetus is to be a patient or not. When she does, recommendations in Step 8 are justifiably directed to the protection and promotion of the fetal patient's social-role interests. Fetal neglect is a more serious matter early in pregnancy, for example, intrauterine growth retardation and the teratogenic and other effects of substance and alcohol abuse. Again, recommendations to protect the fetal patient should involve the spouse or partner, as well, for the same reasons that are set out just above.

Recommendations made in Step 8 should *not* be directive vis-à-vis possible termination of the previable pregnancy. Instead, the physician should be strictly *non*directive in this matter. This is because a decision by the pregnant woman to confer the status of being a patient on the previable fetus is *not* irrevocable before viability. If she does revoke such status and elects termination of her pregnancy, the previable fetus is no longer a patient. Because she is then the only patient, the woman's subsequent care is to be managed under gynecologic ethics, as explained in the previous chapter.

Routine Offering of Antenatal Diagnosis

Antenatal diagnosis is not recommended routinely in the United States. Whether as part of Step 8 antenatal diagnosis, both obstetric ultrasound and invasive genetic diagnosis, should be offered to all pregnant women is considered in this section.

Routine Obstetric Ultrasound

Whether every pregnant woman should have an ultrasound examination is probably the most controversial question in obstetric ultrasound today.[9] All would agree that ultrasound plays a central role in modern obstetric practice and that ultrasound examinations should be recommended when indicated[10] and performed with the woman's consent. The NIH consensus statement has proposed a number of specific indications for obstetric ultrasound.[11] Here we want to identify a new indication for obstetric ultrasound, prenatal informed consent for sonogram (PICS), and to defend it on the basis of an ethical analysis of existing clinical and scientific data regarding routine obstetric ultrasound.[12]

Unfortunately, the present debate about the use of obstetric ultrasound has been shaped by a dichotomy: examine all pregnancies[13] or examine only when indicated.[14] This way of thinking has obscured from view an important and reasonable middle ground. We will defend the view that the standard of care in obstetrics should include informing all pregnant women about the availability of this technology, including a thorough discussion of its advantages and disadvantages. In all cases in which pregnant women request an ultrasound examination it should be performed in a standard manner by appropriately trained personnel.[15] PICS, as a middle ground position on the use of obstetric ultrasound, enhances the autonomy of pregnant women and thus makes a significant contribution toward the goal of humanizing obstetric care.

Everyone would agree that there are advantages to routine obstetric ultrasound examinations done once, at about 18 weeks. It is well appreciated that dating a pregnancy based on menstrual history or early physical examination is notoriously unreliable.

Campbell, et al. have established that ultrasonic measurement of gestational age between 12 to 18 weeks to be superior to an optimal menstrual history in predicting the date of delivery.[16] Any improvement in gestational age assessment might well decrease the morbidity and mortality that accompany an expected premature or postmature birth. Although several age-independent modalities for the detection of intrauterine growth retardation have been described, if information is available concerning an accurate gestational age based on early ultrasound, the diagnosis and hence management of intrauterine growth retardation at a later age is facilitated.[17]

Major structural anomalies can be diagnosed by ultrasound at 18 weeks in the majority of cases.[18] This has the benefit of providing an adequate information base for the pregnant woman so that she can decide about the disposition of her pregnancy in a thoughtful way. While some women will choose to terminate a pregnancy when an anomaly is detected, others will continue to term. In these latter cases, outcome can be optimized by appropriate obstetric management and neonatal care. In addition one can prevent maternal psychological trauma from an unexpected anomalous birth.

There are other potential benefits in pregnancies going to term, such as the detection of multiple gestation or identification of a high risk group for placenta previa. The value of the information is it enables more thorough planning for the management of the pregnancy. In addition, in rare cases, an unexpected hydatidiform mole, other tumors, or fetal death could be detected which would greatly benefit a management plan.[19] There may also be the psychological benefit of increased bonding.[20]

In addition to the benefits just discussed there are thought to be harms associated with routine ultrasound. Some harms can occur when false positive or false negative ultrasound diagnoses are made. As all positive diagnoses should generate an appropriate referral, the false positive rate should be minimized.[21] Nevertheless, maternal anxiety may be caused in the interim. False negative diagnoses are an inherent risk of all diagnostic interventions. In the case of routine ultrasound, this risk can be minimized by adherence to well defined standards.[22]

Other potential harms conceivably might result from routine ultrasound. Kremkau has reviewed four mechanisms by which it is possible to theoretically implicate ultrasound in the causation of fetal anomalies: heat, cavitation, microstreaming, and radiation force.[23] The American Institute of Ultrasound in Medicine in its safety statement has assessed these theoretical beneficence-based harms and concluded that "the benefits to patients of the prudent use of diagnostic ultrasound far outweigh any potential risk."[24]

These beneficence-based harms might have influenced the thinking of the NIH consensus panel when it did not recommend routine ultrasound screening. Implicit in the analysis of the NIH consensus panel seems to be "*Primum non nocere*" or "first do no harm," or the principle of nonmaleficence.[25] This principle was discussed in Chapter 1.

This very narrow principle can be applied successfully to an analysis of routine obstetric ultrasound only under two assumptions. First, routine obstetric ultrasound will cause harms. Second, the harms assumed to be caused by routine ultrasound, even harms of very rare incidence, will outweigh any benefits, even those of great incidence. Therefore, routine obstetric ultrasound should not be performed.

This line of reasoning involves a serious error in medical ethics, discussed in Chapter 1, namely assuming that the principle of nonmaleficence is the primary means by which physicians should evaluate the harms and benefits of clinical intervention. After all, taken to its logical conclusion, "*Primum non nocere*" makes unethical virtually all of contemporary medicine, because the potential for harm cannot be eliminated. Instead, clinical judgment requires: (1) the balancing of harms versus the benefits gained; (2) the recognition that in many circumstances, the benefits outweigh the harms; and (3) the recognition that there is an important role for how the patient weighs benefits against harms when there is clinical uncertainty about how to do so. These three ethical dimensions of clinical judgment pertain to obstetric ultrasound. Therefore we require an expanded, more nuanced ethical analysis, which employs beneficence and respect for autonomy. The implications of both principles must be taken into account in any adequate ethical analysis of routine obstetric ultrasound.

The application of the principle of beneficence to obstetric ultrasound requires the physician to balance benefits against harms, and not simply to avoid harm. One might be tempted to conclude that there is a beneficence-based justification for routine obstetric ultrasound, if one assumes that its benefits can be established. After all, established benefits at the present time outweigh harms, because the harms of false positive and false negative diagnoses can be minimized and the potential harms described by Kremkau may not ever be established.[26] The problem with this line of reasoning is that there is considerable uncertainty about whether the benefits of routine obstetric ultrasound have in fact been definitely established.[27] Elias and Annas' recent admonition that careful validation of the fact that benefits do outweigh harms of prenatal screening tests applies here.[28] Thus, even though there is some benefit to ultrasound screening, a decisive beneficence-based argument in favor of routine obstetric ultrasound cannot be established at the present time.

A beneficence-based argument against routine obstetric ultrasound fares no better. Such an argument must assume that the harms of routine ultrasound will outweigh any benefits (including new benefits that may be discovered in the future). That is, the harms outweigh the benefits of reducing fetal morbidity and mortality. However, the most that can be reasonably assumed at the present time is that some theoretical harms may outweigh some of the benefits. There is no way to know reliably at the present time whether, on balance, *all* of the harms will come to outweigh *all* of the benefits. Yet again, a beneficence-based ethical analysis of the clinical data fails to produce a decisive argument against routine obstetric ultrasound.

Given the absence of conclusive scientific data and the consequent failure of beneficence-based analyses to produce a decisive argument to resolve matters finally one way or the other, physicians can and do reasonably disagree about whether the benefits of ultrasound are worth the price of harms. In short, application of the principle of beneficence does not decide the question whether routine ultrasound should be part of obstetric care.

To subsequently conclude therefore that ethical analysis has nothing to contribute to clinical judgment until more data are collected and analyzed is a mistake for two reasons. First, it assumes that clinical judgment should be based only on the principle of beneficence—in other words, prove that routine ultrasound does not cause harm, or on balance produces a benefit. This is a radically incomplete approach to medical ethics and therefore to an analysis of clinical judgment because it ignores altogether the ethical principle of respect for autonomy.[29] It is for this reason that we find the recent analysis of Ziskin incomplete, because of the exclusive reliance on prudence, which relies only on nonmaleficence and beneficence.[30]

Second, the above conclusion is mistaken because some of its proponents assume that pregnant women are incapable of making the reliable calculations of the reasonable balance of goods versus harms in the absence of conclusive scientific information. The authors can find no scientific evidence to support this view. To the contrary, asking patients to make such calculations is a necessary part of good clinical care because of the rarity of conclusive scientific evidence about so many aspects of clinical judgment and care. Patients may not be qualified to undertake the technical and scientific judgments that we have revealed above, but they are capable of determining whether potential benefits outweigh theoretical harms in the formation of their deliberative interests.

So far our ethical analysis has shown that the principle of nonmaleficence is irrelevant to routine obstetric ultrasound and that the principle of beneficence leads to uncertainty. As a consequence, the interests of the pregnant woman cannot be well determined from a clinical perspective. In such circumstances, it is reasonable to rely on the ethical principle of respect for autonomy to manage clinical uncertainty. The justification for this conclusion is twofold. First, the beneficence-based uncertainty about the balance between harms and benefits of routine ultrasound means that the pregnant woman does not violate present or future beneficence-based obligations to the fetal patient if she decides to have an ultrasound. Conversely, in the absence of the indications identified by the NIH consensus panel,[31] a pregnant woman's decision not to have ultrasound screening does not place the fetal patient at risk for harm. In short, the pregnant woman who decides to have an ultrasound as a routine part of her prenatal care or who refuses ultrasound in the absence of other indications, acts in a way that is not inconsistent with present or future beneficence-based obligation to the fetal patient. The pregnant woman thus confronts no ethically significant constraint on the exercise of her autonomy regarding the use of ultrasound.

Second, the principle of beneficence is properly accented in clinical judgment in those cases in which there is a clear balance of benefits over harms or vice versa. In cases where the balance is uncertain, however, the principle of beneficence necessarily loses this force. Therefore, the principle of respect for autonomy properly becomes the overriding consideration for the physician. This is simply a logical feature of the ways in which the two ethical principles shape clinical judgment, as pointed out in Chapter 4. Making clear this often poorly understood ethical dimension of clinical judgment, in conjunction with the above argument, leads necessarily to the following conclusion: pregnant women should be allowed to choose for themselves whether ultrasound should be a routine part of their obstetric care.

The informed consent process, described in Chapter 4, is the means for implementing the clinical strategy of prenatal informed consent for sonogram (PICS) with every pregnant woman. PICS should be undertaken in several stages, following the description of informed consent in Chapter 4. As part of Step 3, shortly after the pregnancy is diagnosed, every pregnant woman should be provided with information about the actual and theoretical benefits of obstetric ultrasound and about its harms. The pregnant woman should be provided an opportunity to evaluate this information in terms of her own values and beliefs, something every autonomous patient is qualified to do (Steps 4–7). It may be helpful to some women to consider, at this point in the process, the physician's scientific evaluation of the clinical data that have been reported in the literature. Step 7 in PICS is for the pregnant woman to articulate her preference regarding the use of ultrasound in the management of her pregnancy. Step 8 is for the physician to provide the pregnant woman with the physician's own recommendation, if the physician has one. Step 8 involves a thoughtful and sensitive discussion of any disagreement that may emerge. The woman should then make her final decision. This decision should then determine the use of obstetric ultrasound for that pregnant woman. This process provides a significant role for the physician's clinical judgment and experience, as well as any recommendation the physician thinks is in the patient's best interest. Thus, respect for the pregnant woman's autonomy does not devalue the physician's role to that of an automaton.

The authors are aware that PICS may fail the test of a cost-benefit analysis, were it possible to undertake one. Some might object that we are therefore proposing the addition of one more possibly wasteful and probably expensive procedure to the obstetrical armamentarium. This involves the much larger problem of excluding entire categories of medical intervention for which cost-benefit data are not available. This macro-level problem of bioethics and public policy must be resolved through democratic institutions of self-government in our society. The authors are not alone in believing that there is no political consensus for placing rigorous cost-benefit restrictions on health care in the United States. In the absence of such a consensus, it is arbitrary to single out any particular intervention for restriction. It may also be unjustified in the case of PICS because of the negative impact on the exercise of autonomy by pregnant women. Unjustified economic restraints on pregnant women could seriously dehumanize obstetric care and further restrict in an arbitrary way the access of pregnant women to abortion for serious fetal anomalies.

Routine Invasive Genetic Diagnosis

Chromosomal abnormalities are among the most common genetic abnormalities. Autosomal trisomies are often seen in live born neonates while aneuploidies commonly lead to fetal loss. There is a linear correlation between maternal age and the incidence of chromosomal abnormalities. Amniocentesis for prenatal diagnosis has become a common procedure. With the advent of techniques to determine human karyotypes and the demonstration of the relative safety of obtaining amniotic fluid, analysis of cultured fibroblasts by cytogenetic techniques has proven to be a highly reliable, reproducible technique with minimal maternal and fetal risk. Chorionic villus sampling (CVS), either transcervical or transabdominal, has also proven to be reliable although some question of increased incidence of fetal loss and possible association with specific fetal abnormalities have been raised.[32]

Regardless of the controversy surrounding the type of procedure used, genetic diagnostic procedures to determine fetal karyotype are regularly offered to pregnant women who are 35 years and older or who have a medical history giving them greater risk for conceiving a fetus with an abnormal karyotype, a practice that has become the standard of care in the obstetric community. These procedures are offered as diagnostic procedures only and no assumption is made as to the course the patient will follow once a diagnosis of abnormal fetal chromosomal complement is made.

Essential to the discussion of this procedure is the provision of information to the patient in Step 3 of the informed consent process, so that the woman can make an informed decision as to what options she and her family would have if an abnormality were detected. This information would include the following. A degree of mental retardation is universal in trisomies. Other chromosomal abnormalities exhibit a wide spectrum of expression. For example, some patients with Turner syndrome XO may have a normal lifestyle, while some with an XXY karyotype may have an increased chance of future societal and/or psychological problems. Obviously, the informed consent process requires that all options be presented to the patient, including continuation of the pregnancy and assistance with planning for the future, and pregnancy termination.

Because of the potentially profound impact that children and adults with chromosomal abnormalities may have on the family, knowledge of fetal karyotype could be an important influence on a pregnant woman's decision about the disposition of her pregnancy. As a consequence, one investigator, Druzin, made a decision to routinely offer genetic diagnosis, primarily amniocentesis, to all patients in a private obstetric practice.[33] The following items were discussed with each patient in a nondirective manner:

1. the age-related risk of chromosomal abnormalities;
2. the risk of fetal loss with amniocentesis, quoted as 1:200 procedures;
3. the variability of expression of chromosomal aberrations in liveborns, though the uniformity of some degree of mental retardation for trisomies was mentioned;
4. the likelihood of not being reimbursed by commercial third party payor for this procedure and an approximate out-of-pocket cost of $600–1,200; and
5. the necessity for formal genetic counseling by a certified genetic counselor if this procedure was contemplated.

No procedure was performed without this counseling.

This study documents the routine offering of genetic diagnosis to a low-risk population in a private practice setting. The ethical dimensions of the practice involve (1) whether patients are able to resist the "technological imperative," (2) how this strategy enhances the autonomy of pregnant women, (3) whether the likely increased loss of pregnancies that would accompany this practice can be ethically justified, and (4) whether the expected increase in abortion that would follow the adoption of such a practice is ethically troublesome.

Routine offering of genetic diagnosis to this population resulted in a high rate of rejection (77.5%) of the procedure. This rate of rejection is ethically significant; it indicates that offering genetic diagnosis to a low risk population does not appear to be inherently psychologically coercive. If doing so were coercive, one would expect to see a far lower rate of rejection. This population of women, for whatever reasons, resisted the so-called "technological imperative." The commonly voiced concern in the bioethics literature that patients will accept whatever their physicians offer in the way of "high-tech" medicine is not supported by these data. This implies that the routine offering of genetic diagnosis to pregnant women should not be expected to impair their autonomy.

This strategy enhances the autonomy of pregnant women, because it provides access to genetic information that they would otherwise not have. This information is, in effect, denied by the present practice of only offering genetic diagnosis when indicated. Providing patients with information increases the range of alternatives known to them. Doing so is widely acknowledged in the bioethics literature as an autonomy-enhancing strategy. This will especially be the case for new tests and information generated by genome research. There may be attempts to rank-order what information should be part of offering and performing genetic diagnosis. Inevitably, such attempts will wind up appealing to one of two ethically unjustified grounds: either that the fetus is always a patient or that it has independent moral status. Because such grounds fail, only autonomy-based criteria for what information should be tested for and acted on are ethically justified. Any attempt to restrict access to offering or performing genetic testing must defeat this autonomy-based consideration or be considered defective. This has important implications for ethics and policy research that will be funded by the federal government.

There was no loss of pregnancy secondary to amniocentesis in this group. There most likely would have been in a larger study. Some might object to this offering of genetic diagnosis to a low-risk population on the grounds of beneficence. The argument would be that offering an unindicated procedure would result in avoidable loss of pregnancies. Such an argument assumes a balancing of goods over harms in favor of the risk of birth with an anomaly over the risk of a procedure-related death. This is a beneficence-based argument applied to the previable fetus. This line of argument makes the further assumption that the previable fetus is always a patient, that is, always the proper object of beneficence-based clinical judgment. But, as we argued in Chapter 3, this claim is unsupportable. It follows that a beneficence-based objection to routine offering of genetic diagnosis to pregnant women has no force and therefore can be set aside. In other words, the expected increased loss of pregnancies is ethically justifiable.

Routinely offering genetic diagnosis to pregnant women should be expected to increase the rate of abortion for fetal anomalies. This will be seen by some as ethically objectionable. Such a view rests on two assumptions, neither of which can be sustained.

The first assumption is that the fetus possesses independent moral status. For reasons set out in Chapter 3, this cannot be regarded as an ethically valid assumption.

The second assumption is that there are substantial beneficence-based obligations to the previable fetus to avoid unnecessary harm. Obviously, abortion would constitute such a harm. The problem with this line of reasoning is that it assumes that the previable fetus is always a patient, that is, the proper object of beneficence-based clinical judgment. As pointed out above and in Chapter 3, this claim is unsupportable. Because objections to the increased rate of abortion that would probably follow routine offering of genetic diagnosis can be successfully set aside, that increased rate of abortion is not ethically troublesome.

Routinely offering amniocentesis to a low-risk population may fail a test of cost-benefit. If so, some might object that we are proposing one more wasteful and expensive procedure. The ethical issues here involve the much larger problem of excluding, on cost-benefit grounds, an entire population of low-risk patients who, with informed consent, elect genetic diagnosis. This problem must be resolved through the democratic process in our society. We are not alone in our belief that there is no political consensus for placing cost-benefit restrictions on specific issues in health care, especially when the practice in question involves no psychological coercion, enhances the autonomy of pregnant women, involves an ethically justified likely increased loss of pregnancies, and is not ethically troublesome vis-à-vis the abortion controversy. In the absence of such a consensus it appears arbitrary to single out for restriction routine offering of genetic diagnosis to a low-risk population. Moreover, doing so would have a negative impact on the autonomy of pregnant women, which would contribute to the dehumanization of obstetric care.

This study chronicled a population of private patients. For so-called "clinic" patients, there might well be significant financial obstacles encountered in attempting to offer and to perform genetic diagnosis in a low-risk population. The ethical issue here concerns the horizontal allocation of resources, that is, access to health care. The President's Commission on Ethical Issues in Medicine and Biomedical and Behavioral Research took the view that there is a societal obligation to provide universal access to a decent minimum of health care.[34] Because there are no beneficence-based objections to this health care, and because it enhances the autonomy of pregnant women, perhaps the routine offering of genetic diagnosis to pregnant women should be considered part of the decent minimum health standard.

It follows from the ethical considerations that both obstetric ultrasound and invasive genetic diagnosis should routinely be offered to pregnant women as part of the informed consent process described in Chapter 4. These techniques, obviously, should only be performed by qualified physicians and technicians. It goes without saying that genetic diagnosis requires access to qualified laboratory personnel and facilities. Because there is no entailment that antenatal diagnosis itself leads to abortion in all cases, there are no plausible private conscience objections to routinely offering antenatal genetic diagnosis.

Gender Identification

There is considerable controversy surrounding the use of antenatal diagnosis to identify fetal gender.[35] There seems to be strong consensus against doing so.[36] This view cannot be sustained, for the following reasons.

First, the worry seems to be mainly that pregnant woman will prefer male to female offspring and that this will constitute invidious discrimination. But this assumes that the previable fetus always has a right against such discrimination, that is, that it is a person or at least possesses independent moral status. As we showed in Chapter 3, this assumption is groundless. The worry that sex selection would encourage sexual discrimination in society at large is purely speculative. Second, it is objected that gender is not a disease. This is a tautology. The connection between this tautology and the ethical claim that gender identification for its own sake is unjustified is typically left unexplained, as though the connection were self-evident.[37] But it is not self-evident, because this connection is solely beneficence-based. In other words, proponents of this view are in effect taking the position that the presence of a fetal disease or anomaly is the only justification for an abortion. Therefore, abortion for gender identification is frivolous, because there could be no good reason for it. But, this view holds only if one ignores, without argument, autonomy-based considerations. That is, opposition to fetal gender identification for its own sake without an explicit treatment of autonomy-based considerations can only result from a defective approach to obstetric ethics.

This approach also makes the implicit assumption that abortion for gender reasons is not a good enough reason for any physician to perform an abortion. Again, only two assumptions, both unsupportable, sustain such a view: either the fetus possesses independent moral status or is always a patient. Ultimately all objections to fetal gender identification rest on one or both assumptions and so those objections in all cases fail.

Recall from Chapter 3 that the pregnant woman is free to confer, withhold, or having once conferred withdraw the moral status of being a patient on or from the previable fetus. The force of our argument is that whether the previable fetus is a patient or not is a function of the explicit exercise of the pregnant woman's autonomy. Coercion of her choice in any form, as may be the case in some parts of the world, is never justified and we condemn such coercion. Imputing exercise of autonomy to establish that the previable fetus is a patient as an implicit commitment of seeking prenatal diagnosis is therefore not ethically justified. Instead, seeking prenatal diagnosis involves suspension or postponement of a decision to confer such status, pending the woman's evaluation of the results. In short, autonomy-based considerations are decisive in the ethical justification of gender identification.

There may be advantages to gender identification. Principal among these will be giving the patient's spouse or partner time to adjust to the information and to accept it.[38] In this way, the patient can be protected from potential coercion, which is the ethically significant issue in gender identification. That is, the spouse or partner as a third party is bound by the obligation to respect the pregnant woman's autonomy. Physicians can play a useful and important role in this regard.

Again, since gender identification may be followed by abortion, there are plausible grounds for objection in private conscience to abortion on the basis of gender identification. Private conscience in such circumstances justifies referral for the abortion, or the antenatal diagnosis test. However, in offering routine antenatal diagnosis, the physician should ask the pregnant woman whether she wishes to learn the gender of her fetus(es), to the extent permitted by the diagnostic modality being considered.

Antepartum Management of Fetal Anomalies

Management of Fetal Anomalies

Recent advances in antenatal diagnosis permit the detection of a wide variety of fetal anomalies.[39] Prior to viability, abortion is a legally available option, according to the U.S. Supreme Court in *Roe* v. *Wade*,[40] in *Webster* v. *Reproductive Health Services*,[41] and in *Casey* v. *Planned Parenthood of Southeastern Pennsylvania*.[42] After 24 weeks, however, termination of pregnancy is difficult to obtain for a variety of reasons. Moreover, the medical profession has begun to focus on therapeutic aspects of fetal anomalies detected during the third trimester. As a consequence, the concept of the third trimester fetus as a patient has emerged.[43]

At first glance, it would appear to follow from the fetus being a patient that the physician should, after discussing available management strategies, always recommend to the pregnant woman aggressive management of any pregnancy in which fetal anomalies are detected during the third trimester. On closer analysis of the physician's and the pregnant woman's ethical obligations to the viable fetal patient, however, the ethical obligations owed to the fetus are heterogenous, not homogeneous, in character, as discussed generally in the section above, on directive versus nondirective counseling for fetal benefit. Here we provide a clinically comprehensive management strategy for third trimester pregnancies complicated by fetal anomalies. First, we describe the disclosure requirements of Step 3 of the informed consent process. Second, we identify the range of recommendations regarding the management of pregnancy that are justified in Step 8 of the informed consent process by the continuum of ethical obligations owed to the third trimester fetus. We do so in terms of the results of a recent study.[44] (See Tables 6–1 and 6–2.)

The disclosure requirements of the informed consent process are based on those aspects of respect for the autonomy of the pregnant woman that were shown in Chapters 1 through 3 not to involve areas of conflict. Those aspects included respect for the integrity of the pregnant woman's values and beliefs and the obligation to elicit her subjective-interests-based and deliberative-interests-based preferences. The latter obligation cannot be fulfilled if the pregnant woman lacks adequate information. This is especially the case for the formation of her deliberative interests, as explained in Chapter 1. Respect for the autonomy of the pregnant woman thus ethically obligates the physician as part of Step 3 of the informed consent process to disclose information about the range of available management alternatives: aggressive management; nonaggressive management; and termination of pregnancy during the third trimester. (See Table 6–1.) The pregnant woman should be apprised frankly about the very limited access in the United States to termination of pregnancy during the third trimester. These disclosure requirements obligate the physician to be objective in the presentation of this information. That is, the physician is not justified in withholding information about available management alternatives to which the physician might object for reasons of private conscience.

The second part of the proposed clinical management strategy involves the continuum of ethically justified recommendations that the physician

Table 6-1 Summary of Management Recommendations and Actual Management of 72 Fetal Anomalies Diagnosed During the Third Trimester

	Aggressive Management Performed	*Nonaggressive Management Performed*	*Termination of Pregnancy Performed*	*Total*
Aggressive management recommended	49	1	1	51
Aggressive management and nonaggressive management offered	2	13	3	18
Nonaggressive management and termination of pregnancy offered	0	1	2	3
Total	51	15	6	72

Table 6-2 Classification of Fetal Anomalies by Degree of Probability of Antenatal Diagnosis and Degree of Probability of Outcome

Category	*Probability of Antenatal Diagnosis*	*Probability of Death or Absence of Cognitive Developmental Capacity*	*Example*
A	Certainty	Certainty	Anencephaly
B	Certainty	Very high probability	Trisomy 18
B	Very high probability	Certainty	Renal agenesis
B	Very high probability	Very high probability	Thanatophoric dysplasia
C	Less than very high probability	Very high probability or certainty	Lissencephaly
C	Very high probability or certainty	Less than very high probability	Isolated hydrocephalus
C	Less than very high probability	Less than very high probability	Achondroplasia

should make as part of Step 8 of the informed consent process. This is because the ethically significant features of fetal anomalies are that the degree of probability of the diagnosis varies and the outcomes of fetal anomalies vary. (See Table 6–2.)

The authors interpret this clinical continuum in terms of a general approach to obstetric ethics that incorporates beneficence-based obligations to the third trimester fetus. There is a continuum of beneficence-based obligations to such fetuses: (1) from no beneficence-based obligations to the fetus; (2) through minimal beneficence-based obligations to the fetus; (3) to more than minimal beneficence-based obligations to the fetus. The criteria for these obligations and the recommendations that are consistent with these obligations will now be described. (See Table 6–3.)

The three cases in category A represent clear examples of when recommending alternatives to aggressive management is ethically justified, even when one regards the third trimester fetus as a patient. Anencephaly and triploidy are anomalies that can be detected with certainty.[45] These anomalies involve either immediate lethality or, in rare cases of short term survival, the absence of cognitive developmental capacity. The justification for recommending nonaggressive management will be described first, followed by the justification for recommending termination of pregnancy. (See Tables 6–2 and 6–3.)

Recommending nonaggressive management as an option is justified because it does not increase the already unavoidable risk of death: death is usually imminent and almost always inevitable in the immediate postpartum period. Recommending nonaggressive management as an option also does not increase the unavoidable risk of the absence of the capacity for cognitive development, because no such capacity exists for these anomalies. Because both survival and cognitive development are impossible to achieve, there is no beneficence-based obligation to the fetus to undertake medical interventions to prolong fetal life. No ethical principle obligates the physician to attempt the impossible. Thus, nonaggressive management in these cases is justified and can justifiably be recommended.

As a rule, termination of a pregnancy with no detectable anomalies in the third trimester causes a preventable death. This is a prima facie violation of a well understood beneficence-based obligation in clinical practice, to avoid unnecessary mortality for patients. However, the death of fetuses with anencephaly and triploidy is not preventable. Termination of the pregnancy therefore does not introduce death as a new outcome to the pregnancy; death is already in the prognosis with certainty. Because cognitive development is impossible in these cases, fetuses who survive in the short term postpartum period derive no benefit from medical inter-

Table 6-3 An Ethically Justified, Clinically Comprehensive Management Strategy for Third-Trimester Pregnancies with Fetal Anomalies Based on Beneficence-Based Obligations to the Fetus

Category	*Disclosure Requirements Regarding Management Alternatives*	*Beneficence-Based Obligations to the Fetus to Provide Aggressive Obstetric Management*	*Ethically Justified Management Recommendations*
A	All available management alternatives	None	Recommend a choice between nonaggressive management and termination of pregnancy
B	All available management alternatives	Minimal	Recommend a choice between aggressive management and nonaggressive management; recommend against termination of pregnancy
C	All available management alternatives	More than minimal	Recommend aggressive management; recommend against nonaggressive management and termination of pregnancy

vention to prolong life during the neonatal period, because they do not achieve independent moral status.[46] Preventing a future that holds no benefit for a patient does not harm the patient. Thus, beneficence-based obligations to a fetus with a lethal anomaly are not violated by termination of pregnancy. Therefore, recommending termination of pregnancy is consistent with the physician's beneficence-based obligations to the fetus.

The pregnant woman can also be understood to be bound by beneficence-based obligations to the third trimester fetal patient. Based on the immediately preceding ethical analysis, it is clear that the pregnant woman violates no beneficence-based obligations to a fetus with incurable lethal anomalies diagnosed with certainty if she elects nonaggressive management or termination of her pregnancy in the third trimester. Therefore, recommending a choice between termination and nonaggressive management of the pregnancy is consistent with the woman's beneficence-based obligations to the fetus.

To summarize the cases in category A, there is no beneficence-based obligation to the third trimester fetus to provide aggressive management since they involve pregnancies when there is (1) certainty of diagnosis; and either (2a) certainty of death as an outcome of the anomaly diagnosed, or (2b) in some cases of short-term survival, certainty of the absence of cognitive developmental capacity and nonachievement of independent moral status as an outcome of the anomaly diagnosed. (See Table 6–2.) Therefore, recommending a choice between nonaggressive management and termination of pregnancy is justified. When aggressive management contradicts beneficence-based obligations to the pregnant woman, it is justified to go further and recommend against aggressive management should a pregnant woman inquire about this option.

By contrast, for the cases in category B there are minimal beneficence-based obligations to the third trimester fetus to provide aggressive management because there is (1) a very high probability but sometimes less than complete certainty about the diagnosis and, either (2a) a very high probability of death as an outcome of the anomaly diagnosed, or (2b) survival with a very high probability of severe and irreversible deficit of cognitive developmental capacity as a result of the anomaly diagnosed. (See Table 6–2.) When these two criteria apply, both aggressive and nonaggressive management can be justified, from which it follows that a choice between aggressive or nonaggressive management, but not termination, can be recommended. (See Tables 6–2 and 6–3.)

The ethical justification of this approach to the management of pregnancies complicated by fetal anomalies meeting the above two criteria can be summarized as follows. There are some, but only minimal, beneficence-based obligations to the fetal patient to provide aggressive management of the pregnancy. Two main considerations support this conclusion. First, nonaggressive management prevents a course of neonatal intensive care that involves a high probability of potentially harmful and, in many cases, ultimately futile, intervention.[47] Second, medical intervention that results in severe and irreversible cognitive developmental impairment does not confer significant benefit on the infant, because achievement of independent moral status is highly improbable. Because beneficence-based obligations to the fetal patient are minimal in these cases, the pregnant woman does not violate her beneficence-based ethical obligations to the fetal patient by selecting nonaggressive management. Aggressive management is consistent with minimal beneficence-based obligations to the fetal patient, while termination of the pregnancy is inconsistent with those obligations.[48]

In category B, there were two cases in which the pregnant women elected aggressive obstetric management. While at first this may strike some as pointless, this clinical management is consistent with minimal beneficence-based obligations to the fetal patient and autonomy-based obligations to the pregnant woman. By contrast, the three cases in category B in which termination occurred are ethically troublesome. The uncertainty of ultrasound diagnosis of renal agenesis has been documented.[49] Thus, the criteria for no beneficence-based obligations to the third-trimester fetus cannot be satisfied. This is also the case for encephalocele with skeletal dysplasia, because of the absence of certainty about its prognosis. In such cases, the physician should recommend against termination of the pregnancy, because the criteria for category A cannot be satisfied. (See Tables 6–2 and 6–3.)

The anomalies in Category C do not fully satisfy either set of criteria for inclusion into categories A or B, because they have a prognosis following medical intervention of expected survival with no or manageable deficit of cognitive developmental capacity. (See Table 6–2.) Such fetuses can survive to later achieve independent moral status. Therefore, there are more than minimal beneficence-based obligations to such fetuses to provide aggressive obstetric management, because such medical intervention is reasonably expected to confer significant benefit. Aggressive management should not be recommended simply as one alternative among others, as if the others—nonaggressive management and termination of the pregnancy—were ethically justified alternatives. (See Table 6–3.) Rather, aggressive management should be strongly recommended, especially when necessary to persuade a hesitant or reluctant woman. The physician should recommend against nonaggressive management and termination of the pregnancy.

Some of the cases in categories B and C involved the administration of cephalocentesis.[50] Because of its very high fetal mortality rate this procedure is inconsistent with both minimal and more than minimal beneficence-based obligations to the fetal patient.[51] After all, these both include a prohibition against killing patients, as pointed out in Chapter 1. Thus it cannot be used without sufficient ethical justification, which is considered in the next section.[52]

There are three important limitations to our classification system. First, the lines drawn among the three categories should be understood to be thick and gray, not thin and red. This is because the ethical distinctions we have made occur along the continuum of beneficence-based obligations to the third trimester fetus, not between sharply defined break points. Obviously such matters are not to be understood as a simple trichotomy. In addition, even when a thorough fetal evaluation, including karyotyping,[53] is included, it should be recognized that the ability of antenatal diagnosis to determine prognosis is at times imperfect. Second, we will not be surprised—indeed we fully expect—that some readers may reasonably assign particular fetal anomalies to a category other than that we have proposed. In part, this is because we ourselves have potentially erred on the side of being sanguine about the prognosis for some anomalies. Those less sanguine will reach different judgments. For example, some may manage pregnancies complicated by trisomy 18 in terms of category A rather than in terms of category B. Third, gestational age at the time of diagnosis of some anomalies may be an important factor. Idiopathic nonimmune fetal hydrops diagnosed at a later gestational age, for example, 38 weeks, should be placed in category C because there is a possibility of survival, whereas such a diagnosis at 25 weeks[54] should be managed in terms of category B if delivery is imminent because there is little chance of survival.

Cephalocentesis

Cephalocentesis has long been accepted as a destructive procedure to avoid intrapartum morbidity and mortality when fetal hydrocephalus occurs with macrocephaly. This procedure performed either transabdominally or transvaginally saved maternal lives prior to the time of safe cesarean section.[55] Currently, obstetric ultrasound greatly facilitates this procedure by allowing simultaneous guidance of needle placement either transabdominally or transvaginally.[56] Needle placement is directed into the cerebrospinal fluid and enough fluid is drained to permit compression of skull diameters to pass through the birth canal. A 95 percent perinatal mortality has been associated with this procedure. However, if decompression is performed in a controlled manner, this mortality may be reduced by an unknown amount.[57]

It should be obvious that cephalocentesis, a potentially destructive procedure in a term fetus, requires careful justification in beneficence-based clinical judgment, to avoid its ethically unjustified use. Because fetal hydrocephalus presents with varied etiologies having varied outcomes, ethical analysis must be carried out by respecting the heterogeneity of this condition. Therefore, we will consider resolution strategies for two ends of a continuum: (1) isolated fetal hydrocephalus, and (2) fetal hydrocephalus with severe associated abnormalities (those incompatible with postnatal survival or those characterized by the virtual absence of cognitive function.) We then consider (3) fetal hydrocephalus with other associated abnormalities as a middle ground on the continuum. The ethical analysis of each of these will take place in the following steps. First, we will identify the beneficence-based and autonomy-based obligations of the physician to the pregnant woman and to the term fetus. Second, we will identify the sorts of conflicts that can occur among these obligations. Third, we will weigh these obligations against each other in an attempt to arrive at a well-argued priority among conflicting obligations.

Isolated Fetal Hydrocephalus

We begin our ethical analysis of isolated fetal hydrocephalus by noting that there is considerable potential for normal, sometimes superior, intellectual function for term fetuses with even extreme isolated hydrocephalus.[58] However, as a group, infants with isolated hydrocephalus experience a greater incidence of mental retardation and early death than the general population.[59] In addition, associated anomalies may go undetected and a fetus may be incorrectly diagnosed to have isolated hydrocephalus.[60]

There are compelling beneficence-based reasons for concluding that continuing existence of term fetuses with isolated hydrocephalus is in their social-role interest. The probability of mental retardation does not diminish the social-role interest of a viable fetus with isolated hydrocephalus in continuing existence, because it is impossible to predict which fetuses with isolated hydrocephalus will have mental retardation, and because the degree of mental retardation cannot be predicted in advance. Hence, isolated fetal hydrocephalus does not rule out later achieving independent moral status.

In light of this ethical analysis of the social-role interest of the viable fetal patient, the beneficence-based obligation of the physician to the term fetus with isolated hydrocephalus is to perform a cesarean delivery, because this clinical intervention clearly involves the least risk or mortality, morbidity, and handicap for the fetus as opposed to the alternative of cephalocentesis to permit subsequent vaginal delivery. Even when performed under maximal therapeutic conditions under sonographic guidance, cephalocentesis cannot reasonably be regarded as protecting or promoting the social-role interest of the at-term fetal patient in avoiding a death that would be both premature and unnecessary. This procedure is followed by a high rate of perinatal mortality, fetal heart-rate deceleration, and pathological evidence of intracranial bleeding.[61] As a consequence, cephalocentesis cannot reasonably be construed as an ethically justifiable mode of management, insofar as it is inconsistent with beneficence-based obligations to avoid increased mortality and morbidity risks for the fetal patient. Cephalocentesis, employed with a destructive intent is altogether antithetical to these beneficence-based obligations.[62] The risks of cesarean delivery to the pregnant woman's social-role interests are minimal. Therefore, for the management of isolated fetal hydrocephalus the physician should recommend, strongly, cesarean delivery as part of Step 8 of the informed consent process.

Hydrocephalus with Severe Associated Abnormalities

Some abnormalities that occur in association with fetal hydrocephalus are severe in nature for the child afflicted with them. We define "severe" abnormalities as those that either (1) are incompatible with continued existence, for example, bilateral renal agenesis[63] and cloverleaf skull with thanatophoric dysplasia[64] or, (2) although compatible with survival in some cases, result in virtual absence of cognitive function, for example, trisomy 18[65] and alobar holoprosencephaly.[66] Because there is no available intervention to prevent postnatal death in the first group, beneficence-based obligations of the physician and the pregnant woman to attempt to prolong the fetus's life are nonexistent. No ethical theory obligates anyone to attempt the impossible. For the second group, beneficence-based obligations of the physician and the pregnant woman to sustain the fetus's life are minimal. This is because the handicap imposed by the abnormality is severe. In these cases, the potential for cognitive development and therefore, the potential to promote the social-role interests of the child such a fetus can become, are virtually absent.

In these circumstances, the woman is released from her fiduciary role because no significant goods can be achieved by cesarean delivery for the term fetus or the child it will become. There remain only the autonomy-based and beneficence-based obligations of the physician to the pregnant woman. Following the preceding analysis of these obligations, we conclude that the physician's overriding moral obligations are to the pregnant woman's voluntary and informed decision. Because there are no weighty beneficence-based obligations to the fetus, the physician may therefore justifiably recommend cephalocentesis to enable vaginal delivery of such fetuses, as part of Step 8 of the informed consent process.

Hydrocephalus with Other Associated Abnormalities

On the continuum between the cases of isolated hydrocephalus and hydrocephalus with severe associated abnormalities, there is found a variety of cases of hydrocephalus associated with other abnormalities of varying degrees of impairment of cognitive and physical function. These range from hypoplastic distal phalanges[67] to spina bifida[68] to encephalocele.[69] Because these conditions involve varying prognoses, it would be clinically inappropriate and, therefore, ethically misleading to treat this third category as homogeneous. Therefore, the authors propose a working distinction between different kinds of prognoses.

The first we call "probably promising," by which we mean that there is a significant probability the child will experience cognitive development, with learning disabilities and physical handicaps that perhaps can be ameliorated to some extent. The second we call "probably poor." By this phrase, we mean that there is only a limited probability for cognitive development, because of learning disabilities and physical handicaps that cannot be ameliorated to a significant extent. We propose these definitions as tentative. Therefore, they are subject to revision as clinical and ethical investigation of such associated anomalies continues in the future. As a consequence, our ethical analysis of these two categories cannot be carried out as completely as those in the previous two sections. In essence, we propose that the clinical continuum in these cases is paralleled by an ethical continuum of progressively less weighty, beneficence-based obligations to the fetus.

When the prognosis is probably promising (for example, isolated arachnoid cyst[70]), there are serious beneficence-based obligations to the term fetus, because there is some probability that independent moral status can later be achieved. However, these are not necessarily on the same order as those that occur in cases of isolated hydrocephalus. (It has recently been suggested that any associated anomaly may increase the possibility of a poor outcome.[71]) Therefore, in cases with a prognosis of probably promising, the authors propose that the physician recommend cesarean section as part of Step 8 of the informed consent process, although perhaps not as vigorously as in cases of isolated hydrocephalus.

In cases when the prognosis, even though uncertain, is probably poor (for example, encephalocele[72]), beneficence-based obligations to the viable fetal patient are less weighty than those owed to the term fetus with a promising prognosis, because there is a low probability of later achieving independent moral status. Thus, these cases resemble ethically those of hydrocephalus with severe anomalies, with the provision that some, albeit limited, benefits can be achieved for the fetus by cesarean section and aggressive perinatal treatment. Thus, the recommendation of a choice between aggressive or nonaggressive management seems justified, as part of Step 8 of the informed consent process.[73]

Fetal Therapy Versus Fetal Experimentation

Fetal therapy is increasingly emerging as a response to the diagnosis of fetal anomalies. Whether invasive fetal therapy can be judged to be standard of care on ethical grounds depends on the clinical implications of the concept of the fetus as patient.[74] Recall from Chapter 1 that a human being is a patient when two conditions are fulfilled: (1) one is presented to a physician (2) for the purpose of applying clinical interventions that are reliably expected to protect and promote the interests of that individual—in the case of the fetal patient, its social-role interests.

Recall, now from Chapter 3, that (1) the previable fetus is a patient only when the pregnant woman confers that status upon the fetus and (2) the viable fetus is a patient only when the pregnant woman is obligated to present it for care. The pregnant woman is therefore under no ethical obligation to confer the status of being a patient on her previable fetus simply because there exists a fetal intervention that might protect and promote the interests of a previable fetal patient, because the fetus has such interests only when the pregnant woman confers the status of being a patient on it. Whether such fetal intervention is, on ethical grounds, to be judged standard of care for her previable fetus, and thus fetal *therapy,* is entirely a function of the pregnant woman's autonomy.

The same is true for fetal interventions on the viable fetus. This is because of a factual consideration—fetal therapy necessarily involves physical (and, perhaps, mental health) risks to the pregnant woman—and an ethical consideration—she is ethically obligated only to accept reasonable risks to herself in order to attempt to benefit her fetus.

The preceding helps to distinguish an ethical from a legal standard of care for fetal therapy. An ethical standard must take account not only of beneficence-based considerations applied to the fetus but also of both beneficence-based and autonomy-based considerations applied to the pregnant woman. A legal standard of care tends to focus on efficacy and safety, which are beneficence-based considerations applied to both the fetus and, perhaps, the pregnant woman. The legal standard of care tends to ignore autonomy-based considerations applied to the pregnant woman. This constitutes the fundamental differences between a legal and an ethical standard of care for fetal therapy.

Therapy for the Viable Fetus

There is no simple algorithm by which a pregnant woman—or her physician—can reach the judgment that she is obligated to accept risk to herself on behalf of her viable fetus. In the authors' view, such an ethical obligation—which should *not* be automatically equated with a legal obligation—exists when three criteria are satisfied. The first criterion concerns the outcome of the procedure for the fetus and its later achieving independent moral status. The other two criteria concern risks of harm for the viable fetus, as well as the pregnant woman. The three criteria are the following:

1. when invasive intervention on the viable fetus has a very high probability of being life-saving or of preventing serious and irreversible disease, injury, or handicap for the fetus;
2. when such therapy involves low mortality risk and low or manageable risk of serious and irreversible disease, injury, or handicap to the viable fetus;[75] and
3. when the mortality risk to the pregnant woman is very low and when the risk of disease, injury, or handicap to the pregnant woman is low or manageable.

The justifications for these criteria are both beneficence-based and autonomy-based. When the first two criteria are satisfied there is a clear and substantial net benefit to the viable fetus. When the third criterion is satisfied there is no clear and substantial net harm to the pregnant woman. Given the expected net benefit to the viable fetus and the low risk of harm to the pregnant woman, the latter are risks she should reasonably be expected to accept, for example, in the case of intravascular transfusion for severe isoimmunization. This moral fact shapes how she should exercise her autonomy in response to her beneficence-based fiduciary, ethical obligations to her viable fetus.

Under beneficence-based and autonomy-based clinical judgment, therefore, treatment of the viable fetus is warranted when these three criteria are satisfied. The burden of ethical proof seems to rest with those who would propose further ethical obligations when one or more of these three criteria cannot be satisfied. This should be a matter of further careful investigation and debate in the ethics of fetal therapy.

When the pregnant woman is ethically obligated to accept fetal intervention of her viable fetus, such management is ethically, not necessarily legally, judged to be standard of care. Any forms of fetal intervention for which an ethical obligation on the part of the pregnant woman to accept them cannot be established must be regarded as experimental. For example, because open abdominal fetal surgery involves risks that no pregnant woman can be understood, at this time, to be *obligated* to accept on behalf of an attempt to benefit her viable fetus, all such surgery must, on ethical grounds, be regarded as experimental. This would only change if the risks to the pregnant woman of such surgery someday satisfy the third criterion.

In the case of the viable fetus the physician is ethically justified in recommending invasive fetal intervention that meets the ethical standard of care, as part of Step 8 of the informed consent process. There is a vital role in this process for the exercise of the woman's autonomy in assessing the risks and benefits to herself and to her fetus. These matters should be explained carefully to the pregnant woman as part of Step 3 of the informed consent process. The benefits and risks of both invasive and noninvasive fetal intervention should be explained without bias, to the extent humanly possible, to the pregnant woman. She should be given time to reflect, to consult with those close to her or other physicians, and to reach her own decision.

Experimental therapy (that is, situations in which one or more of the above mentioned criteria are not satisfied) of the viable fetus can only be offered to the pregnant woman. That is, unlike the case of standard of care therapy, there is no ethical justification to *recommend* experimental fetal intervention because there is no clear net benefit to the fetus or there is a clear net harm to the pregnant woman. Moreover, experimental intervention can be offered with ethical confidence only if there is a formal, scientifically sound protocol for the research and that protocol has been approved by the appropriate institutional review process. In such circumstances, for the sake of future patients there may be an obligation to offer enrollment in trials. Obviously, discussion of experimental invasive fetal intervention with the pregnant woman should be rigorously nondirective.

Therapy for the Previable Fetus

There are two subgroups of previable fetuses. The first comprises those upon whom the pregnant woman has conferred the status of being a patient. When she has done so, and the above mentioned ethical criteria are also satisfied, it is ethically justified to recommend invasive fetal intervention. This situation is directly analogous to informed consent to therapy for the viable fetus and the strategies discussed above apply.

When the pregnant woman withholds or withdraws the status of being a patient from her previable fetus, the situation is directly analogous to experimental fetal intervention. This is so because there is no ethical obligation on the part of the pregnant woman or the physician to regard the previable fetus as a patient. It follows that any discussion of experimental invasive fetal intervention must be strictly nondirective.

The authors are aware that some physicians may take the view that a standard of care for fetal intervention that is based in large part on respect for the pregnant woman's autonomy is unrealistic, because of the strong, perhaps even coercive, psychological pressure pregnant women may experience when confronted with an imperiled pregnancy and the availability of invasive fetal interventions, therapeutic and experimental. To the contrary, the authors are well aware of such a phenomenon and have sought to address its main ethical implication, namely, the possible impairment of the exercise of the pregnant woman's autonomy. Indeed, our emphasis on the place and importance of nondirective counseling is meant precisely as the most powerful antidote to such impairment. In other words, there is no reason whatever to believe, and substantial ethical stakes in not acting on the belief, that such self-imposed, psychological pressure is in all cases irreversible and therefore irresistible. Physicians should beware the unjustified paternalism implicit in such a belief, because it can become a self-fulfilling prophecy, not a clinical observation.

Management of Prematurity

Recommendations concerning the management of prematurity differ. One set of recommendations is appropriate for prematurity after viability and another for "near viable" fetuses.

Prematurity of the Viable Fetus

Recommendations concerning the management of prematurity of the viable fetus find their basis in the more-than-minimal beneficence-based obligations to the viable fetal patient. Such obligations exist for two reasons. First, given access to level III neonatal care, there exists a range or continuum of management strategies that protect and promote the interests of the fetal patient to some degree and are thus variously in that patient's social-role interests. Second, also given access to level III neonatal care, there is less than a high probability of either premature death before the end of the neonatal period and less than high probability of near-term survival with severe central nervous system impairment. The latter is especially important, because it excludes as unreasonable the view that beneficence-based obligations to the viable fetal patient are only minimal.

It is presently believed that the beneficence-based interests of the viable fetus not at term are best protected and promoted by its remaining in utero. Tocolysis by various agents is believed to be an effective means to attempt to achieve this goal.[76] However, its efficacy is presently being challenged and there are significant beneficence-based risks for the pregnant woman in the use of tocolysis. There will be clinical situations in which tocolysis is justifiably recommended in Step 8 of the informed consent process, that is, when the risks of tocolysis to the pregnant woman are reliably thought to be outweighed by the potential benefits to the fetus. At the same time, because tocolysis can result in significant risk to the pregnant woman's social-role interests, informed refusal of tocolysis should be respected. This is because aggressive neonatal management, as described just below, following delivery protects and promotes the neonate's interests to a reasonable degree. Hence, refusal based on the woman's assessment of her wishes does not violate her fiduciary obligations to the fetal patient. This may not be the best alternative at, for example, 25 weeks gestational age, but it is, given the outcomes of aggressive neonatal management, still a good alternative for the fetal patient.

Cesarean delivery can be employed as part of the management of prematurity of viable fetal patients only on the basis of a reliable expectation that this mode of delivery will protect and promote the fetal patient's social-role interests. Given the uncertainty of outcomes from cesarean versus vaginal delivery of just viable fetuses, such a reliable expectation cannot be claimed at the present time, as we pointed out above (p. 199). Aggressive obstetric management cannot therefore be reliably expected to protect and promote the social-role interests of the viable fetal patient. Thus, the recommendation for management of the premature just-viable fetus should be a choice between cesarean delivery and vaginal delivery, followed by neonatal intensive care.

Aggressive neonatal management in a level III facility does provide, at least initially, for the protection and promotion of the neonatal patient's social-role interests. That this is the case at the beginning of neonatal care does not mean that it will remain the case throughout the course of such care. This is because neonatal care may become so burdensome that the infant's death is no longer unnecessary, although it will be premature. At this point, neonatologists should offer parents the choice between aggressive and nonaggressive neonatal management. That is, neonatal care, as a form of critical care, should be understood—as should all forms of critical care—as a trial of intervention to determine if continuing critical care will protect and promote the infant's social-role interests.

On the basis of the foregoing, for prematurity of viable fetuses after 24 weeks gestational age, the physician's recommendation in Step 8 of the informed consent process should be for aggressive neonatal management as a trial of critical care intervention. Such management should include transfer of the pregnant woman, if possible, to a level III facility, to protect and promote the viable fetal patient's interests.

Prematurity of the "Near-Viable" Fetus

Recommendations concerning the management of prematurity of the near-viable fetus, 22–24 weeks gestational age, find their basis in two factors. The first is the recognition that the near-viable fetus is a patient if and only if the pregnant woman confers that status on it, something she is not obligated to do, even in the case of prematurity. Hence, institution of tocolysis is solely the pregnant woman's decision. Second, there can be no reliable expectation that either aggressive obstetric management in the form of cesarean delivery or aggressive neonatal management will prevent premature death, inasmuch as present data are only anecdotal. Thus, both aggressive obstetric management and aggressive neonatal management of the "near-viable" fetus should be regarded as forms of fetal experimentation. There is no obligation on the part of the pregnant woman to authorize any fetal experimentation, as we argued above. In short, there are no beneficence-based obligations on the part of the pregnant woman or her physician to undertake to prevent stillbirth or death shortly after birth.

Thus, the recommendation in Step 8 of the informed consent process for the management of prematurity of the "near-viable" fetus should be for nonaggressive obstetric management, that is, vaginal delivery, and nonaggressive neonatal management. If the woman accepts this recommendation, neonatology should be involved, if at all, only as a consultant to the obstetrician, not to take over the care of the fetus/infant.

It is also permissible, though not ethically obligatory, to offer aggressive neonatal management as an experiment, provided the following conditions are met.[77] First, there are consulting neonatologists who are willing to conduct such an experiment. Second, these neonatologists are conducting such clinical research under a protocol that has approval of the institution's Institutional Review Board for research with human subjects. Third, that protocol should have very clear stopping rules. In particular, the role and authority, including sole authority, of the parents to stop research on their infant should be clearly spelled out. Fourth, all of this must be clearly and carefully explained to the parents at a level that insures their understanding—too much is at stake to accept "rough" understanding. Fifth, they should consent to such experimentation on their child.

HIV Infection During Pregnancy

HIV infection during pregnancy poses a number of ethical challenges to the physician in obstetric practice. These include whether a recommendation to terminate the pregnancy is ethically justified and whether to offer or recommend pharmacologic therapy to the pregnant woman that may pose risks for her fetus.

Not all pregnant women with HIV infection will transmit the virus to the fetus and the child it can become. Moreover, life expectancy for infants who are HIV+ exceeds that of other fetal complications, for example, trisomies 13 and 18, Tay-Sachs disease, and anencephaly. Before viability there is no compelling justification for recommending termination of the pregnancy in the latter sorts of circumstances. It follows that, as with any pregnancy, the pregnant woman should be informed about the alternatives for managing her pregnancy. Whether the previable fetus is to become a patient is, as we have consistently argued, a function of her autonomy. After viability, there is a strong beneficence-based prohibition against killing the fetal patient and so termination of pregnancy cannot be offered. Since the rate of transmission of HIV is not 100 percent and since HIV seropositivity in infants does not count as a lethal condition in the sense of this term used in our discussion of fetal anomalies, a recommendation of nonaggressive management cannot be justified either. In short, recommendations for the management of a pregnancy complicated by HIV infection of the pregnant woman should be the same as in any other pregnancy.

Prophylactic pharmacologic therapy may benefit the HIV-infected pregnant woman, by providing secondary prevention. At the same time, such pharmacologic agents pose uncertain levels of risk to the fetal patient and the child it will become. The CDC presently recommends that the use of such agents is "inadvisable."[78] Recently Minkoff and Moreno have criticized this position and have argued, instead, that pregnant women with HIV infection should be informed about the availability of pentamidine because "the risks presented to the fetus are . . . , at this time, highly uncertain."[79]

This conclusion is, we believe, insufficiently nuanced. Before viability, as we have argued just above, the pregnant woman who is HIV+ should be informed about the availability of abortion *in a strictly nondirective fashion*. She is free to exercise her autonomy regarding the disposition of her pregnancy as she sees fit, just as in any pregnancy. In particular, she is free to elect termination of her pregnancy before undertaking prophylactic drug therapy.

When the fetus is a patient, the ethical analysis is more complicated. The central question is this: Is the pregnant woman obligated to the fetal patient (and the child it will become) to undertake the risks of not taking prophylaxis in order to benefit the fetal patient by not subjecting it to uncertain risks of exposure to possibly teratogenic medications? On the one hand, not taking the drug benefits the fetal patient by avoiding possible risks of the drug, while subjecting the pregnant woman to a level of risk that, as matter of her deliberative interests, she may reasonably find to be unacceptable. She forgoes significant benefit to herself to avoid theoretical risk to her fetus and, on the face of it, this seems not to be obligatory. On the other hand, taking the drug, as Minkoff and Moreno point out, involves uncertain risks for the fetal patient and potential, significant benefit for the pregnant woman. To conclude decisively that the woman is *obligated* to forgo significant benefit for herself for the sake of avoiding risk to the fetal patient requires that the risk to the fetus be well-established, occur with a significant incidence, and involve serious setbacks to its social-role interests. These conditions seem not to be satisfied, given our present knowledge about the teratogenetic risks of prophylaxis for HIV infection. It follows that the pregnant woman who is HIV infected is not obligated to the fetal patient to forgo prophylaxis; she is free to take prophylaxis or not. Thus, it is ethically justified to offer drug prophylaxis to HIV-infected pregnant women.

Critical Care Obstetrics

Critical care obstetrics involves a level of complication not found in any other sort of critical care: there *may be* two patients involved. Moreover, the pregnant woman's life is at stake; otherwise critical care intervention would neither be contemplated nor initiated.

In Chapter 3 we argued that whether or not the viable fetus is presented to the physician is, in part, a function of the woman's ethical obligation to do so. The strength of this obligation, recall also from Chapter 3, turns on whether there is good reason to think that the risks involved to the pregnant woman in an attempt to benefit the viable fetus are reasonable. If such attempts risk the life of the pregnant woman, they are unreasonable in beneficence-based clinical judgment, because her death would be premature and unnecessary. The only way to deny the latter is to assert an independent-moral-status-based fetal right to life, an assertion that cannot be sustained. If beneficence-based clinical judgment were the whole of the story, the recommendation in Step 8 of the informed consent process regarding critical care obstetrics would be in favor of a trial of intervention to save the pregnant woman's life.

Of course, as we have argued throughout, this beneficence-based clinical judgment is *not* the whole of the story; respect for autonomy must also be considered. This ethical principle of respect for autonomy requires the physician to give the choice about the goals of critical care intervention to the pregnant woman. The choice is fundamental and beneficence-based clinical judgment is incompetent to answer it: whose life shall be saved if both cannot?

Thus, the physician cannot justifiably make a definitive recommendation, as part of Step 8 of the informed consent process, of critical care obstetrics. This form of clinical management, including its nature as a trial of intervention, should be explained to the patient as part of Step 3 of the informed consent process in all cases. It will be a crucial part of this process to support the pregnant woman in what can be stressful circumstances, to maximize her opportunity to exercise her autonomy.

The Case of In Re A.C.

The recent case, *In re A.C.*, should be addressed in this context. The facts of this much-publicized and commented upon case appear to be the following.[80] Ms. Angela Carder, 27 years of age at the time of the case, had a history of cancer, which had been in remission. She married and became pregnant. On a routine prenatal visit, Ms. Carder was noted to have back pain and shortness of breath and had a chest film taken, which revealed a lung tumor that was judged inoperable. Two days later she was admitted to the hospital. At that time, 25 weeks pregnant, she was reported to have said that she wanted to have her baby. On day 6 of hospitalization her condition worsened and she was informed that her condition was terminal. She agreed to palliative care and attempted to reach 28 weeks gestational age, to improve fetal outcome. When asked whether she wanted her baby, she was equivocal. The hospital sought a declaratory judgment. Counsel for both Ms. Carder and the fetus were appointed. The court of original jurisdiction ordered that a cesarean section be performed. It was performed and both Ms. Carder and her baby died. The Court of Appeals vacated this order, even though the case was moot.

The fetus in this case was what we have termed just-viable. As such, the pregnant woman and her physicians owe more minimal than beneficence-based obligations to such a fetus, if it is a fetal patient. But, this depends on whether the pregnant woman, Ms. Carder, was obligated to accept the risks of cesarean delivery. There are two decisive reasons why she could not be understood to do so.

First, there is no documented efficacy of cesarean delivery of just-viable fetuses. Thus, the more than minimal beneficence-based obligations to the fetus are equally served by cesarean delivery and vaginal delivery. Moreover, any claim that waiting until Ms. Carder could be declared dead, followed by cesarean delivery, was clearly not in the fetus' social-role interests is anecdotally supported, at best.[81]

Second, cesarean delivery for a patient with Ms. Carder's medical history involves far higher risks of mortality than those associated with cesarean delivery at term. The greater the risks to the pregnant woman's social-role interests, the stronger is the beneficence-based obligation not to place them at risk. The beneficence-based logic of critical care as trial of intervention surely prohibits gratuitous risks to the patient's social-role interest in preventing premature death. Given the unsubstantiated nature of alleged fetal benefit of immediate cesarean delivery, Ms. Carder's social-role interest in preventing unnecessary death—here death that is not necessary to protect and promote alleged fetal interests—would be seriously set back by cesarean delivery.

In summary, there was in this case no beneficence-based justification for a recommendation of cesarean delivery, until Ms. Carder was dead. Indeed, the ethically justified recommendation to her surrogate should have been against immediate cesarean delivery. There was, therefore, no beneficence-based justification for treating this case as a crisis, much less a conflict, and seeking a court order. The views of some commentators notwithstanding,[82] *In re A.C.* has no value as a precedent for the management of maternal-fetal conflict, especially concerning the intrapartum management of at-term pregnancies of otherwise healthy pregnant women. This is because there was no ethical conflict in the first place. Indeed, the "conflict" would have been and should have been prevented, had this moral fact been recognized.[83]

Conclusion

Because of possible differences between the physician's beneficence-based and autonomy-based obligations to the pregnant woman and beneficence-based obligations to the fetal patient, there is an inherent potential for ethical conflict in obstetric practice. This is surely true of the topics addressed in this chapter. In our view this potential is realized in clinical practice too frequently. The informed consent process, especially information disclosed in Step 3 and recommendations made in Step 8, is an underutilized clinical strategy to prevent ethical conflict and crisis in obstetric practice. In this chapter, we have attempted to provide concrete and comprehensive preventive ethical proposals for obstetric practice. What to do when strategies of preventive ethics in gynecologic and obstetric practice fail, and ethical crisis occurs, is the subject of the next and final chapter.

NOTES

1. For a valuable account of the issues involved see Howard W. Jones, Jr., "Assisted Reproduction," *Clinical Obstetrics and Gynecology* 35 (1992):749–57. For a guide to the literature see Mary C. Coutts, "Ethical Issues in In Vitro Fertilization" (Washington, D.C.: National Reference Center for Bioethics Literature, Kennedy Institute of Ethics, 1988), and Sue A. Meinke, "Surrogate Motherhood: Ethical and Legal Issues" (Washington, D.C.: National Reference Center for Bioethics Literature, Kennedy Institute of Ethics, 1988).
2. Frank A. Chervenak and Laurence B. McCullough, "An Ethically Justified, Clinically Comprehensive Management Strategy for Third Trimester Pregnancies Complicated by Fetal Anomalies," *Obstetrics and Gynecology* 75 (1190):311–316; and Frank A. Chervenak and Laurence B. McCullough, "Does Obstetric Ethics Have any Role in the Obstetrician's Response to the Abortion Controversy?," *American Journal of Obstetrics and Gynecology* 163 (1990):1425–29.
3. Frank A. Chervenak and Laurence B. McCullough, "Nonaggressive Obstetric Management: An Option for some Fetal Anomalies during the Third Trimester," *Journal of the American Medical Association* 261 (1989):3439–30.
4. See note no. 3.
5. M. Hack and A.A. Fanaroff, "Outcomes of Extremely-Low-Birth-Weight Infants between 1982 and 1988," *New England Journal of Medicine* 321 (1989):1642–47.
6. ibid.
7. ibid.
8. ibid.
9. S.B. Thacker, "Quality of Controlled Clinical Trials. The Case of Imaging Ultrasound in Obstetrics: A Review," *British Journal of Obstetrics and Gynecology* 92 (1985):437–44.
10. R.E. Sabbagha, *Diagnostic Ultrasound Applied to Obstetrics and Gynecology* (Philadelphia: J.B. Lippincott Co., 1987).
11. *Diagnostic Ultrasound Imaging in Pregnancy. Report of a Consensus Development Conference Sponsored by the National Institute of Child Health and Human De-*

velopment, the Office of Medical Applications of Research, The Division of Research Resources, and the Food and Drug Administration (Bethesda, Md.: U.S. National Institutes of Health, 1984).

12. Frank A. Chervenak, Laurence B. McCullough, and Judith L. Chervenak, "Prenatal Informed Consent for Sonogram (PICS): An Indication for Obstetrical Ultrasound," *American Journal of Obstetrics and Gynecology* 161 (1989):857–60.

13. Royal College of Obstetricians and Gynecologists, *Report of RCOG Working Party on Routine Ultrasound Examination in Pregnancy* (London Royal College of Obstetricians and Gynaecologists, 1984).

14. See note no. 11.

15. American Institute of Ultrasound in Medicine, *Official Statement of Antepartum Obstetrical Ultrasound Examination Guidelines* (Bethesda, Md.: American Institute Ultrasound in Medicine, 1985); American Institute of Ultrasound in Medicine, *Official Statement on Guidelines for Minimum Post-Residency Training in Obstetrical and Gynecological Ultrasound* (Bethesda, Md.: American Institute of Ultrasound in Medicine, 1982).

16. Stuart Campbell, S.L. Warsof, D. Little, et al., "Routine Ultrasound Screening for the Prediction of Gestational Age," *Obstetrics and Gynecology* 65 (1985):613–20.

17. See note no. 10.

18. See notes nos. 10 and 13, Frank A. Chervenak and Glenn Isaacson, "Diagnosing Congenital Malformation in Utero: Ultrasound," *Clinics in Perinatology* 13 (1986):593–607, and Lyn S. Chitty, Gaye H. Hunt, Jennifer Moore, et al., "Effectiveness of Routine Ultrasonography in Detecting Fetal Structural Abnormalities in a Low Risk Population," *British Medical Journal* 303 (1991):1165–69.

19. See note no. 13.

20. Stuart Campbell, A.E. Reading, D.N. Cox, et al., "Ultrasound Scanning in Pregnancy: The Short Term Psychological Effects of Early Realtime Scans," *Journal Psychosomatic Obstetrics and Gynecology* 1 (1982):57–61.

21. R.E. Sabbagha, Z. Sheikh, R.F. Tamura, et al., "Predictive Value, Sensitivity and Specificity of Ultrasonic Targeted Imaging for Fetal Anomalies in Gravid Women at High Risk for Birth Defects," *American Journal of Obstetrics and Gynecology* 152 (1985): 822–27.

22. See note no. 15.

23. F.W. Kremkau, "Biological Effects and Possible Hazards," *Clinical Obstetrics and Gynecology* 10 (1983):395–405.

24. American Institute of Ultrasound in Medicine Bioeffects Committee, *Journal of Ultrasound Medicine* 2 (1983): R14.

25. See note no. 11.

26. See notes nos. 23 and 24 and E.A. Lyons, C. Dyke, M. Toms, et al., "In-Utero Exposure to Diagnostic Ultrasound: A 6-Year Follow-Up," *Radiology* 166 (1988): 687–90.

27. See notes nos. 9, 11, and 13.

28. Sherman Elias and George J. Annas, "Routine Prenatal Genetic Screening," *New England Journal of Medicine* 317 (1987):1407–9.

29. Bernard Ewigman, Michael LeFevre, Raymond P. Bain, et al., "Ethics and Routine Ultrasound in Pregnancy," *American Journal of Obstetrics and Gynecology* 163 (1990):256–57; and Frank A. Chervenak and Laurence B. McCullough, "Ethics and Routine Ultrasound in Pregnancy," *American Journal of Obstetrics and Gynecology* 163 (1990):257–58.

30. M.C. Ziskin, "The Prudent Use of Diagnostic Ultrasound," *Journal of Ultrasound in Medicine* 6 (1987):415–16.

31. See note no. 11.

32. C.H. Rodeck, "Fetal Development after Chorionic Villus Sampling," *The Lancet* 241 (1993):468–69.

33. Maurice L. Druzin, Frank Chervenak, Laurence B. McCullough, Robert N. Blatman, and Julie Neidich, "Should All Patients Be Offered Prenatal Diagnosis Irrespective of Age?," *Obstetrics and Gynecology* 81 (1993):615–18.

34. President's Commission for the Study of Ethical Problems in Medicine and Biomedical and Behavioral Research, *Securing Access to Health Care, Volume One: Report* (Washington, D.C.: U.S. Government Printing Office, 1983).

35. Tabitha M. Powledge, John C. Fletcher, et al., "Guidelines for the Ethical, Social and Legal Issues in Prenatal Diagnosis: A Report from the Genetics Research Group of the Hastings Center, Institute of Society, Ethics and the Life Sciences," *New England Journal of Medicine* 300 (1979):168–72; John C. Fletcher, "Ethics and Amniocentesis for Sex Identification," *New England Journal of Medicine* 30 (1979):550–53; and Dorothy C. Wertz and John C. Fletcher, "Fetal Knowledge? Prenatal Diagnosis and Sex Selection," *Hastings Center Report* 19 (1989):21–27.

36. Mark I. Evans, A. Drugan, S.F. Bottoms, et al., "Attitudes on the Ethics of Abortion, Sex Selection, and Selective Pregnancy Termination among Health Care Professionals, Ethicists, and Clergy likely to Encounter such Situations," *American Journal of Obstetrics and Gynecology* 164 (1991):1092–99.

37. See, for example, John C. Fletcher and Mark I. Evans, "Ethics in Reproductive Genetics," *Clinical Obstetrics and Gynecology* 35 (1992):763–782.

38. Jonathan D. Moreno, "Ethical Indications for Fetal Sexing," unpublished manuscript.

39. See note no. 10.

40. *Roe* v. *Wade,* 410 US 113 (1973).

41. *Webster* v. *Reproductive Health Services,* 492 U.S. 490 (1989).

42. *Casey* v. *Planned Parenthood of Southeastern Pennsylvania* 60 U.S. 4795 (1992).

43. Michael Harrison, Mitchell Golbus, R. Filly, *The Unborn Patient* (New York: Grune & Stratton, 1984). See also Chapter 3, *passim.*

44. Frank A. Chervenak and Laurence B. McCullough, "An Ethically Justified, Clinically Comprehensive Management Strategy for Third Trimester Pregnancies Complicated by Fetal Anomalies," *Obstetrics and Gynecology* 75 (1990):311–16.

45. Frank A. Chervenak, Margaret A. Farley, LeRoy Walters, et al., "When is Termination of Pregnancy During the Third Trimester Morally Justified?," *New England Journal of Medicine* 310 (1986):501–4; and J. Sherard, C. Bean, B. Bove, et al., "Long-Term Survival in a 69, xxy Triploid Male," *American Journal of Genetics* 25 (1986): 307–312.

46. ibid.

47. Richard A. McCormick, "To Save or Let Die: The Dilemma of Modern Medicine," *Journal of the American Medical Association* 229 (1974):172–76; and Laurence B. McCullough and Catherine Myser, "Recent Developments in Perinatal and Neonatal Medical Ethics: A U.S. Perspective," *Seminars in Perinatology* 11 (1987):216–23.

48. Frank A. Chervenak and Laurence B. McCullough, "Nonaggressive Management—An Option for Some Fetal Anomalies During the Third Trimester," *Journal of the American Medical Association* 261 (1989):3439–40.

49. R. Romero, M. Cullen, P. Grannum, et al., "Antenatal Diagnosis of Renal Anomalies with Ultrasound. III. Bilateral Renal Agenesis," *American Journal of Obstetrics and Gynecology* 151 (1985):38–43.

50. Frank A. Chervenak, Richard L. Berkowitz, M. Tortora, et al., "The Management of Fetal Hydrocephalus," *American Journal of Obstetrics and Gynecology* 151 (1985):933–42; Frank A. Chervenak and Laurence B. McCullough, "Ethical Challenges in Perinatal Medicine: The Intrapartum Management of Pregnancy Complicated

by Fetal Hydrocephalus with Macrocephaly," *Seminars in Perinatology* 11 (1987):232–39.

51. Frank A. Chervenak and Laurence B. McCullough, "Ethical Analysis of the Intrapartum Management of Pregnancy Complicated by Fetal Hydrocephalus with Macrocephaly," *Obstetrics and Gynecology* 68 (1986):720–24.

52. See also, Carson Strong, "Ethical Conflicts between Mother and Fetus in Obstetrics," *Clinics in Perinatology* 14 (1987):313–28; and Carson Strong, "Delivering Hydrocephalic Fetuses," *Bioethics* 5 (1991):1–22.

53. K.R. Nicolaides, C.H. Rodeck, C.M. Gosden, "Rapid Karyotyping in Non-Lethal Fetal Malformations," *Lancet* 1 (1986):283–87.

54. H.M. Andersen, J.H. Drew, N.A. Beischer, "Non-Immune Hydrops Fetalis: Changing Contribution to Perinatal Mortality," *British Journal of Obstetrics and Gynaecology* 90 (1983):636–39.

55. Frank A. Chervenak and R. Romero, "Is There a Role for Fetal Cephalocentesis in Modern Obstetrics?," *American Journal of Perinatology* 1 (1984):170–73.

56. Frank A. Chervenak, Richard L. Berkowitz, M. Tortora, et al., "The Management of Fetal Hydrocephalus," *American Journal of Obstetrics and Gynecology* 151 (1985):933; B. Chayen and M.D. Rifkin, "Cephalocentesis: Guidance with an Endovaginal Probe and Endovaginal Needle Placement," *Journal of Ultrasound in Medicine* 6 (1987):221–23.

57. R.K. Silver and R.W. Huff, "Intrapartum Management of the Fetus with Idiopathic Hydrocephalus," *American Journal of Perinatology* 4 (1987):16–19.

58. David C. McCullough and L.A. Balzer-Martin, "Current Prognosis in Overt Neonatal Hydrocephalus," *Journal of Neurosurgery* 57 (1982):378–83; Frank A. Chervenak, C. Duncan, and L.R. Ment, "The Outcome of Fetal Ventriculomegaly," *Lancet* 2 (1985):179–82; D.B. Shurtleff, E.L. Floz, J.D. Loeser, "Hydrocephalus: A Definition of its Progress and Relationship to Intellectual Function, Diagnosis, and Complications," *American Journal of Disabled Child* 125 (1973):688–93; and E.H. Kovnar, W.S. Coxe, and J.J. Volpe, "Normal Neurological Development and Marked Reconstitution of Cerebral Mantle after Postnatal Treatment of Intrauterine Hydrocephalus," *Neurology* 34 (1984):840–41.

59. See note no. 58.

60. See notes nos. 54, 55, 56 and Frank A. Chervenak, Richard L. Berkowitz, R. Romero, et al., "The Diagnosis of Fetal Hydrocephalus," *American Journal of Obstetrics and Gynecology* 147 (1983):703–16.

61. D.N. McCrann and B.S. Schifrin, "Heart Rate Patterns of the Hydrocephalic Fetus," *American Journal of Obstetrics and Gynecology* 117 (1973):69–74.

62. Frank A. Chervenak and Laurence B. McCullough, "Perinatal Ethics: A Practical Method of Analysis of Obligations to Mother and Fetus," *Obstetrics and Gynecology* 66 (1985):442–46.

63. See note no. 58.

64. Frank A. Chervenak, K. Blakemore, Glenn Isaacson, et al., "Antenatal Sonographic Findings of Thanatophoric Dysplasia with Cloverleaf Skull," *American Journal of Obstetrics and Gynecology* 146 (1983):984–85.

65. See note no. 55.

66. Frank A. Chervenak, Glenn Isaacson, Maurice J. Mahoney, et al., "The Obstetric Significance of Holoprosencephaly," *Obstetrics and Gynecology* 63 (1984):115–21. See note no. 54.

67. See note no. 56.

68. Frank A. Chervenak, D. Duncan, L.R. Ment, et al., "Perinatal Management of Meningomyelocele," *Obstetrics and Gynecology* 63 (1984):376–80.

69. Frank A. Chervenak, Glenn Isaacson, Maurice J. Mahoney, "The Diagnosis and Management of Fetal Cephalocele," *Obstetrics and Gynecology* 64 (1984):86–91.

70. See note no. 56.
71. See note no. 56.
72. See note no. 56.
73. Despite his attempt to differentiate his position from ours, Strong in essence adopts our position. See Carson Strong, "Delivering Hydrocephalic Fetuses," *Bioethics* 5 (1991):1–22.
74. Frank A. Chervenak and Laurence B. McCullough, "An Ethically Justified Standard of Care for Fetal Therapy," *Journal of Maternal-Fetal Investigation* 1 (1991): 175–80.
75. See note no. 51.
76. Denise M. Main and Elliott K. Main, "Preterm Birth," in Steven G. Gabbe, Jennifer R. Niebyl, and Joe Leigh Simpson (eds.), *Obstetrics: Normal and Problem Pregnancies,* 2nd ed. (New York: Churchill Livingstone, 1991), pp. 829–80.
77. The provisions of the so-called "Baby Doe" law do not apply here, because reasonable medical judgment does not view experimentation as standard of care. Child Abuse Prevention and Treatment and Adoption Reform Act Amendments of 1984, Public Law 98–457, 42 U.S.C. 5101 *et seq* (1984). For a useful discussion of this law and its history, see Mary Ann Gardell and H. Tristram Engelhardt, Jr., "The Baby Doe Controversy: An Outline of Some Points in its Development," in Richard C. McMillan, H. Tristram Engelhardt, Jr., and Stuart F. Spicker (eds.), *Euthanasia and the Newborn* (Dordrecht, The Netherlands: D. Reidel Publishing Co., 1987), pp. 293–99.
78. Centers for Disease Control, "Guidelines for Prophylaxis against *Pneumocystis carinii* pneumonia for persons infected with human immunodeficiency virus," *Morbidity and Mortality Weekly* 38 (1989):1–9.
79. Howard L. Minkoff and Jonathan D. Moreno, "Drug Prophylaxis for Human Immunodeficiency Virus-Infected Pregnant Women: Ethical Considerations," *American Journal of Obstetrics and Gynecology* 163 (1990):1111–14. See also Jonathan D. Moreno and Howard Minkoff, "Human Immunodeficiency Virus Infection During Pregnancy," *Clinical Obstetrics and Gynecology* 35 (1992):813–20.
80. *In re A.C.*, 573 A.2d 1235 (DC Ct App 1990).
81. Indeed, Ms. Carder's physicians seem to have thought that postmortem delivery was reasonable. See Margot L. White, "Reflections on the Case of Angela Carder: A Tragedy of Decision Making," *BioLaw: A Legal and Ethical Reporter on Medicine, Health Care, and Bioengineering* 39 (1990):S:433–S:442.
82. Carson Strong, "Court-Ordered Treatment in Obstetrics: The Ethical Views and Legal Framework," *Obstetrics and Gynecology* 78 (1991):861–68; and William J. Curran, "Court-Ordered Cesarean Sections Receive Judicial Defeat," *New England Journal of Medicine* 323 (1990):489–92.
83. See Dena S. Davis, "Reflections on A.C.," *BioLaw* 39 (1990):S:448–S:451.

III *The Management of Ethical Conflict and Crisis in Gynecologic and Obstetric Practice*

7 | The Management of Ethical Conflict and Crisis in Gynecologic and Obstetric Practice

The strategies of preventive ethics described in the previous chapter may fail. When they do, one of the following occurs: (1) the female or pregnant patient refuses to move from subjective to deliberative interests, when the patient's, including the fetal patient's, social-role interests are vitally at stake; (2) the female or pregnant patient refuses any longer to be a patient; (3) the female or pregnant patient remains a patient but refuses all of the alternatives within the range or continuum of reliable beneficence-based clinical judgment, or (4) a third party acts in such a way that neither beneficence-based nor autonomy-based obligations of the physician to the patient(s) can be fulfilled. These four possible outcomes of preventive ethics strategies will, we are confident, be rare. Nonetheless, each must be addressed.

Clinical Strategies for When the Female or Pregnant Patient Refuses to Move From Subjective to Deliberative Interests When the Patient's, Including the Fetal Patient's, Social-Role Interests are Vitally at Stake

One outcome of the failure of preventive ethics strategies is that the female or pregnant patient expresses only subjective-interests-based preferences and will not move to the expression of deliberative-interests-based preferences, when the patient's, including the fetal patient's, social-role interests are vitally at stake. The first response to such ethical conflicts between beneficence-based obligations to the woman or fetal patient and autonomy-based obligations to the woman that are based on the patient's subjective interests is to recycle such conflicts through the strategies of preventive ethics. The justification for doing so is the following.

As pointed out in previous chapters, when the woman or the fetal patient's social-role interests are vitally at stake the woman has an ethical obligation to the physician to be a *serious* partner in the decision making process. To be serious means she needs to take into account the fact that her and/or the fetal patient's social-role interests are at risk for being set back in a serious, far-reaching, and irreversible fashion. To insist that she indeed take things seriously and thus to recycle the strategies of preventive ethics, is an ethically acceptable means, in our view, for enforcing within the clinical setting the patient's ethical obligation to the physician to attend to, participate in, and be serious about clinical decision making and, when they exist, the pregnant woman's beneficence-based obligations to the fetal patient. The alternative is to disrespect women as persons by reducing respect for their autonomy as patients to a mere legal self-determination. This may not even be appropriate in the law, given the physician's fiduciary role. In any case, not obliging her to be serious, when it is necessary to be serious, in ethics reduces respect for the autonomy of the female and pregnant patient to little more than a slogan.

This recycling effort will result either in a mutually agreed upon plan of care, or in the second or third outcome described above. We turn, therefore, to a consideration of these outcomes.

Clinical Strategies for When the Female or Pregnant Patient Refuses any Longer to be a Patient

Typically, it is held in the bioethics literature that autonomous refusal of health care interventions by a patient must be respected. The patient is simply insisting on the exercise of a negative right, the right to be left alone. Any intrusion into the zone of privacy created by that right is an unwarranted intrusion against autonomy, which operates as a side-constraint against just such unwanted, unconsented to or nonconsensual intrusions. We believe that this standard account of refusal of medical intervention is simplistic, and applies only when neither the woman's nor the fetal patient's social-role interests are vitally at stake. When either of those interests is vitally at stake, a more nuanced, clinically realistic account is justified. There are important implications of this account for how the problem of paternalism should properly be understood.

A more accurate account of refusal of medical interventions when social-role interests are vitally at stake distinguishes two kinds of refusals. In the first, the refusal is a negative right *simpliciter*—a negative right without any qualification or a "pure" negative right. Such a right is being exercised when the refusal of medical intervention takes the form of the individual in question refusing any longer to be a patient. This is because that individual's physician needs only do nothing to respect the patients' right to noninterference. Thus, when the autonomous patient with uterine cancer, for example, discharges herself from the hospital against medical advice, she is asserting the negative right to be left alone by her hospital physician.

When a patient refuses medical intervention, but does not withdraw from the role of being a patient, matters are more complex, particularly in the case where the patient insists on a mode of management that is unreasonable in beneficence-based clinical judgment concerning her and/or the fetal patient. When this occurs, a negative right is being asserted in combination with a positive right. In the case of refusing any longer to be a patient, the woman asserts only a negative right. Thus, we distinguish the second from the third outcome of the failure of preventive ethics strategies.

A negative right is usually understood in ethics as a right of noninterference in decision making and behavior. A negative right, therefore, generates duties on the part of others to leave the individual in question alone. In law, the rights to privacy and to self-determination, both of which are grounded in autonomy as legal self-determination, are negative rights not to be subject to nonconsensual bodily invasion. By contrast, positive rights involve a claim on the resources of others to have some need, desire, or want met. Such rights obligate others to act in specified ways in response, as illustrated in the above examples. As a rule, positive rights are in all cases understood to be liable to limits by their very nature. This feature of positive rights contrasts sharply with negative rights, for which the burden of proof is on others to establish limits, for example, on the basis of preventing serious harm to innocent others.

There are a number of ethically justified responses to a negative right *simpliciter,* that is, a negative right alone, exercised in the refusal any longer to be a patient. Before ultimately respecting that refusal, the typical approach endorsed in the bioethics literature, the following strategies are reasonable to consider.

The first is to recycle the strategies of preventive ethics, with a view to obliging the patient to reconsider her refusal. This strategy has two separate applications. When neither her nor the fetal patient's social-role interests are vitally at stake (because either there is no fetal *patient* or the social-role interests of the viable fetus are not vitally at stake), this is a not overly burdensome enforcement within the clinical setting of her ethical obligation to be a partner in the informed consent process. If she still refuses any longer to be a patient, her refusal should be respected, for two reasons. First, beneficence-based clinical judgment is not competent to insist that the female or pregnant patient present herself for care. Hence, the physician is not competent, qua physician, to insist that she remain a patient. Second, since the social-role interests of the fetal patient are not vitally at stake, such as the pregnant woman smoking, the harm to the fetal patient is not something that the pregnant woman is strongly obligated to prevent, especially if she incurs significant risks to herself in doing so. Hence, the physician cannot justifiably invoke serious, far-reaching, and irreversible harm to the fetal patient as the basis for insisting that the pregnant woman has an overriding obligation to remain a patient, and thus protect and promote the social-role interests of the fetal patient.

When either the woman's or the fetal patient's social-role interests (which applies to both previable and viable fetal patients) are vitally at stake, such as acute intrapartum fetal distress, recycling the strategies of preventive ethics is ethically justified, again either to enforce within the clinical setting in a nonburdensome way the female patient's or pregnant patient's ethical obligation to the physician to be serious, or to enforce in a nonburdensome way the pregnant woman's beneficence-based obligation to the fetal patient.

When the fetal patient's social-role interests are vitally at stake, it also seems justified to go one step further, in the case of the refusal of a pregnant woman to remain a patient, to refer the case to the physician's hospital or other institutional ethics committee. In doing so, the committee should be asked to review the record of strategies of preventive ethics for quality assurance.[1] If the committee is satisfied as to quality assurance, it would be justified to ask that pregnant woman to appear before the committee, to explain her refusal and to engage her, one last time, in negotiation and respectful persuasion. In this process, the committee should appoint one member or ask the institution's patient advocate or ombudsman to be the pregnant woman's advocate, to manage to a minimum the potentially coercive nature of this role for an ethics committee.

The pregnant woman may consent to such a process. If she does and this last attempt at preventive ethics results in a mutually agreed upon care plan, the physician should implement it. If she refuses to meet with the committee or if she does not agree with the committee on a care plan, the only resort is a court order for management of the conflict, to require the woman to present herself (and the fetal patient) for care. Because court orders are also a possible response to the third outcome of the failure of preventive ethics strategies, court orders will be considered after this third outcome is addressed.

Clinical Strategies for When the Female or Pregnant Patient Remains a Patient but Refuses All of the Alternatives Within the Range or Continuum of Beneficence-Based Clinical Judgment

When the female or pregnant patient refuses all of the alternatives within the range or continuum of beneficence-based clinical judgment, the typical response in the bioethics literature is to insist on respect for such a refusal because any interference with that refusal would constitute a form of paternalism, which is unjustified. In the case of refusal of intervention necessarily coupled to a positive right to an alternative that is patently unreasonable in beneficence-based clinical judgment, the standard construal of medical paternalism is inaccurate. It fails to distinguish refusal that is an unqualified negative right from refusal that is a negative right coupled to a positive right. The correct analysis, we believe, is the following: the negative right of the patient against nonconsensual bodily invasion together with a positive right to intervention or management is asserted against the clinician's negative right against nonconsensual practice of patently unreasonable medicine, because the positive right of the patient to an unreasonable alternative threatens the clinician's autonomy. Here the clinician's autonomy should be understood in terms of the ethical integrity of medicine, which has been recognized by the courts[2] and in the literature[3] and was discussed in Chapter 1.

It would seem that these rare cases of medical paternalism do not therefore involve a clash between beneficence and autonomy, but between autonomy and autonomy. Indeed, it may be correct to see the clash in terms of a clash between autonomy as a side constraint[4] of both the patient and the physician. "How should such clashes be resolved?," seems a question best addressed on the basis of an analysis of the harms that would ensue from the violation of the autonomy of the patient on the one hand, and of the physician on the other, and arguments about how those harms should be rank-ordered.

For the most part, rank-orderings in the bioethics literature strike us more as a function of de facto public policy than of rigorous analysis and argument. Thus, for example, it is a matter of public policy in the United States, in virtue of the First Amendment to the United States Constitution and the body of law based on the First Amendment, that the integrity of religious beliefs is given a protection not accorded the integrity of medicine. But this public policy is an accident of our history, not of a well worked-out philosophical account of how harms should be ranked.

The same would seem to be the case for the near-absolute character of the legal right of self-determination, as articulated in *Schloendorff* v. *Society of New York Hospital*[5] and other informed consent cases. In *Schloendorff* Judge Cardozo, not surprisingly, was unaware of the sort of analysis we suggest here. Moreover, he simply lays down without argument the right of self-determination of the patient regarding health care decisions. Neither the accidents of history nor the dicta of judges count as sustained philosophical analysis and argument. Perhaps it is time to reconsider accepted views about medical paternalism.

The first element of this reconsideration is that the choice for the physician is, in the language of James,[6] live, forced, and momentous, particularly in the case of intrapartum refusal of cesarean delivery when the social-role interests of the fetal patient are vitally at stake. This situation involves a live choice because there are two ethically compelling alternatives: (1) respect the patient's autonomy and sacrifice the intellectual and moral integrity of medicine; and (2) protect the intellectual and moral integrity of medicine at the price of egregiously violating the female or pregnant patient's autonomy. This situation involves a forced choice, because, the woman having remained a patient, the physician must either employ aggressive obstetric management, cesarean delivery, or nonaggressive obstetric management, assisting (an attempt at) a vaginal delivery. This situation involves a momentous choice, because aggressive management is reasonable in reliable beneficence-based clinical judgment, and nonaggressive management is unreasonable in beneficence-based clinical judgment. Such live, forced, and momentous choices go beyond mere ethical conflicts; they constitute ethical crises.

Again, the appropriate utilization of an institutional ethics committee is justified, along the same lines described above. First, the committee should be asked to engage in quality assurance of the preventive ethics strategies. Second, if the committee is satisfied on this score, it should ask the pregnant woman to make her case to the committee, following the process described above. This seems especially justified when the woman does not move from the expression of subjective interests to the expression of deliberative interests. After all, when the fetus is a patient, the pregnant woman must as a matter of intellectual and moral integrity take account of her obligations to the fetal patient. The outcome will be either a mutually agreed upon plan of care or persistent refusal of all reasonable beneficence-based management. Again, seeking a court order is a last resort in such circumstances.

Seeking Court Orders

Seeking court orders to force aggressive obstetric management on a pregnant woman in the intrapartum period is a serious matter and thus should be approached in a serious manner.[7] Several considerations seem requisite.

Institutional Considerations of Due Process

The first consideration concerns the hospital. The hospital in which the situation is occurring is necessarily involved for two reasons, in our view. First, the hospital acts as an institutional moral fiduciary of the social-role, subjective, and deliberative interests of the pregnant woman and the social-role interests of the fetal patient. Second, the hospital also has legitimate interests in its relationship to pregnant patients and their families, for example, in avoiding civil action for wrongful death (of the fetal patient) or for battery (of the pregnant woman). These legitimate interests are surely at stake in seeking court orders.

Thus, at a minimum no court order should be sought without institutional review and approval, as a first step in due process, because the physician is not a free agent. The institutional ethics committee, having undertaken quality assurance of the preventive ethics strategies directly with the pregnant patient, should make a recommendation as to whether court orders should be sought. In doing so, it should seek the advice of institutional legal counsel about whether there exist precedents for court orders that apply to the situation at hand. If there are none, legal counsel should be asked frankly to assess the probability that a court order for aggressive obstetric management would be forthcoming. If existing precedents or legal counsel's advice do not indicate that such an order is highly probable to be forthcoming, the ethics committee should be very reluctant to recommend seeking a court order. This will almost always be the case for female patients.

Moreover, the committee should be very sensitive to evidence that court orders for aggressive obstetric management have been more frequently issued in cases where the pregnant woman is a member of a racial minority group or lacks English as a first language.[8] These are serious matters, because they raise the specter of invidious discrimination, which, obviously, cuts against the grain of every theory of justice. Therefore, the committee should recommend seeking a court order only if it can satisfy itself, after careful consideration, that no invidious discrimination is involved in the case at hand.

Legal Considerations of Due Process

Virtually all commentators on the subject of court-ordered aggressive obstetric management have correctly criticized legal cases in which there was a lack of due process, in particular, the failure to see to it that the pregnant woman is represented by competent legal counsel.[9] The authors propose that, given the crucial importance of adequate legal representation in an adversarial civil proceeding, the hospital should be prepared to provide legal counsel for patients who cannot afford it. If a hospital is unwilling to do so, we believe, it is not fully committed to legal due process and should not seek court-ordered aggressive obstetric management.

Judges have also been criticized for leaving the courtroom and making such decisions at the bedside.[10] Given that many pregnant patients in the intrapartum period, especially high-risk patients, cannot be safely transported to a courtroom, this criticism strikes us as unreasonable. Hospitals can assure an adequate meeting space for a court proceeding in the hospital.

The Substantive Issue: Can Court-Ordered Aggressive Obstetric Management be Ethically Justified?

If the preceding two procedural requirements are met, the physician and hospital confront the substantive ethical issue: Can court-ordered aggressive obstetric management be ethically justified? The answer to this crucial question involves two stages. The first is the provision of a "negative" argument, to show that the most formidable objections to court-ordered aggressive obstetric management, cesarean delivery in particular, can be defeated, that is, to show that such court orders are not ethically unjustified. The second is a "positive" argument that whether such orders are indeed ethically justified is at least an open question.

The "Negative" Argument That Court Orders for Cesarean Delivery Are Not Ethically Unjustified

The literature opposing court orders fails to appreciate the heterogeneity of cases involved. Thus, we distinguish court orders for well-documented, complete placenta previa[11] from court orders for fetal distress. Here, we address well-documented, complete placenta previa.

WELL-DOCUMENTED, COMPLETE PLACENTA PREVIA. Consider, first, well-documented, complete placenta previa. First, spontaneous resolution of the condition or an erroneous diagnosis are highly unlikely. Second, the outcome of vaginal delivery for the fetus is that there is a very substantial risk, approaching certainty, of fetal death. That is, fetal survival with very high probability will not occur.[12] Third, the outcome of cesarean delivery for the pregnant woman vis-à-vis vaginal delivery is a dramatic reduction of risk of mortality.

Can the physician say unconditionally that the fetus will not survive vaginal delivery? No. However, the issue for prognostic clinical judgment, as we argued in Chapter 1 (see pp. 42–45), is its reliability, not its truth. The ethical issue regarding reliability here is this: Can any physician competently claim to have documented evidence of a significant rate of intact fetal survival from vaginal delivery? No. Indeed, such a claim would properly be regarded as an irrational basis for obstetric management. Moreover, to study the question via a randomized clinical trial would be judged unethical by any Institutional Review Board for human subjects research asked to review such a proposal, because of grave risk to fetuses in the vaginal delivery arm of such a clinical trial. It follows from this ethical analysis that the physician is correct to conclude that the only obstetric management strategy consistent with promoting the social-role interests of the fetus is cesarean delivery, because vaginal delivery dooms the social-role interests of the fetus, while cesarean delivery dramatically protects and promotes those interests.

With regard to the pregnant woman's social-role interests, the reliability of prognostic clinical judgment here means that any clinical judgment that well-documented, complete placenta previa is most likely self-limiting and most likely to resolve spontaneously is unfounded and probably irrational. The only rational assumption to make is that vaginal delivery places the pregnant woman at grave risk for exsanguination. The gravity of such a risk is underscored by the long-standing obstetric dictum never to perform a vaginal examination on a third-trimester patient who is experiencing vaginal bleeding, because of the rapidity with which uncontrollable blood loss might result from disruption of a placenta previa.[13]

Should bleeding occur, massive blood replacement may save some women.[14] However, this intervention may not be sufficient to prevent maternal death. In addition, there are significant risks of morbidity and mortality associated with massive blood transfusion, risks that greatly exceed those of cesarean delivery. Finally, no one would seriously propose that studying this issue via a clinical trial is ethically justified, because the maternal risks are so well defined.

The implication of this clinical-ethical analysis is that vaginal delivery carries grave risks of maternal mortality that can only infrequently be managed successfully. By comparison, cesarean delivery, despite its morbidity and mortality risks for the woman and despite its invasiveness, unequivocally produces net benefit for the pregnant woman. Any clinical judgment to the contrary borders on the irrational and cannot, therefore, be consistent with promoting the beneficence-based interests of the woman. Therefore the clinician who recommends cesarean delivery to protect the pregnant woman is making a recommendation with the highest reliability that can be applied to clinical judgment: No competent, rigorous clinician will undertake her management on the basis of a clinical judgment of expected spontaneous resolution, because doing so will virtually doom the pregnant woman's beneficence-based interests. Hence, the risks of cesarean delivery are those the pregnant woman ought reasonably be expected to take. Hence also, the fetus in the case of well-documented, complete placenta previa clearly benefits from cesarean delivery.

The ethical implications of this level of reliability of clinical judgment and of refusal of cesarean delivery are the following: (1) no physician is justified in accepting such a refusal because doing so would be based on patently unreliable clinical judgment; and (2) the physician is justified in resisting a patient's exercise of a positive right when fulfilling that positive right contradicts the most highly reliable clinical judgment and dooms the beneficence-based interests of the pregnant woman and fetal patient. Patients do not have a positive ethical right to obligate physicians to practice medicine in ways that are patently inconsistent with the most reliable clinical judgment.[15]

Because of their thoroughness and because the arguments of others in effect rely on them, Rhoden's objections[16] to court-ordered cesarean delivery must be addressed and defeated to justify limiting the refusal of cesarean delivery for well-documented, complete placenta previa. First, we consider Rhoden's claim that court-ordered cesarean delivery necessarily treats the pregnant woman solely as an instrument or means by which the fetus is benefitted but by which she is not benefitted at all, but only placed at risk. In Rhoden's terms, court orders treat the pregnant woman as a "mere means" to the benefit of her fetus. To defeat this objection, we must show that forced cesarean delivery does indeed benefit the pregnant woman.

Cesarean delivery produces significant benefit for the pregnant woman, the dramatic reduction in maternal mortality risks, and significant benefit for the fetus, essentially complete elimination of risks of fetal mortality. That is, cesarean delivery for well-documented, complete placenta previa produces two *causally independent* effects: benefit for the pregnant woman and benefit for the fetus. Both of these promote social-role interests, the social-role interests of the pregnant woman in particular. Thus, the pregnant woman is not a "mere means" to the benefit of her fetus, in the sense that benefit to her is not considered relevant. Instead, she is an end and is, therefore, in no way whatever reduced to being simply a "fetal container," the dramatic but, in this context, totally misleading phrase of Annas.[17] The pregnant woman is, and remains throughout the procedure, a patient in her own right, a status that is never compromised, because her interests are indeed protected and promoted—to a highly significant degree and in a clear-cut fashion.

This argument does not imply that cesarean delivery is risk-free. To the contrary, because it is major abdominal surgery, it implicates risks, albeit small and usually manageable, of morbidity and rare incidence of mortality. The key feature in the present context of cesarean delivery for well-documented, complete placenta previa is that the *net effect* of cesarean delivery for the pregnant woman is to produce benefit. Because the risks involved in cesarean delivery are a means to benefit the pregnant woman, while at the same time benefitting the fetus, the pregnant woman is not a "mere means" for benefitting the fetus. By aggregating all cases of cesarean delivery—in particular fetal distress and complete placenta previa—Rhoden is prevented from identifying this unique ethical feature of cesarean delivery for well-documented, complete placenta previa.

Rhoden's next objection is that forced cesarean delivery treats pregnant woman as a "means merely." That is, her autonomy, i.e., her negative right against bodily invasion, is violated without sufficient justification. This objection can be defeated by establishing that the pregnant woman is ethically obligated to accept cesarean delivery for the management of well-documented, complete placenta previa. If this is the case, her autonomy is already constrained and no new constraint is introduced by forced cesarean delivery.

We argued in Chapter 3 that the pregnant woman, in a pregnancy being taken to term, is ethically obligated to accept reasonable risks on behalf of the fetus in the management of her pregnancy. Robertson argues for a similar legal obligation.[18] Nelson and Milliken,[19] as well as Rhoden,[20] accept an ethical obligation. If this view is reasonable in obstetric ethics, then it is all the more reasonable to hold that the pregnant woman is ethically obligated to accept obstetric interventions that benefit the fetus *while also benefiting her.* If she is obligated to accept reasonable *risks,* she is surely obligated to accept well-documented *benefits* for herself. That is, her negative right is inherently subject to the limitation imposed by this obligation. It is therefore not the case that the pregnant woman in such moral circumstances possesses an unconditioned negative right against nonconsensual bodily invasion. The courts, and the literature on court-ordered cesarean delivery, have failed to appreciate this key ethical consideration.

Another justification exists for constraining autonomy in these cases: the harm principle. According to this well-understood tenet of ethical theory, an individual's exercise of rights, negative and positive, can justifiably be limited to prevent virtually certain, preventable, serious, and far-reaching harm to innocent others. This justification becomes even stronger when imposing such limits also benefits the individual subject to those limits.

On the basis of the above analysis, another of Rhoden's objections fails, namely, the objection based on analogies to forced donation of tissue, such as bone marrow, or one of a matched pair of solid organs.[21] Rhoden argues that, just as courts have refused to order family members (more precisely, distant family members, namely, cousins) to donate tissue or organs, so too, courts should not order cesarean deliveries.

At first glance, these analogies possess a powerful intuitive appeal. On closer examination, that appeal fails in the case of well-documented, complete placenta previa. In cases of tissue and organ transplantation, the donor is subject to significant harms: the risks of morbidity and mortality of the medical procedures, of hospitalization, and—in the case of organ donation—subsequent life without the donated organ. There may be psychological benefits in being a donor.[22] In the case of bone-marrow transplantation, the benefits to the pediatric recipient are not uniformly significant, given the high failure rate of this therapy.[23] In the case of pediatric kidney transplantation, it is regarded as the preferred management of end-stage renal failure, although it has persistent, not insignificant rates of failure.[24] Moreover, even though independence is increased, pediatric renal transplantation can involve diminished quality of life in other respects.[25]

Cesarean delivery for well-documented, complete placenta previa produces clear-cut benefit for the pregnant woman (the analogue of the tissue or organ donor) and clear-cut benefit for the fetus (the analogue of the pediatric recipient of tissue or an organ). Thus, the alleged analogies fail. Indeed, there is no such analogy in pediatrics to cesarean delivery for well-documented, complete placenta previa. Hence, Rhoden's objection to interference with the pregnant woman's negative right on this score fails.

Rhoden next considers at some length differences in beliefs about outcome between pregnant women and their physicians and understandable fears about major surgery on the part of patients. In the present context a belief on the part of the pregnant woman that vaginal delivery would be more beneficial for her or for her fetus than cesarean delivery is a matter of empirically very poorly founded belief, not a difference between two equally empirically valid beliefs. Fear of the cesarean delivery is, therefore, in all likelihood, an irrational fear. False beliefs and irrational fears are properly understood in bioethics not to be an expression of autonomy, but as factors that can significantly disable autonomy.[26] Thus, neither demonstrably false belief nor irrational fear should be treated as expressions of autonomy. Rather, they should be addressed as obstacles to the exercise of autonomy via the strategies of preventive ethics. Rhoden's argument on this score, therefore, fails.

Rhoden also considers and supports religious objections to forced cesarean delivery. Here we believe that there is an analogy to overriding parental refusal on religious grounds of well-documented, life-saving interventions for children who are patients, an analogy that defeats Rhoden's view. Rhoden points out that one reason that the courts are correct to protect pediatric patients in these circumstances is that no physical burden is imposed on the parents by a court order to treat their child. To be sure, cesarean delivery is invasive, major abdominal surgery. In the case of well-documented, complete placenta previa, invasiveness should not be the sole criterion for assessing physical burdens, because invasiveness in this case is not associated with net harm. To the contrary, it is associated with net benefit, because it dramatically reduces the risk of maternal mortality. To be sure, in the pediatric cases, parents may take moral, religious, or psychological offense in being overridden, but the courts apparently do not regard this as a significant invasion of their autonomy. The same would hold true in the present instance. The net effect, therefore, of cesarean delivery for this complication is to benefit the pregnant woman, not burden her. This would seem to complete the analogy to court orders to override religiously-based objections of parents for well-documented, life-saving interventions for pediatric patients. Hence, Rhoden's support of religious objections to cesarean delivery also seem to fail. We conclude that court orders are not ethically unjustified when strategies for preventive ethics fail to alter refusal of cesarean delivery for well-documented, complete placenta previa.

The "Positive" Argument that Court Orders for Cesarean Delivery Are Ethically Justified

The preceding "negative" argument has important implications for how the "positive" argument to ethically justify court orders must proceed. The issue is *not* the use of the state's power to resolve a conflict between the pregnant woman's unqualified negative right against nonconsensual bodily invasion and fetal benefit.[27] The central issue is, instead, twofold: (1) the use of the state's power to enforce the pregnant woman's beneficence-based obligation to the fetal patient when the net risk to her is nonexistent, as is the case for cesarean delivery for well-documented, complete placenta previa; and (2) the priority that ought to be given in public policy to the autonomy of the pregnant woman as a side-constraint against nonconsensual bodily invasion and to the autonomy of the physician as a side-constraint against nonconsensual practice of patently unreasonable, in reliable beneficence-based clinical judgment, clinical management. To date, no court has addressed this twofold central issue and we conclude that court orders—for at least well-documented, complete placenta previa, as we have defined it in this book—constitute an open question, to which intensive research should be devoted by physicians, ethicists, legal scholars, policy experts, and judges.

The case of *In re A.C.*,[28] discussed in Chapter 6, and an earlier case, also from the District of Columbia, *In re Madyun*,[29] both illustrate the failure of the courts to frame the issues properly. The court in *In re A.C.* found that "in virtually all cases the question of what is to be done is to be decided by the patient—the pregnant woman—on behalf of herself and the fetus."[30] The *Madyun* court ordered cesarean delivery, over the religiously-based objections of the pregnant woman, after failure of labor to progress 60 hours after rupture of membranes.

In essence, both courts framed the issues in the same way. First, "any person has the right to make an informed choice, if competent to do so, to accept or to forego medical treatment."[31] Autonomy as legal self-determination requires this, as explained in Chapter 1. The patient's right to bodily integrity is not constrained by obligations the patient may have to others.[32] The woman "may not be concerned exclusively with her own welfare"[33] but the court does not state that she is under an *obligation* to be so concerned.[34]

Second, this right is not absolute and can be constrained by probability of harm to third parties, "even in the fetal state."[35] The state can assert an interest in protecting third parties from gratuitous, serious, preventable harm.

Judge Belson, concurring in part and dissenting in part, claims that

> . . . a woman who carries a child to viability is in fact a member of a unique category of persons. Her circumstances differ fundamentally from those of other potential patients for medical procedures that will aid another person, for example, a potential donor of bone marrow for transplant. This is so

> because she has undertaken to bear another human being, and has carried an unborn child to viability. Another unique feature of the situation we address arises from the singular nature of the dependency of the unborn child upon the mother. A woman carrying a viable unborn child is not in the same category as a relative, friend, or stranger called upon to donate bone marrow or an organ for transplant. Rather, the expectant mother has placed herself in a special class of persons who are bringing another person into existence, and upon whom that other person's life is totally dependent. Also, uniquely, the viable unborn child is literally captive within the mother's body. No other potential beneficiary of a surgical procedure on another person is in that position.[36]

Judge Belson's choice of terms is unfortunate, especially "mother" and "unborn child." These matters notwithstanding, his claim is interesting for what it does not say and what needs to be said to make his claim compelling: the primary moral relationship of a pregnant woman to the fetal patient is one of obligation, not unrestrained freedom. That is, the pregnant woman carrying a fetal patient is analogous to a parent, not an organ donor. Childress has convincingly shown that the latter analogy is to someone whose action is "voluntary, charitable, altruistic, and not enforceable by law."[37] Instead, like a parent, the pregnant woman carrying a fetal patient is someone whose action is obligatory and therefore enforceable by law, depending on priority that ought to be assigned to the autonomy-as-a-side-constraint of the pregnant woman versus that of the physician. The court in *In re A.C.* does not turn "the law in the proper direction,"[38] but continues in the same wrong-headed direction.

There are several important implications of this alternative, ethically sound framing of the issues. First, coerced cesarean delivery involves ethical, institutional, legal, and policy questions that medicine is not competent to address conclusively. As a consequence, when there is time to get a court order, there is no ethical justification for bypassing institutional and legal considerations of due process, as well as court review, and simply forcing aggressive obstetric management on the pregnant woman within the clinical setting. Physicians, in short, lack social sanction for simply acting on their own when the outcome of failure of the strategies of preventive ethics is moral crisis for which time is available to obtain court review.

For some cases of well-documented, complete placenta previa there may not be time to obtain a court order (at all or under conditions of due process set out above). This occurs, for example, when a woman with well-documented, complete placenta previa is actively bleeding or with severe persistent fetal bradycardia at term. May the physician simply tell the pregnant woman that a cesarean delivery is required to protect the fetal patient/infant and take her to surgery in the hope that she will not physically resist? Such behavior by the physician seems at first to be coercive and therefore unjustified violation of autonomy-based obligations to the pregnant woman (as defined in Table 1–3, Chapter 1, p. 57, and in Table 3–2, Chapter 3, p. 120). Such behavior could also be interpreted as urgently, although not disrespectfully, persuasive, to which the woman's acquiescence is to some (unknown) degree autonomous. In other words, the woman's acquiescence to such behavior by the physician is not necessarily nonautonomous. Hence, autonomy-based obligations to the pregnant woman may not be violated if she acquiesces. Hence, also, telling the woman that a cesarean delivery is required and taking her to surgery may be ethically justified for well-documented, complete placenta previa when there is no time to get a court order.

If the woman does not acquiesce and physically resists cesarean delivery when there is no time to get a court order, one cannot claim that the woman may have autonomously acquiesced and so the argument above does not apply. Moreover, the physician's ethical obligation is to respect nonacquiescent, physical resistance of cesarean delivery when there is no time to obtain court review, in order to protect the social-role interests of the pregnant woman and the fetal patient. The damage to these interests dramatically and unacceptably increases when surgery is performed on a physically resistant patient when an intravenous line is not in place.

Second, medicine has two crucial contributions to make to the public policy debate: (1) the identification of situations in which it is reasonable to seek civil enforcement of a pregnant woman's ethical obligations to the fetal patient during the intrapartum period; and (2) the precise sense in which the intellectual and moral integrity of medicine and hospitals as social institutions is at stake in moral crises of this sort.

Third, there can be no objection in principle to a public policy of moral enforcement of the pregnant woman's obligations to the fetal patient.[39] We have provided ample argument for the gravity of those obligations in the case of well-documented, complete placenta previa. In addition, as noted above, there are relevant analogies in the law, in particular, the enforcement of parental obligations in matters of child abuse and neglect.

Fourth, in making such an analogy, we are not suggesting that the public policy debate be framed in terms of the criminal law. Because the civil law has not developed on the basis of an adequate ethical understanding of the issue involved, the civil law cannot be judged as inadequate—it has not yet been adequately tested, much less found wanting. Thus, there is no urgency of the sort required to turn to the far more powerful—and therefore worrisome—resort of the criminal law.

Courts that address the correctly framed question of enforcing ethically justified obligations would be well advised, we believe, to keep in mind the following considerations in addressing what must be regarded as an open question in the civil law. First, a request to enforce an ethically justified, well-founded obligation is not a new legal issue. Indeed, it is a staple of the common law. Second, the primary relationship of all parties to the fetal patient is one of obligation, not unrestrained freedom. Third, fulfilling one's obligations is intrinsically burdensome, in the sense that obligation, by design, limits freedom. Hence, the burdensomeness of obligations does not count as a strong objection to enforcing obligations. Excessive burden does.

Fourth, Nelson and Milliken have criticized us for being unclear in our earlier work about what risks a pregnant woman should be reasonably expected to take on behalf of the fetal patient,[40] that is, when the burden of obligation to the fetus is excessive. Tests of reasonableness are a staple of the common law, so the objection of Nelson and Milliken cannot be an objection in principle. We argued in Chapter 6 (see p. 224) that there are reliable criteria for distinguishing fetal therapy from fetal experimentation. These criteria shape the contours of reasonableness: (1) when invasive intervention on behalf of the at-term fetus has a very high probability of being life-saving or of preventing serious and irreversible disease, injury, or handicap for the fetus and child it is about to become; (2) when such therapy involves low mortality risk and low or manageable risk of serious and irreversible disease, injury, or handicap to the fetus; and (3) when the mortality risk to the pregnant woman is very low and when the risk of disease, injury, or handicap to the pregnant woman is low or manageable.[41]

Fifth, the pregnant woman has a legitimate interest in avoiding unreasonable burdens in the fulfillment of her obligations. In this respect, she is like the physician and so there are limits on the moral demands of the virtue of self-sacrifice in her case, analogous to those we discussed in Chapter 1. Thus, any attempt to go beyond criterion (3) above faces a considerable, perhaps daunting, burden of proof. As a consequence, the worry that court orders will be so routinely issued as to drive many women away from antenatal care cannot be generated by this conservative criterion.

The question of the enforceability of ethically justified obligations of pregnant women to fetal patients is thus an open one and the preceding considerations ought to frame future court opinions. This is also the case for drug and substance abuse during pregnancy. Criminal penalties are not acceptable,[42] but civil remedies may be.[43] These could include, for example, the woman seeking a restraining order to keep people, including men, away from her who want to give or supply her with drugs that she wants to avoid or restraining orders prohibiting her from entering premises where drugs are known to be used or sold.

None of these remedies, of course, are as urgently needed as interventions to prevent drug and substance abuse during pregnancy as a priority in public health practice and policy. This point can be generalized. The resort to court orders to manage ethical crises in the intrapartum period is, in part, a function of such factors as poverty and social disorganization, including lack of universal access to prenatal care in American society. Preventive ethics requires that, as a public health matter, these and other social barriers to prenatal care be identified and effectively addressed. The obstetric community should be in the forefront of advocacy for change in public policy, to assure such access and thus to eliminate the conditions that give rise to ethical crises in the first place.

Clinical Strategies for When a Third Party Acts in Such a Way That Neither Beneficence-Based nor Autonomy-Based Obligations of the Physician to the Patient Can Be Fulfilled

We come now to the final sort of ethical crisis, a situation in which a third party acts in such a way as to make it impossible for the physician to fulfill any beneficence-based or autonomy-based obligations to the patient. We address this problem in two contexts: (1) third parties that are institutions of health care;[44] and (2) third parties that own or manage resources consumed in the care of patients.

Crises With Institutions of Health Care

The response to crises with institutions of health care finds its justification in the ethical nature of such institutions. These institutions are properly understood, we believe, to be the moral fiduciaries of their patients. As a consequence, institutions of health care are bound by the same beneficence-based and autonomy-based action guides that physicians are. Moreover, institutions of health care are not any freer to abrogate those obligations than physicians are, lest these institutions sunder themselves by undermining their own moral integrity. But then they would destroy themselves. Thus, the ethically justified response to ethical crises generated by institutions of health care is to call those institutions back to their mission, to serve patients as their fiduciary. The physician should point out to the institution's managers that the relationship of the institution and, therefore, of the managers to the patient is primarily one of obligation, not freedom—just as is the case for the physician.

We come now to the heart of the issue: must institutions of health care sacrifice themselves *ad infinitum* for patients? If self-sacrifice is not an absolute obligation of physicians, as we argued in Chapters 1 through 3, neither is self-sacrifice an absolute obligation of institutions of health care. Institutions of health care, like physicians, are therefore justified in setting limits on who will be allowed to be or to remain a patient for particular services. That is, the institution is obligated not to doom the patient's social-role or deliberative interests, subjective interests (as pointed out in Chapter 1) being too unstable to command the respect of institutions. But, an institution can justifiably opt for the less or even least expensive of alternatives consistent with protecting and promoting the patient's social-role and deliberative interests to some reasonable degree. In this respect, the business values of efficiency, controlling costs, and predicting costs are not inherently inconsistent with the institution's fiduciary obligations to the patient. Ethical crisis, therefore, seems to be a function of the institution's managers or the physician losing sight of this moral fact. In short, in health care institutions there is always a common moral ground for managing ethical crises, because the ethical obligations of the institution directly parallel those of the physician and, like the latter, can be justifiably subjected to reasonable limits.

Crises with Third Parties That Own or Manage Resources Consumed in the Care of Patients

Crises with third parties that own or manage resources consumed in the care of patients must be managed differently, because such parties are not always fiduciaries of patients. Private insurance plans must be distinguished from public payment plans, because the two are ethically heterogenous.

Private Insurance Plans

As pointed out in Chapter 4, private insurance plans have contractual obligations to the patient. Presumably, the patient understands the limits and exclusions of her private plan, the vast majority of which are provided by employers as part of employee benefit packages. Employers have only limited obligations in justice to provide payment for employees (present and retired) and their dependents. Employers, it also seems, are justified in expecting that employees will be prudent savers to cover the costs of deductibles, copayments, and noncovered services.

The patient is therefore not wronged if her plan does not cover the cost of a service necessary to protect and promote her social-role and deliberative interests, the subjective interests of the patient being too unstable to warrant justice-based obligations on the part of any employer. Morreim puts this point well, using the example of experimental interventions:

> If [the patient's] plan explicitly refuses to cover experimental care then [the patient] is not wronged if, when later [the patient's] unexpected major illness can only be treated by an experimental drug, his insurer refuses to pay for it. The reality may seem harsh, yet it is the only way in which to make, and adhere to, an economically and medically rational health care system.[45]

That is, patients need to pay close attention to the provisions of their private insurance and plan accordingly. If they are imprudent, the physician is not accountable; the patient is.[46]

At the same time, the physician has a fiduciary obligation not to doom the patient's social-role and deliberative interests. Thus, the physician cannot abandon the patient and neither can a health care institution, for the reasons noted in the previous section. It may be unfair of patients to their physicians and health care institutions to fail to plan prudently for the costs of health care, but that unfairness leaves the fiduciary relationship to the patient of the physician and the health care institution intact.

Public Payment Plans

Public payment plans create, by statute, entitlement to health care. The central issue is what entitlement to health care does a society owe to its citizens. Spurred by the President's Commission's recommendation,[47] there is much talk in the bioethics literature of a basic, decent minimum standard of care that is obligatory in justice. Whether such an obligation exists and, if it does, are hotly disputed matters. Nonetheless, this much can, we think, reliably be said.

First, the ethical frameworks set out in Chapters 1 through 3 allow us to give some concrete meaning to the concept of a basic, decent minimum standard of care. Such a standard never dooms any patient's social-role or deliberative interests and such a standard protects and promotes those interests to some reasonable degree. As noted above, the latter is consistent with the business values of efficiency, controlling costs, and predicting costs. Any society that did less would seem to place the moral integrity of medicine and of institutions of health care systematically at risk, something any society does at its grave peril.

How should physicians respond if this is what they *reliably* believe to be the case? Morreim's emphatic rejection of "gaming the system" is apropos. To game the system is "to bypass those rules [of resource use] while still appearing to honor them and thereby to secure resources that were not, technically at least, intended for this patient."[48] If society is failing to provide a decent minimum such that the moral integrity of medicine and health care institutions is threatened, subterfuge, "fudging," or "deception"—for example, putting down reimbursable payment or insurance codes that are not clinically accurate—are not ethically justified. This is because private responses to public injustice are not adequate to the moral gravity of public injustice, although they may be adequate to meet a particular patient's needs. In these circumstances, a public response is also required in the form of open admission of "gaming the system" and subjecting oneself to peer review.

Public responses also take a variety of other forms: publicizing the plight of poor pregnant women and the outcomes of inadequate or inaccessible prenatal care for women and their children; lobbying for political change; or even civil disobedience. Grumbling to colleagues is simply inadequate, inarticulate anger even less so. Ethical crises with public payers are public crises and must therefore be brought to *and kept in* a public forum. The responsibility to do so is among the physician's public health ethical obligations.

Conclusion

We are confident that the frameworks that we have provided for identifying ethical conflict and the clinical strategies for preventing ethical conflict will make the occurrence of moral crises in gynecologic and obstetric practice very rare indeed. Moreover, the institutional and legal considerations of due process that we have set out should reduce still further any resort to court orders. The issues involved here concern the macro-level of bioethics, what morality ought to be for health care institutions and health care policy. We have taken here the first steps, we believe, toward a fully comprehensive account of ethics in gynecologic and obstetric practice.

NOTES

1. Quality assurance of preventive ethics strategies includes the following: review of informed consent process, especially whether the full range of beneficence-based alternatives was described in Step 3 and included in the recommendation of Step 8 of the informed consent process; review of negotiation, especially whether common values went unidentified; and review of respectful persuasion, especially whether a good faith-effort was made to reach a mutually agreed-upon care plan.

2. See, for example, *Superintendent of Belchertown* v. *Saikewicz*, 373 Mass. 728. 370 N.E.2d 417 (1977), and *Satz* v. *Perlmutter*, 362 So.2d 160, affirmed 379 So.2d 359 (1978).

3. See The Hastings Center, *Guidelines on the Termination of Life-Sustaining Treatment and the Care of the Dying* (Briarcliff Manor, N.Y.: The Hastings Center, 1987), *passim*. Our main claim here is that beneficence-based clinical judgment involves intellectual integrity when that judgment has been reached in a rigorous fashion. Physicians cannot claim ethical integrity for clinical judgment in the absence of such rigor, especially for clinical impressions that are held by only an individual physician. We acknowledge that the ethical integrity of medicine—in this and other respects—is arguably fragile at the present time. Indeed, this recognition played a powerful motivating role in our argument in Chapter 1 for the centrality of the virtue of integrity as a fundamental virtue of physicians.

4. H. Tristram Engelhardt, Jr., *The Foundations of Bioethics* (New York: Oxford University Press, 1986).

5. *Schloendorff* v. *Society of New York Hospital*, 211 N.Y. 125, 105 N.E. 92 (1914). See discussion of this case in Chapter 1, pp. 49–50.

6. William James, "The Will to Believe," in Ralph Barton Perry (ed.), *Essays on Faith and Morals, by William James* (Cleveland, Ohio: The World Publishing Company, 1965), pp. 32–62.

7. For a useful, concise account of the legal issues involved in court-ordered cesarean delivery, see Lawrence J. Nelson, "Legal Dimensions of Maternal-Fetal Conflict," *Clinical Obstetrics and Gynecology* 35 (1992):738–48.

8. V. Kolder, J. Gallagher, and M.T. Parsons, "Court-Ordered Obstetrical Interventions," *New England Journal of Medicine* 316 (1987):1192–96.

9. See, for example, Lawrence J. Nelson and Nancy Milliken, "Compelled Medical Treatment of Pregnant Women: Life, Liberty, and Law in Conflict," *Journal of the American Medical Association* 259 (1988):1060–66.

10. See, for example, Nancy K. Rhoden, "The Judge in the Delivery Room: The Emergence of Court-Ordered Cesareans," *California Law Review* 74:1951 (1986), 1950–2030. A shorter version of this article appeared as Nancy K. Rhoden, "Cesareans and Samaritans," *Law, Medicine and Health Care* 15:3 (1987), 118–25.

11. By this phrase, we mean the following: Transabdominal or transvaginal ultrasound examination is performed by individuals competent in the technique and interpretation of its results, and the placenta is clearly visualized on ultrasound examination to cover the cervical os completely. To maximize reliability, ultrasound examination should be performed shortly before delivery. [W.J. Ott, "Placenta Previa," in F.A. Chervenak, S. Campbell, and G. Isaacson (eds.), *Textbook of Ultrasound in Obstetrics and Gynecology* (Boston: Little, Brown, 1993), pp. 1493–1502; D. Farine, H.E. Fox, and I.E. Timor-Tritsch, "Placenta Previa: Transvaginal Approach," in *Textbook of Ultrasound in Obstetrics and Gynecology*, pp. 1503–8.] The reliability of the examination varies indirectly with the length of time remaining before expected date of delivery. In addition, there should be no uterine contractions and the maternal bladder should be empty, because, if these factors are not taken into account, false positive diagnosis can occur. Satisfaction of these criteria makes a false positive diagnosis of complete placenta previa highly unlikely. In two legal cases, complete placenta previa would appear either to have been

misdiagnosed (in our view the more likely explanation) or to have spontaneously resolved. See *Jefferson* v. *Griffin Spalding County Hospital Authority,* 274 Ga. 86, 274 S.E. 2d 457 (1981) and *In Re Baby Jeffries,* No. 14004 (Jackson County, Mich. P. Ct. May 24, 1982). Neither of these cases, we want to emphasize, fits the definition of well-documented, complete placenta previa.

12. C. Crenshaw, D.E.D. Jones, and R.T. Parker, "Placenta Previa: A Survey of Twenty Years Experience with Improved Perinatal Survival by Expectant Therapy and Cesarean Delivery," *Obstetric Gynecologic Survey* 28 (1973), 461–70. See also note no. 9.

13. J.A. Pritchard, P.C. MacDonald, and N.F. Gant (eds.), *Williams Obstetrics* 17th ed. (Norwalk, Conn.: Appleton-Century-Crofts, Norwalk, 1985), p. 409.

14. D.B. Cotton, J.A. Read, R.H. Paul, et al., "The Conservative Aggressive Management of Placenta Previa," *American Journal of Obstetrics and Gynecology* 137 (1980), 687–95.

15. Allen Brett and Laurence B. McCullough, "When Patients Request Specific Interventions: Defining the Limits of the Physician's Obligations," *New England Journal of Medicine* 315 (1986), 1347–51.

16. See note no. 10. See also Laurence J. Nelson, B.P. Buggy, and C.J. Weil, "Forced Medical Treatment of Pregnant Women: 'Compelling Each to Live as Seems Good to the Rest'," *Hastings Law Journal* 37 (1986):703–63.

17. George J. Annas, "Pregnant Women as Fetal Containers," *Hastings Center Report* 12 (1982):16–17; 45. Annas wishes to claim that women are "fetal containers" because of court-ordered cesarean deliveries. He takes this phrase from Margaret Atwood's *The Handmaid's Tale* (Boston: Houghton Mifflin Company, 1986), a story about women who are tyrannized in virtually every respect of their lives, including being raped by their masters and then forced to bear them children. The horror of the phrase, "fetal container," in the book draws on the total subjugation of women. Court-ordered cesarean delivery does not involve the total subjugation of women to their male masters; at least Annas nowhere shows that this is the case. Thus, his use of this metaphor is on its own terms defective and also undermines the moral force of Atwood's extraordinary novel.

18. John A. Robertson, "The Right to Procreate and in Utero Fetal Therapy," *The Journal of Legal Medicine* 3:3 (1982), 333–66. See also John A. Robertson, "Legal Issues in Prenatal Therapy," *Clinical Obstetrics and Gynecology* 29:3 (1986), 603–611.

19. See note no. 9.

20. See note no. 10.

21. These analogies play a significant role in the arguments of those opposed to court-ordered cesarean section. Robertson (See note no. 18) believes that a legal justification can be developed for court-ordered tissue or organ donation. That argument is irrelevant in the present context, because of the irrelevance of the analogies.

22. Robert M. House and Troy L. Thompson, "Psychiatric Aspects of Organ Transplantation," *Journal of the American Medical Association* 260: 4 (1988), 535–39.

23. C. Philip Steuber, "Bone-Marrow Transplantation," in Frank A. Oski (ed.-in-chief), Catherine D. DeAngelis, Ralph D. Feigin, and Joseph B. Warshaw (eds.), *Principles and Practice of Pediatrics* (Philadelphia: J.B. Lippincott Company, 1990), pp. 1578–79.

24. Edward C. Kohaut, "End-Stage Renal Disease," in Frank A. Oski (ed.-in-chief), Catherine D. DeAngelis, Ralph D. Feigin, and Joseph B. Warshaw (eds.), *Principles and Practice of Pediatrics* (Philadelphia: J.B. Lippincott Company, 1990), pp. 1619–24.

25. Larry M. Gold, Beverly S. Kirkpatrick, F. Jay Fricker, and Basil J. Zitelli, "Psychosocial Issues in Pediatric Organ Transplantation," *Pediatrics* 75: 5 (1986), 738–44; House and Thompson, "Psychiatric Aspects of Organ Transplantation."

26. Ruth R. Faden and Tom L. Beauchamp, *A History and Theory of Informed Consent* (New York: Oxford University Press, 1986), especially Chapter 7.

27. This misconception of the legal issue is widespread. It can be found, for example, in American College of Obstetricians and Gynecologists, Committee on Ethics, "Patient Choice: Maternal-Fetal Conflict" (Washington, D.C.: American College of Obstetricians and Gynecologists, 1987, Technical Bulletin No. 55); American Academy of Pediatrics, Committee on Ethics, "Fetal Therapy: Ethical Considerations," *Pediatrics* 81 (1988):898–99; H.M. Cole, "Legal Interventions During Pregnancy," *Journal of the American Medical Association* 264 (1990):2663–70; Thomas E. Elkins, H. Frank Andersen, Mel Barclay, et al., "Court-Ordered Cesarean Section: An Analysis of Ethical Concerns in Compelling Cases," *American Journal of Obstetrics and Gynecology* 161 (1989):150–54; Carson Strong, "Court-Ordered Treatment in Obstetrics: The Ethical versus Legal Framework," *Obstetrics and Gynecology* 78 (1991):861–68; and George J. Annas, "Protecting the Liberty of Pregnant Patients," *New England Journal of Medicine* 316 (1988):1213–14.

28. *In re A.C.,* 573 A.2d 1235 (DC Ct App 1990). We quote from a reproduction of the opinion in *Bio-Law: A Legal and Ethical Reporter on Medicine, Health Care, and Bio-Engineering* 2 (1990):S:367–S:420. For brief account of the case, see Chapter 6, pp. 231–232.

29. *In re Madyun* 114 Daily Wash. L. Rptr. 2233 (1986), affirmed on appeal to the Court of Appeals in the District of Columbia by unpublished order.

30. *In re A.C.* S:369–S:370.

31. ibid.: S:383.

32. ibid.: S:392; S:397; S:401–S:402.

33. ibid.: S:401.

34. ibid.: S:401–402.

35. ibid.: S:391.

36. ibid.: S:414.

37. James F. Childress, "Analogical Reasoning: Organ/Tissue Donation and Cesarean Sections," *BioLaw* 2 (1990):S:447.

38. William J. Curran, "Court-Ordered Cesarean Sections Receive Judicial Defeat," *New England Journal of Medicine* 323 (1991):492. By contrast, see Norman F. Fost, "Maternal-Fetal Conflicts: Ethical and Legal Considerations," *Annals of the New York Academy of Science* 562 (1989):248–54.

39. Strong seems to object to enforcement of ethical obligations in law and public policy, an odd view. See Carson Strong, "Court-Ordered Treatment in Obstetrics: The Ethical versus Legal Framework." Strong has gone so far as to call our views "neither ethically nor legally justifiable." See Carson Strong, "Court-Ordered Treatment in Obstetrics: The Ethical Views and Legal Framework," *Obstetrics and Gynecology* 79 (1992): 479 (letter) in response to our letter, *Obstetrics and Gynecology* 79 (1992):476–77. Strong's errors in his letter and his article of the same title are subtle and disabling. First, he ignores legal scholarship that takes opposing views, notably Robertson's important work. (See note no. 18.) Second, he criticizes some courts for being too brief, correctly, but ignores the extensive arguments given in *Madyun,* a case he cites. (See note no. 29). Third, he distorts *In re A.C.,* a crucial case for his view. (1) He ignores the court's claim that no maternal-fetal conflict existed in this case, yet he wants the ruling to apply to maternal-fetal conflict. (2) He omits Judge Belson's reservations about the court's dictum on the primacy of treatment refusal and that, indeed, the state's interests in protecting a viable fetus must at least be given some weight. (3) He claims that the dictum in *In re A.C.* will be important for future cases, but cites only one commentator in support of a claim that is largely speculative. This speculation is undermined by the neutrality of the court in *In re A.C.* to *Madyun,* a dimension of *In re A.C.* that Strong ignores as well. Fourth, in his reliance on *Thornburgh* v. *American College of Obstetricians and Gynecologists,* 476 US 747, 90 LEd2d 779, 106 SCT 2169 (1986), he makes

several errors. (1) He provides no argument to show that abortion cases are analogous to maternal-fetal conflicts. (2) He cites *Cruzan* v. *Director, Missouri Department of Health,* 111 LEd2d 224, 110 SCT 2841 (1990) in support of a constitutionally protected right to refuse medical treatment, when the language of the court in *Cruzan* on this subject is far from unequivocal. (3) He ignores Judge Belson's doubts in *In re A.C.* (fn. 12, p. 52) that *Thornburgh* applies in cases of cesarean delivery at-term. (4) Strong ignores his own insistence that there is a strong prohibition against killing at-term fetuses. (See Carson Strong, "Delivering Hydrocephalic Fetus," *Bioethics* 5 (1991):1–22.) He does not show how this squares with the application of *Thornburgh* to maternal-fetal conflicts. In short, Strong fails utterly to show that our views lack legal and ethical justification.

40. See note no. 9.

41. Mathieu agrees that the issue should be framed in terms of the enforceability of the pregnant woman's duty to the fetus. She rejects the concept of the fetus as patient, however. The whole force of our book is that this is a mistake, in part because Mathieu is left with no conceptual basis for criteria for enforcing such a duty. As she lamely puts it, ". . . my guess is that most people would consider such sacrifices of autonomy and bodily integrity—with the concomitant pain and risk (albeit small) of death—to go well beyond the range of what should be legally required of a parent," a conclusion reinforced by ineliminable uncertainty in clinical prognostic judgment. (Deborah Mathieu, *Preventing Prenatal Harm* (Dordrecht, The Netherlands: Kluwer Academic Publishers, 1991), p. 92.) Mathieu's errors are serious and totally disable her claim. First, if it is an empirical claim, she offers no evidence for it. Even if she did, it would be nothing more than a consensus view and subject to all of the serious difficulties associated with consensus as a methodology for bioethics. (See Chapter 1, pp. 68–69.) Second, it may be an intuition, but she offers no explanation of its plausibility. Third, we must conclude that it is an unsupported assertion, a "mere opinion" and so it can be dismissed. Fourth, Mathieu fails to understand the uncertainty of clinical prognostic judgment in terms of its reliability and so this assertion is, ultimately, empty.

42. Sandra Anderson Garcia, "Birth Penalty: Societal Responses to Chemical Dependence," *The Journal of Clinical Ethics* 1 (1990):135–40; Wendy Chaokin, "Jennifer Johnson's Sentence: Common on Birth Penalty," *The Journal of Clinical Ethics* 1 (1990):140–42; Michelle Oberman, "Sex, Drugs, and Pregnant Addicts: an Ethical and Legal Critique of Society Responses to Pregnant Addicts," *The Journal of Clinical Ethics* 1 (1990):145–52; Carol Levine and David M. Movick, "Expanding the Role of Physicians in Drug Abuse Treatments: Problems and Perspectives," *The Journal of Clinical Ethics* 1 (1990):152–56; and Judith Berkendorf and Kevin FitzGerald, "Genetic Counseling for Addicted Obstetric Patients," *The Journal of Clinical Ethics* 1 (1990):156–57.

43. Frank A. Chervenak and Laurence B. McCullough, "Preventive Ethics Strategies for Drug Abuse During Pregnancy," *The Journal of Clinical Ethics* 1 (1990):157–58.

44. We use "institution" deliberately broadly, to cover everything from the solo, fee-for-service physician in private practice, through group practices and hospitals, to large-scale private delivery (e.g., private insurance) and public delivery (U.S. Department of Veterans Affairs) and payment (e.g., Medicare and Medicaid) schemes.

45. E. Haavi Morreim, *Balancing Act: The New Medical Ethics of Medicine's New Economics* (Dordrecht, The Netherlands: Kluwer Academic Publishers, 1991), p. 147.

46. ibid., Chapter 7, *passim.*

47. President's Commission on Ethical Problems in Medicine and Biomedical and Behavioral Research, *Access to Health Care, Volume I: Report* (Washington, D.C.: U.S. Government Printing Office, 1983).

48. E. Haavi Morreim, *Balancing Act,* p. 72.

Glossary

Beneficence action guides that translate the social-role interests of the patient into clinical practice.

Bioethics the disciplined study of morality in health care (the morality of physicians, patients, institutions of health care, and health care policy).

Compassion a virtue that requires the physician to acknowledge and respond to the suffering of the patient.

Deliberative interests those things in which the patient has a stake because they are valued in a settled way, after adequate information is obtained and carefully considered.

Dependent moral status possession of moral status dependent on some factor other than the properties of the individual.

Ethical principles action guides that translate the interests of the patient into clinical practice.

Ethics the disciplined study of morality (right and wrong conduct; good and bad character).

Independent moral status possession of moral status independent of any factor other than the properties of the individual, for example, being a person.

Integrity a virtue that sustains the physician's life-long commitment to excellence in the care of patients.

Interests stakes that individuals have in the outcome or issues of events.

Justice action guides that translate fairness to the interests of third parties into clinical practice.

Legitimate interests of the physicians meeting the conditions for learning and practicing medicine well; fulfilling obligations to individuals other than the patient; living a coherent and meaningful life.

Moral status the property of being a human being to whom obligations are owed.

Paternalism overriding the patient's wishes or intentional actions for beneficent reasons.

Patient an individual human being who (1) is presented to a physician (2) for the purpose of applying clinical interventions that are reliably expected to protect and promote the interests of that individual.

Respect for autonomy action guides that translate subjective and deliberative interests of the patient into clinical practice.

Self-effacement a virtue that negates the adverse impacts on the physician's attitude and behavior of distracting differences between the physician and the patient.

Self-sacrifice a virtue that requires the physician to accept risk to self and to be calm in that acceptance.

Social role interests those things in which one has a stake in virtue of being a patient.

Subjective interests those things in which the patient has a stake because they happen, perhaps unreflectively, to be valued by the patient.

Vices traits of character that unleash mere self-interest so that the physician becomes blinded to the interests of the patient.

Virtues traits of character that blunt mere self-interest and therefore direct the physician's concern to the interests of the patient.

Viability The ability of the fetus to survive ex utero with full technological support through the neonatal period and into the second-year of life during or near the end of which independent moral status comes into existence.

Index